Handbook of Music, Adolescents, and Wellbeing

Handbook of Music, Adolescents, and Wellbeing

Edited by

Katrina McFerran
Professor, University of Melbourne, Australia

Philippa Derrington
Senior Lecturer, Queen Margaret University, UK

Suvi Saarikallio
Senior Researcher, University of Jyväskylä, Finland

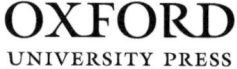
OXFORD
UNIVERSITY PRESS

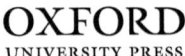

Great Clarendon Street, Oxford, OX2 6DP,
United Kingdom

Oxford University Press is a department of the University of Oxford.
It furthers the University's objective of excellence in research, scholarship,
and education by publishing worldwide. Oxford is a registered trade mark of
Oxford University Press in the UK and in certain other countries

First Edition published in 2019

Impression: 1

Published in the United States of America by Oxford University Press
198 Madison Avenue, New York, NY 10016, United States of America

British Library Cataloguing in Publication Data

Data available

Library of Congress Cataloguing in Publication Data

Data available

ISBN 978–0–19–880899–2

Printed and bound by
CPI Group (UK) Ltd, Croydon, CR0 4YY

Oxford University Press makes no representation, express or implied, that the
drug dosages in this book are correct. Readers must therefore always check
the product information and clinical procedures with the most up-to-date
published product information and data sheets provided by the manufacturers
and the most recent codes of conduct and safety regulations. The authors and
the publishers do not accept responsibility or legal liability for any errors in the
text or for the misuse or misapplication of material in this work. Except where
otherwise stated, drug dosages and recommendations are for the non-pregnant
adult who is not breast-feeding

Links to third party websites are provided by Oxford in good faith and
for information only. Oxford disclaims any responsibility for the materials
contained in any third party website referenced in this work.

Foreword

I am not a music therapist, music psychologist, music educator, or musician. I am a social worker who has worked with children and adolescents, often in groups in a variety of settings, since 1974. Music played a role in many of my groups. I didn't have to invite it. It invited itself. All I had to do was welcome it.

The first adolescent group I formed was composed of 14–18-year-old Mexican American boys and girls living in a low-income agrarian community in the Midwestern United States. At the time I had no professional credentials or schooling in child development or clinical practice. I was part of a national service programme known as VISTA or Volunteers in Service to America. The focus I brought to that first group was the members' Mexican identity and heritage. It entailed incorporating traditional Mexican American music and dance into our group meetings and, ultimately, public performances to the wider membership of this close-knit community—performances that the elders loved and which helped to strengthen communal and inter-generational bonds.

I was fortunate to come into this experience ignorant of professional scholarship or convention. I learned inductively and avoided the spiritual incarceration that plagued others whom I've met over the years. I knew nothing but my heart; and I had a fairly steady ethical compass. Consequently, I felt free to experiment, improvise, innovate, and create. It was a good way to begin.

Looking back

When I was a child, almost every Sunday morning my father drove me to the bar and grill he managed in Newark, New Jersey. It was called the P.O.N., which stood for the Pride of Newark. One of the things I remembered best about the P.O.N. was its jukebox. My father gave me coins and I played my favourite song, over and over, week after week. The song was Lloyd Price's 'Personality'.

My only public solo musical performance as a child in the 1950s was at a 'swim club' (a place with a huge swimming pool and social-recreational activities for adults and kids) that my parents took me to during my childhood summers. I attended a day camp there. My counsellor was a dancer who decided that his campers would put on a dance show for the entire membership of the club, probably a couple of hundred parents and kids.

I didn't want to participate in the dance project. Instead I convinced the counsellor to let me give a solo performance of Jerry Lee Lewis' 'Great Balls of Fire'. I practised and practised, listening to the song over and over on a 45 rpm vinyl turntable record player, performing in front of my mother who helped me to transcribe the lyrics from the 45.

Although I rarely talk about any of this today, listening and singing along with 'Personality' on the jukebox on Sunday mornings in the bar with my dad; and, practising

'Great Balls of Fire' in the 1950s with my mom are among the enduring memories of my childhood years.

Moving forward

Now I am a father of two boys, young men today, who played instruments in school and garage bands throughout all of their school age and teenage years. There was never a time I can recall them not listening to music. Jamie, my older son, played trumpet in jazz and Dixieland bands. My younger son Darren played the drums. Together with a few class-mates, they formed a punk rock band, DIY-style. Because he was the drummer and we had the drum set in our den, the band practised for many years on the first floor of our two-storey house in Long Beach, New York.

One autumn day, when Darren was about 14 years old, he asked my wife and I if his band and some of their fellow bands could have a concert in our side yard. We con-ferred and then said, 'Sure, okay', providing he sought and received consent from our neighbours. On concert day scores of kids flocked to our yard, spilling out into the street. My wife Dale, a high school art teacher, and I served as 'security' for the concert. One neighbour (there's always one) called the police. A uniformed police officer rolled up in a cruiser and told me that we had to 'shut it down'. I offered to approach the com-plainant and make an appeal to him. I cajoled him into backing off and rescinding his complaint. The neighbour told me, 'Just ask them to turn down the volume, my house is shaking'.

I promised the neighbour, but then, as I turned to walk back down the street to my house, a van pulled up in front and some older teenage boys proceeded to cart out a set of speakers four times the size of the ones that were already in use. Needless to say, it was a memorable Sunday afternoon.

Darren's closest band mate and lifelong friend Kaitlyn Eldridge went on to form the band Big Eyes, which has produced a number of albums and tours the United States and abroad, including one tour with C.J. Ramone.

All of which brings me back to my role as a social worker and my intuitive if not in-tellectual knowledge about the importance of music in young peoples' lives. 'Is everyone musical?' ask Alexandra Lamont and David Hargreaves. Probably so.

Back in the field

Some years ago I was working with a pre-adolescent group and, as we approached the end of our time together the group members made a decision to sing songs as a parting ritual, as the group was about to end its time together. Most of the group members chose contemporary songs with themes that had to do with 'saying goodbye'. The group mem-bers, boys and girls, performed despite their various talent levels. Some chose silly songs that brought laughter; including parodies by 'Weird Al' Yankovic, the most renowned performer of the genre. No attempt was made to interpret the lyrics. They created a spir-ited and meaningful ending ritual that I did not wish to step on, control, or contaminate.

One 'performance' floored me. Charley (a pseudonym) came to the group some time after he had witnessed his mother's murder. I advocated for including Charley to be in the group, although some of my more experienced colleagues cautioned me against that. They said, as I recall, that the other group members, all of whom had experienced loss, would not be able to 'handle' the details of Charley's story should he choose to reveal them in the group. I reasoned why Charley shouldn't be isolated from his peers, who I trusted were stronger than they were given credit for. One of my credos is to invite the whole person to participate, not just the broken, troubled, and hurt parts. For his parting song Charley performed an old-time tune that struck a different chord in me and the other group members than any of the other songs. As I listened I imagined that it was a song that his deceased mother had sung to him, and his grandmother to her. As Charley started to sing, the others grew quiet and gave Charley the space that he needed. He seemed to choke on the word 'mother' in the first stanza, but continued through until the end. With his sweet smile and sorrowful eyes he sang 'Play a Simple Melody'. It was an old time song written by Irving Berlin and performed by Bing Crosby. It was hardly Demi Lovato or Snoop Dogg, but the group gave him the respect that he needed and deserved. They stepped up.

Kat and the band

My long-distance friend Kat McFerran invited me to write the Foreword to this book despite the fact that I haven't nearly the credentials or musical 'chops' of the wonderful authors who fill this incredible compendium on working with adolescents to promote their wellbeing using music. As Kat asserts, which gives me a glimmer of 'street cred' for my years using music as a clinical social worker, 'the pairing of music and emotions is natural and to a certain degree, unavoidable'.

Kat is from Australia and I'm from the United States. We got to know one another first through e-mail correspondence about our mutual interest in adolescent groups. It was my pleasure to meet Kat face to face when she visited New York. I took her on a tour of my agency North Shore Child and Family Guidance Center, a 65-year-old children's mental health centre located on Long Island. We've continued to stayed in touch ever since. And, now, through this book she has introduced me to all of her music therapy band mates. And, she's allowed me to play an opening number with this awesome band.

A final thought

This book offers readers the opportunity to balance the value placed in verbal product with the meaning and impact of nonverbal activity, including silent moments. After all, good music is appreciated for the spaces between the sounds—silent intervals—as well as the sounds themselves.

I recently read Bruce Springsteen's autobiography, *Born to Run*, which blends many elements of his life, from early family experiences to first steps as a musician to forming a band to becoming a rock star, husband, and parent. At the core of the book is the enduring and troubling impact of his relationship with his father Doug. Springsteen reveals a dream in which he is performing on stage. His then deceased father is sitting in the audience. Bruce approaches him in the dream and says: 'Look dad ... that guy on stage ... that's you, that's how I see you'. I was struck with the overwhelming feeling that he wrote the book in its entirety in the voice of vulnerable young boy, as opposed to world-renowned music icon. The boy has been fighting the isolation and loneliness of living with mental illness in the family his whole life.

In this book, Tia De Nora writes that 'age is a flexible construction' with inherent plasticity and that, 'to the extent that it is always possible within music to be "young", music affords connection and reconnection with all of our aged-selves, all our days'.

Springsteen epitomizes that. His life story is not only about rising to music stardom; it is a story about debilitating depression, mental illness, and adverse childhood experiences. And, it is a story of hope. He shows that despite his most troubling childhood experiences that were lived in relative silence, resilience and healing are possible.

In these troubled and troubling times, we need to look closely at our practice in field and classroom and find what we do that contributes to silencing young people and what we do that helps to 'break the silence' in a meaningful way. This book goes a long way in showing us how to understand and use music to do just that.

Andrew Malekoff
North Shore Child and Family Guidance Center

Acknowledgements, hopes, and dreams

Both together and separately, we each acknowledge the elders of the far-flung lands on which we work and write, the indigenous cultures of Australia, Scotland, and Finland. We pay our respects to the long cultures of music and healing that have existed before our disciplines and aspire to contribute a particular contemporary perspective to this conversation. To achieve this task, we have endeavoured to include authors from a range of countries, including South Africa, Canada, Germany, Norway, England, and the United States as well as authors with diverse cultural and religious backgrounds and heterogeneous sexual and gender identities. We acknowledge the limits of our attempts, particularly with regards to non-white cultures and less privileged social states and countries. We hope for change and desire the creation of more mutually empowering relationships between diverse persons from around the world, and we believe that music may be one way of achieving this dream. This text is one part of our contribution to this end.

We have chosen to integrate a range of perspectives on the topic of music, adolescents, and wellbeing into the text. This has included music therapy, which is both a profession and a discipline, and within which the active facilitation of people's wellbeing through musical engagement is the primary focus of both. We have also privileged music psychology, a discipline and body of research, which is sometimes used by professionals but is only a career within the academy. Music educators have also been sought for the task of deliberating this topic, which is particularly pertinent since schools are the primary context in which we meet young people in order to engage them in music. In addition, we have solicited texts from authors who identify as music sociologists and community musicians to gather intersecting perspectives on this fascinating topic.

We approached authors who were known to us by their writing and/or their professional practices and so the book blends research and practice orientations. We asked the music therapy scholars to include stories in their chapters to illustrate the ways that theories are applied by trained professionals. The stories further give voice to the young people themselves, but the names of all individuals that are mentioned in the stories, and throughout the text, have been changed to ensure their anonymity. We asked all writers to position themselves respectfully towards diverse bodies of knowledge and to avoid generalizing about beliefs that may be held in some disciplines but not in others; for example, the value of information that can be extracted from brain scans, or the truth of statements that can be made based on the results of randomized controlled trials. We also asked authors to use the first names of people they quoted in texts, with the intention of offering some further glimmers of gender and culture to the people who have influenced them—rather than being assumed to be white men, which surnames can sometimes, unintentionally, imply. Therefore, we have not only included multiple perspectives, but have also asked our colleagues to represent their views with respect and an inclusive attitude to others.

The result of this is a text that is diverse in content and style, emphasizing practical, ideological, theoretical, and empirical perspectives—all of them couched within a political frame that favours multiplicity over binaries, gender equality over patriarchy, and contextual sensitivity over extreme objectivity. Nonetheless, we are three white Western women who are employed by university systems and therefore have access to more than our fair share of world resources and limited networks beyond the academic sector. We hope that this text has implications that reach beyond there, however, and have endeavoured to produce a text that brings together a range of ideas so they can be used and applied by people in education, health and community care, and welfare, and in families around the globe.

Structure of the book

The complex relationship between music, adolescents, and wellbeing could be divided into many categories. We chose processing emotions, performing identity, and being connected as our structure for this text.

Emotions has been placed first because it is often the beginning point of interest for those who have discovered the fascinating scholarship on this topic. It has been explored most voraciously by music psychologists, and therefore much of the research has adopted an objective lens, addressing music as a stimulus or correlate that can explain various wellbeing outcomes. In this book, we include a range of chapters from music psychologists (Genevieve Dingle, Leah Sharman, and Joel Larwood, Australia; Margarida Baltazar, Finland) as well as some insightful recommendations about future music psychology research on this topic (Tan-Chyuan Chin, Australia/Singapore). We also include contributions from three music therapists who work with young people whose emotional uses of music occur in the context of violence, anger, and depression—topics that are not often addressed with depth in the wider literature. This includes chapters from Andreas Wölfl (Germany), Andeline dos Santos (South Africa), and Jospehine Geipel (Germany).

Identity is another important area that is often investigated in music studies with an adolescent lens. Our position is that music can be an agency promoting resource in this context, offering adolescents empowering experiences of being the actors in their life, even if the fundamentals of their selves are changing and need to be renegotiated. This section integrates viewpoints from music psychology (Dave Miranda, Canada), music sociology (Tia De Nora, UK), and music education (Alexandra Lamont and David Hargreaves, UK) to discuss how music serves as a resource for adolescents' identity construction. Three music therapists—Viggo Krüger (Norway), Daphne Rickson (New Zealand), and Elly Scrine (Australia)—further contemplate and illustrate how this becomes visible in the practical work with the young people.

Connectedness is now a much more fascinating area than in previous decades, with new forms of connectivity constantly emerging. We believe that music is an extraordinary medium for connecting with others, and it is being accessed and shared both face to face and online in increasingly diverse ways. In this section, we include chapters from music scholars from a range of disciplines such as sociology (Lisa Nikulinksy and Andy Bennett, Australia), philosophy and education (Susan O'Neill, Canada), and media studies (Roseann Pluretti and Piotr Bobkowski, USA) whose comprehensive and differing perspectives examine the breadth of this topic. We also include chapters by music therapists—Helen Oosthuizen (South Africa), Michael Viega (USA), and Carmen Cheong-Clinch (Australia)—whose exploration of connectedness within the context of their work contributes a wide view of music therapy practice with young people to this book.

Conclusion

Our hopes and dreams for this text is that it provides perspectives, theories, research, and practice ideas that may inspire the reader to connect with young people using music and to appropriate those opportunities to encourage wellbeing. As the overlapping fields of music, adolescence, and wellbeing continue to intersect, we are confident that their connections will be better understood and increasingly utilized, and we encourage readers to support this possibility with whatever resources they have available to them.

Katrina McFerran
Philippa Derrington
Suvi Saarikallio

Contents

Contributors

Margarida Baltazar
University of Jyväskylä, Finland

Andy Bennett
Griffith University, Australia

Piotr S. Bobkowski
University of Kansas, USA

Carmen Cheong-Clinch
University of Melbourne, Australia

Tan-Chyuan Chin
University of Melbourne, Australia

Tia De Nora
University of Exeter, UK

Philippa Derrington
Queen Margaret University, UK

Genevieve Dingle
University of Queensland, Australia

Andeline dos Santos
University of Pretoria, South Africa

Josephine Geipel
SRH University Heidelberg, Germany;
University of Heidelberg, Germany

David Hargreaves
University of Roehampton, UK

Viggo Krüger
University of Bergen, Norway

Alexandra Lamont
Keele University, UK

Joel Larwood
University of Queensland, Australia

Katrina McFerran
University of Melbourne, Australia

Dave Miranda
University of Ottawa, Canada

Lisa Nikulinsky
Griffith University, Australia

Susan A. O'Neill
Simon Fraser University, Canada

Helen Oosthuizen
University of Melbourne, Australia

Roseann Pluretti
Hamilton College, USA

Daphne Rickson
Victoria University of Wellington,
New Zealand

Suvi Saarikallio
University of Jyväskylä, Finland

Elly Scrine
University of Melbourne, Australia

Leah Sharman
University of Queensland, Australia

Michael Viega
Montclair State University, USA

Andreas Wölfl
Freies Musikzentrum, Germany

Part 1

Emotions

Chapter 1

Crystallizing the relationship between adolescents, music, and emotions

Katrina McFerran

Introduction

The topic of music, adolescents, and emotions is one that excites many researchers, practitioners, and lay persons. We all relate to the connection between these three complex and interwoven facets of life. The point at which they intersect is almost unbearably interesting and an increasing amount of scholarship has been focused there. In the following chapters, we offer six different perspectives on this intersection with contributions from music therapists and music psychologists. These views are not easy to integrate, since music psychologists typically focus on the influence of music on emotions, while music therapists tend to prioritize the emotional experience of individuals in various musical conditions. Therefore, in this chapter I will attempt to honour these diverse perspectives using the lens of crystallization, which illuminates the topic from different angles in a way that hopefully highlights points of connection as well as divergence.

What is crystallization?

The scholarship on adolescents, music, and emotions demands an openness to different perspectives on the relationship between music and emotions, since the creators of knowledge draw variously on music practices, laboratory-based research, and theorizing about what they claim to know. I have chosen to employ the notion of 'crystallization' as a frame for this endeavour, inspired by how it has been used in qualitative research to capture the multiple and slippery ways in which knowledge is constructed from a variety of angles (Ellingson, 2017). Crystallization emphasizes the varied perspectives of writers and researchers who use different methods and allow for multiple meanings rather than seeking to integrate different ideas into simplistic and singular truths. According to Laurel Richardson (2000), who originally coined the term, 'the central imaginary is the crystal, which combines symmetry and substance with an infinite variety of shapes, substances, transmutations, multidimensionalities, and angles of approach' (p. 234). This seems very appropriate for representing the infinite variety of ways we can understand adolescents, music, and emotions.

Why crystallization?

The notion of crystallization allows me to explore the rich world of adolescents and their emotions without trying to simplify or generalize from one teenager's experience to another's. In my own experience of working with young people, the unique and complex circumstances in which each is embedded has an enormous influence on the ways they are willing and able to use music. Whether they are living at home, or in foster care; whether they are older adolescents about to become independent, or younger teenagers who still have years in their family home; whether they have high- or low-level intellectual abilities; their gender; their sexual identifications—all of these things interact with how each chooses to use music in relation to their emotions. From my perspective, young people's musical preferences and uses in relation to emotions can only be understood at the intersection of all these 'variables'. In the following six chapters, each author presents a particular perspective on this relationship, and my role is to propose a way of seeing that allows for them all. As Richardson (2000) says, 'Crystallization provides us with a deepened, complex, thoroughly partial, understanding of the topic. Paradoxically, we know more and doubt what we know. Ingeniously, we know there is always more to know' (p. 934).

What do we think we know about music, adolescents, and emotions?

When asked, many adolescents will passionately describe the ways they use music to match and meet their emotions to make them feel better (McFerran and Saarikallio, 2013). A range of studies have also shown that this connection is intensified when young people are struggling emotionally (McFerran et al., 2016) and, indeed, the same has been shown for adults (Saarikallio, 2011). These adolescent accounts affirm what appears obvious to most of us who have experienced adolescence and who observe adolescents. However, what we mean by emotions is vast and diverse, as the six chapters show, since authors variously describe dealing with complex emotions related to aggression (Chapter 2), violence (Chapter 7), and depression (Chapter 5), both in music therapy and independently, as well as using strategies such as immersing in music (Chapter 3) and regulating affect with music (Chapter 6). As Chin describes in Chapter 4, this vast terrain leads to the need for complex and clearly rationalized research approaches and Chin's elegant and systematic suggestions canvas many possibilities that bear consideration by researchers in the future.

Resisting dichotomies: continuums of understanding

The use of a continuum can be valuable for resisting dichotomous understandings (Ellingson, 2011) and the continuum of wellbeing used in Table 1.1 attempts to illuminate a territory that we all traverse over the course of our lives, many times. It moves beyond boxing young people into being healthy or unhealthy, mentally well or mentally ill; this is an avoidance that is particularly important to young people who often fear that one stage

Table 1.1. Emotional uses of music described in the literature presented across a wellbeing continuum

Distressed	Pessimistic	Optimistic	Flourishing
Isolating	Conforming	Rebelling	Connecting
Alienating	Withdrawing	Modelling	Inspiring
Triggering	Negatively comparing	Diverting	Entertaining
Ruminating	Escaping	Improving	Enhancing
Intensifying	Avoiding	Modifying	Sensation-seeking
Worsening	Immersing	Reappraising	Relaxing
Venting	Maintaining	Regulating	Energizing
	Comforting	Calming	
		Reviving	

of their life will somehow define how they will be forever. I have learned from experience that binary notions restrict ways of seeing and describing, as in my previous depiction of healthy and unhealthy ways of using music (Saarikallio et al., 2015). Although we used this framework as a way of drawing attention to the potentially harmful ways that young people sometimes use music, this strategy was ultimately unsatisfying because readers would tend to focus on one or the other. In addition, a binary does not adequately convey the multifaceted ways that young people use the same music for different emotional purposes and outcomes on different days and in different states. I hope that continuums allow for a more nuanced range of possibilities.

Emotional states

In this handbook we ask the reader to accept that the pairing of music and emotions is natural and, to a certain degree, unavoidable. Much has been written about the existence and nature of the relationship (for example Bunt and Pavlicevic, 2001; Juslin, 2009; Pellitteri, 2009; Sloboda and O'Neill, 2001) and a vast range of sources are referenced by the authors in this text. Based on this foundational scholarship, the positive potential inherent in the relationship between music and emotion is assumed by our authors. At our request, they have taken this opportunity to tackle some of the more complex uses of music for emotional purposes, from the perspective of therapists, psychologists, and researchers. It is important to note that our emphasis on depression, aggression, and violence does not suggest that we find this more prevalent than positive uses of music for relaxation, affirmation, and connection. Rather, we are choosing to explore less common uses which need to be better understood in order to ensure that young people are not naïve in their reliance on music for wellbeing, a phenomenon that we have discovered when collaborating with young people (McFerran and Saarikallio, 2013). The power of music can certainly be used in many emotional directions, particularly by those who are struggling with depression and other challenging life events and conditions, and a review of literature on adolescence, music, and depression shows this has been investigated from a number of angles (McFerran et al., 2016). One way of understanding the variety of ways in which young people use music is across a wellbeing continuum, as young people move between distress, pessimism, optimism, and flourishing. My conceptualization of emotions referenced in the literature linking music and adolescents used this continuum to map no fewer than 31 references to emotional uses in only 23 articles (16 music psychology/7 music therapy), all of which may be experienced by any single adolescent at a different moment in their life, although some may find themselves more frequently in one state of being and using (see Table 1.1).

To illustrate, when discussing helpful and unhelpful uses of music with young people, I have often heard stories that sound like the following.

Oh, this is my absolute favourite song. I listen to it all the time. I don't know what I would do without it. It used to be the song my boyfriend and I loved together, but then after we broke up, it really became my tragedy song. I would listen to it and cry and cry. At the same time, I went into a really deep depression that was related to a lot of things that had been going on in my life both then and when I was young. So, I really did listen to it a lot and in lots of ways. I was often using it to bring up my own sadness and keep the connection with that. But since we started talking about helpful ways of using music, I've managed to change up the way this song makes me feel, and it has taken on new meanings, yet again. Now I use it as a way of thinking about how strong I am for having survived that break up and all the sadness at the same time. Now it's become like a survival anthem for me and I listen to it to remind myself that I can handle anything. It doesn't make me cry anymore, but it reminds me that I have cried and survived.

This vignette explains why binaries do not work in understanding the intersection between adolescents, music, and emotions. It shows how young people come to rely on music, and how their passionate commitment to certain songs and genres of music can flexibly move from one association (being a love song), to another (a break-up song), and another (a song of triumph). This young woman's experiences challenge a range of simplistic binary understandings, the most common of which is the assumption that certain music (either genre or song) has a predictable effect on the emotions of young people and that the musical qualities of the song reliably elicit a consistent response.

Emotional intentions

The assumption that certain types of music have a particular effect has been the basis of many studies about the relationship between adolescents, music, and emotions. Although problematic, it is conveniently well-matched with quality standards in objectivist research that rely on controlling variables. In these models, playing a particular type of music and then analysing young people's reactions to it makes logical sense, based on the assumption that if it is the qualities of the music causing the emotion, it would be the same on a different day. While we may learn a great deal from examining young people's emotional reactions to a piece of music, this approach fails to acknowledge the emotional intentions

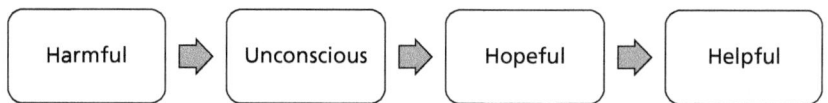

Fig. 1.1 Continuum of music use.

and agency that young people frequently refer to in describing their reactions of music. I believe this is a critical dimension to understanding the intersection between adolescents, music, and emotions, and without it young people are dangerously relegated to a role as passive recipient rather than active agent. As long as we focus on a passive relationship with music, we fail to encourage the more powerful potential that music can have in relation to emotional wellbeing. Music can be used with intention, and if that intention is bought into consciousness, it can be a source of emotional strength. However, if it is used unconsciously during difficult times, music can equally serve to reinforce negative emotional states rather than be used to regulate them. Another vignette captures this assumption in the words of a young person.

My best friend eventually just deleted the song off my phone. I was so angry at him that I didn't talk to him for two days, and if it was anyone else, I would have literally killed them. But he knows me really well, and he's been there for me through all of this crap, and so I had to forgive him. And actually, he was right. I thought that listening to that song over and over was going to make me feel better, but it didn't. It just made me feel worse and worse, but somehow, I didn't notice it. I kept hoping that if I listened enough times, and cathartically expressed my feelings, then I would pass through them and feel better in the end. But it just didn't work like that. I did put the song back on my phone in the end. But now I'm more conscious of what I'm doing with it.

Given the interaction between emotional states and emotional intentions, a different continuum might focus on whether music use is helpful, hopeful, unconscious, or harmful (Fig. 1.1).

Once again, this does not suggest that any particular adolescent should be pigeonholed into only one of these intentions, or even that a particular song might be used to fulfil only one of these emotional functions. Embedded in the proposed continuum is an idea that young people move fluidly between these intentions, and that raising their consciousness about their (often unexpressed) intentions might have benefits for their wellbeing. By acknowledging varying intentions that young people have when using music for emotional work, we might encourage more helpful uses of music and raise the consciousness of young people about how they use music to cope with different experiences in their lives.

Emotions in context

Both the emotional states we are in and our intentions (conscious or not) for using music occur *in situ*, and sensitivity to that context adds a further layer of depth to the intersection between adolescents, emotions, and music. It is not enough to focus only on intrapersonal experience and motivations, since these are profoundly influenced by the place where they occur and how much emotion is allowed in that space by the people who control it.

Schools are the sites where many young people spend the greatest amount of their time and in this context the combination of music and emotions can be considered problematic. This might be the case when music teachers are focused on the kinds of neoliberal goals that lead to the development and testing of musical skills, with less attention being paid to the expressive potentials of music (McFerran et al., 2018). When emotions are allowed or encouraged in the school context it can be quite uncomfortable for the adult players, since our emotional worlds can be quite loud when sounded out. Whether it is joyful celebration or cathartic expression of rage, the noise produced is hard to ignore, both within the room and beyond its walls, which can challenge the school establishment.

Emotions have more place in the social lives of young people, but there is no less complexity in the impact of their expression. When alone, uses of music for emotional work are well-enough captured in Table 1.1 and undoubtedly intersect with the expression of identity, as discussed in the following section of this handbook. When connecting with others, the differences between online and face-to-face expression of emotion are significant, as explored in the final section of the handbook. In fact, it is difficult to extract emotions from identity and relationships in the context of everyday life since they are entwined and embedded.

However, emotions come to the fore in some contexts where we meet young people, particularly when struggling with emotion has become a central focus of their lives. Hospital contexts are one example of this situation, whether the setting is for mental or physical illness. Here, young people may well be *distressed* and *pessimistic*, but are often attempting to use music in *helpful* or *hopeful* ways, accessing it as a resource for coping under difficult circumstances. The best shape for those intentions is perceived quite differently by music therapists and psychologists, according to a critical review of the literature (McFerran, 2016).

Psychologists appear to focus young people's attempts at using music for controlling, regulating, and stabilizing their emotions. The language used in the literature reveals a consistent orientation to cognitively controlled uses of music in order to manage difficult emotions and emphasize positive ones. Music therapists offer a different emphasis, including management but also focusing on expressing and becoming aware of emotions, often by the music therapist holding and containing volatile and intense emotions during shared musical experiences (as seen throughout chapters in this handbook). This difference may be partially mediated by the medium used by these different professionals. While music therapists tend to use music and creative processes as the means of connection, psychologists are more likely to use words and cognitive processes as a way of working with the emotional content. This has a significant impact on the nature of the therapeutic encounter, as the following vignette illustrates.

Sarah was admitted to an acute mental health unit following a period of severe paranoia and delusion. When the music therapist first met her on the ward she undertook an assessment of Sarah's current uses of music to identify both her preferred music and her ways of using that music to make herself feel better or worse. During this time, Sarah made a number of lavish statements about her love of music and her passionate commitment to it, but was unable to focus on answering questions about whether she often felt worse after listening repeatedly to certain songs, or whether she used music to isolate herself from others, which seemed likely. Having completed the assessment, the music therapist then moved in to a less cognitive and more creative process, inviting Sarah to choose an instrument and to join her in a therapeutic improvisation. Sarah's choice of the xylophone afforded her a number of melodic opportunities to express her emotions, and she began to play timidly on the chime bars, staying within a small number of tones and repeating her initial patterns. The music therapist began to accompany her, matching her small range and offering the containment that she seemed to be seeking. From that basis, Sarah began to attempt a more expressive range of notes and striking patterns, while the music therapist provided the stable base from which she could explore and return. After the improvisation finished, Sarah described what it felt like to be given permission to explore her emotions and how feeling safe and held had allowed her to be more honest about how she was really feeling.

Different contexts afford different uses of music for emotional work, as do different professionals and adults involved in the lives of young people. While emotional control might be the priority for some, freedom of emotional expression may be more of a focus for others. This reflects not only the professional occupations of those surrounding the young person, but also their own capacity to tolerate and be with difficult emotions. Perhaps most importantly, the context has an enormous influence over what is considered to be acceptable and helpful, with more hierarchical structures tending to emphasize self-control where creative contexts might actually value greater connection with emotions of all kinds. Music therapists sometimes attempt to bridge the potentials of both these approaches, by balancing expressivity with containment, and experience with cognitive processing. Ultimately, however, it is the young person who decides when, where, how much, and how often they will use music for emotional work, and in what ways.

Forms of musicking

Christopher Small (1998) introduced the verb 'musicking' into academic music discourse as a way of emphasizing the action qualities of music, rather than focusing on music as an object—be it a recording or a score. This kind of emphasis is relevant to a discussion about adolescents, music, and emotions since different ways of musicking afford different potentials for emotional work. To feel that one's emotions are reflected in the music is not the same as expressing one's emotions through music making. Depending on the young person's emotional state, intentions, and context, the same form of musicking can be experienced very differently, as the following vignette highlights.

Stefan had a talent for music and was able to recall and play long pieces of repertoire after hearing them only once. He also had Asperger's Syndrome. When he attended piano lessons, Stefan often spent a lot of time playing and the school staff agreed that it made a difference to his day when he had the opportunity to spend some time at the piano; he was calmer and less likely to get over-stimulated in class. Some of the school team began to wonder whether playing the piano could become even more meaningful and questioned whether it might be valuable to try and connect with him during his music making, rather than simply relying on it to make him feel more relaxed. His piano teacher began to participate with Stefan when he was playing the piano, gently interrupting his playing with playful strikes at the opposite end of the keyboard to get his attention. Initially, Stefan was distressed by the interruptions, but over a number of weeks of gentle offers by his teacher, he began to look for them, turning towards his teacher when he was playing, as if to invite him to play. Over time, the two pianists began to improvise quite playfully on the keyboard, sometimes spending more than five minutes throwing ideas back and forth and interacting together. The content and the experience became emotionally meaningful for both of them, whereas previously it had felt void of emotional content and fixated on the structural or performative dimensions. Staff also reported that Stefan seemed more open to communication in the classroom and would now look to be included in some activities, rather than always distancing himself from group work.

The binary distinction between playing and listening is challenged by this vignette. It illustrates how it is possible to be emotionally distant as well as emotionally engaged when making music. Equally, it is possible to have strong emotional connections with recorded music, and for those emotions to be shared. For example, studies of metal music have consistently shown that listening is a powerful way to connect to intense emotions and that feeling a part of a worldwide community of fans also enhances a sense of connectedness and feeling understood (Snell and Hodgetts, 2007). It is therefore too simple to say that the distinction in emotional affordances is purely related to the different forms of musicking. It is more closely related to young people's abilities to appropriate music, which is impacted by cultural expectations and opportunities (DeNora, 2006).

However, different forms of musicking can be suggested by adult professionals to encourage young people to discover new ways of using music in relation to their emotions. Listening to music with young people readily promotes reflection on emotional content for example. Writing songs and song lyrics with young people encourages the articulation of different emotions and feelings and gives them a narrative and culturally appropriate context for expression. Improvising on instruments avoids any existing connotations that might be associated with songs or genres and allows for a more pure and novel expression and discovery of emotions that might be difficult to uncover through other forms of musicking. This is equally true in groups as it is in individual work, as the following vignette illustrates.

Giovanni struck the bass drum with a huge thump that made some of the other group members jump in their seats. The therapist responded with an accelerating beat on the snare drum and two of the other group members began to strum their electric guitars quickly as they moved their hand up and down the frets, creating wild and intense soundscapes. One of the young women began to call into the microphone in screamo style, perhaps offering words, although they were indecipherable. The improvisation climaxed swiftly and then settled back into a groove, then climaxed again, this time for longer, before settling back down to almost silence. Angela maintained a steady bass guitar ostinato throughout, seemingly untouched by the sounds around her. She then maintained her steady crotchet repeating note for a further minute before ceasing and bringing the improvisation to a close. After some silence, the music therapist asked for reflections from the bereaved young people who were members of the group. 'It felt great to express that rage' said one young man. 'You really rocked that drum kit!' said another. 'Yeah, I feel better after that', replied one more group member, which made everyone laugh. 'Better, huh?' the therapist responded, 'What was it that made you feel better—being connected, being heard, expressing a particular emotion?' 'I dunno ...' they all reply.

This vignette, and the therapist's response, show how it is possible to share emotions with others through music in ways that are non-specific, even to the person who is playing them. And yet, distressed young people repeatedly report that they appreciate the opportunities for creative expression in a safe context that allows for emotional work without letting it get out of control (McFerran, 2011). This has also been shown to occur when using live singing of people's preferred songs, although this often relates to emotions that could more easily be predicted in advance, because the individual has an association with the song (Bibb and McFerran, 2018). The impact of music on other group members is less predictable though, and a research study of using songs in groups with mental health consumers clearly shows that it is common for participants to be triggered emotionally by other people's choices. This obviously requires careful therapeutic handling, especially within the mental health context, but in many ways provides further opportunities for emotional processing in the hands of a therapist.

Why is it important?

Increased access to music

There has been an extraordinary increase in the amount of access young people have to music since the introduction of the Internet and related music apps and streaming services. Studies have shown that young people are taking full advantage of this opportunity and are frequently listening while multitasking with games, using social media, and while studying (Krause et al., 2015). Although there is reason to be concerned about the impact of new technologies, it is also an opportunity to significantly enhance the ways that young people can use music in their everyday lives to promote emotional wellbeing. Since the interaction between emotions and music is so complex, this is no simple task and both music therapists and music psychologists, along with our health professional colleagues, have a role to play in ensuring that music is used to its full potential.

Our studies have shown that young people who are the most distressed are the least able to use music to feel better (Garrido et al., 2017; McFerran et al., 2014). Instead, they are more likely to use music to intensify their emotional state and to increase their sense of emotional isolation (Garrido and Schubert, 2015). This is a natural consequence of the understanding that music and emotions intersect at the axes of states, intentions, contexts, and forms of musicking. A distressed state, combined with an unconsciously ruminative intention that occurs in the context of being isolated and bullied might easily deepen a young person's sense of emotional distress. However, a change in any of these conditions can lead readily to a positive change. For example, moving from being distressed to optimistic can lead to a more helpful choice of musicking, where the young person might choose to participate with others in sharing music rather than isolating themselves with their music. The possibilities are endless, but what is critical is that young people understand the importance of their own agency in benefiting from the emotional power of music, or they will tend to assume that the music will help them with no effort and no positive intention, which is not always the case. This public health message is a critical one for music therapists and others to disseminate.

Increased awareness of mental illness

Studies continue to suggest that young people are increasingly likely be struggling with mental illness and associated emotional challenges by comparison to previous decades (Rickwood et al., 2014). Whether this is due to increased acknowledgement, increased diagnosis, or increased pressures on young people is a theoretical question. However, the need for preventative and early intervention strategies is clear and music is an obvious strategy for this development.

More and more online forums and apps are being developed that help young people to use music as a way to work with their emotions when they are struggling. Some of these are mentioned in the Connectedness section of this handbook (see Chapter 21), and many more are emerging around the globe. If developers provide information about how to use music effectively and encourage young people to recognize the emotional affordances of music, the potentials are enormous. On the other hand, if developers reinforce a sense of passive dependence on music as a pill that will fix problems, apps could be problematic and exacerbate uses of music that reduce emotional wellbeing instead of enhancing it.

Need for non-pharmaceutical prevention

The Recovery movement, which acknowledges the failure of psychotropic drugs to cure mental illness, has resulted in a greater call for non-pharmacological interventions, potentially combined with moderate amounts of medications (Gates et al., 2015). Mental health consumers have expressed a desire to have more control of their own wellness–illness trajectories, and often report that music is an engaging and helpful medium (Solli, 2015). Since emotions are often a barrier and an enabler for more successful personal and social experiences, and pharmaceuticals have not been able to support emotional recovery, it seems likely that music may have a role to play as an accessible and engaging alternative.

Conclusion

Crystallization seems to be a more useful lens for understanding the intersection between adolescents, music, and emotions than more reductive strategies such as triangulation (Richardson, 2000). Although researchers strive to find simple and elegant solutions to problems, this particular combination of forces may not be amenable. Embracing and celebrating the complexity of the many ways that young people can use music for emotional wellbeing may be the most graceful solution. It is certainly true that avoiding binary assumptions about how music works, when it works, what kind of musicking works, and where it works will be critical to the achievement of positive outcomes by individuals and groups.

Despite this complexity, it is an exciting time for posing musical solutions to the pressing challenges facing our youth and our society who are experiencing increasing levels of depression and anxiety. Never before has it been possible to access such diverse forms of music and to communicate so widely with young people about the potentials of music via online and technological mediums. Music has potential to be used for personal and public health outcomes where emotional dimensions are implicated, and the chapters in this handbook speak to many solutions, as well as raising still further questions for researchers to pursue.

References

Bibb, J. and McFerran, K. S. (2018). Musical recovery: The role of group singing in regaining healthy relationships with music to promote mental health recovery. *Nordic Journal of Music Therapy*, **27**(3), 235. doi: 10.1080/08098131.2018.1432676.

Bunt, L. and Pavlicevic, M. (2001). Music and emotion: Perspectives from music therapy. In P. N. Juslin and J. A. Sloboda (Eds.), *Music and Emotion: Theory and Research* (pp. 181–201). Oxford: Oxford University Press.

DeNora, T. (2006). Music and self-identity. In A. Bennett, B. Shank, and J. Toynbee (Eds), *The Popular Music Studies Reader* (pp. 141–147). Oxon, UK: Psychology Press.

Ellingson, L. L. (2011). One introduction to crystallization. In *Engaging Crystallization in Qualitative Research* (pp. 1–28). Thousand Oaks, CA: SAGE Publications.

Ellingson, L. L. (2017). Crystallization. *The International Encyclopedia of Communication Research Methods*, 1–5. doi:10.1002/9781118901731.iecrm0055.

Garrido, S., Eerola, T., and McFerran, K. S. (2017). Group rumination: Social interactions around music in people with depression. *Frontiers in Psychology*, **8**, 490. doi:10.3389/fpsyg.2017.00490.

Garrido, S. and Schubert, E. (2015). Music and people with tendencies to depression. *Music Perception*, **32**(4), 313–321.

Gates, J., Killackey, E., Phillips, L., and Álvarez-Jiménez, M. (2015). Mental health starts with physical health: Current status and future directions of non-pharmacological interventions to improve physical health in first-episode psychosis. *The Lancet Psychiatry*, **2**(8), 726–742.

Juslin, P. N. (2009). Emotional responses to music. In S. Hallam, I. Cross, and M. Thaut (Eds), *The Oxford Handbook of Music Psychology* (pp. 131–140). New York: Oxford University Press.

Krause, A. E., North, A., and Hewitt, L. Y. (2015). Music listening in everyday life: Devices and choice. *Psychology of Music*, **43**(2), 155–170. doi:10.1177/0305735613496860.

McFerran, K. S. (2011). Music therapy with bereaved youth: Expressing grief and feeling better. *Prevention Researcher*, **18**(3), 17–20.

McFerran, K. S. (2016). Contextualising the relationship between music, emotions and the wellbeing of young people: A critical interpretive synthesis. *Musicae Scientiae*, **20**(1), 103–121.

McFerran, K. S. and Saarikallio, S. (2013). Depending on music to make me feel better: Who is responsible for the ways young people appropriate music for health benefits. *The Arts in Psychotherapy*, **41**(1), 89–97. doi:10.1016/j.aip.2013.11.007.

McFerran, K. S., Garrido, S., O'Grady, L., Grocke, D., and Sawyer, S. M. (2014). Examining the relationship between self-reported mood management and music preferences of Australian teenagers. *Nordic Journal of Music Therapy*, **24**(3), 187–203. doi:10.1080/08098131.2014.908942.

McFerran, K. S., Garrido, S., and Saarikallio, S. (2016). A critical interpretive synthesis of the literature linking music and adolescent mental health. *Youth and Society*, **48**(4), 521–538. doi:10.1177/0044118X13501343.

McFerran, K. S., Crooke, A. H. D., and McPherson, G. (2018). Navigating school arts program provision within a neoliberal paradigm: A grounded theory in the Australian context. *Research Studies in Music Education*, in press.

Pellitteri, J. (2009). *Emotional Processes in Music Therapy*. Gilsum, NH: Barcelona Publishers.

Richardson, L. (2000). Writing: A method of inquiry. In N. K. Denzin and Y. S. Lincoln (Eds), *Handbook of Qualitative Research* (2nd edn, pp. 923–943). Thousand Oaks, CA: SAGE Publications.

Rickwood, D. J., Telford, N. R., Parker, A. G., Tanti, C. J., and McGorry, P. D. (2014). Headspace— Australia's innovation in youth mental health: who are the clients and why are they presenting. *Medical Journal of Australia*, **200**(2), 1–4.

Saarikallio, S. (2011). Music as emotional self-regulation throughout adulthood. *Psychology of Music*, **39**(3), 307–327. doi:10.1177/0305735610374894.

Saarikallio, S., McFerran, K. S., and Gold, C. (2015). Development and validation of the Healthy-Unhealthy Uses of Music Scale (HUMS). *Child and Adolescent Mental Health*, **20**(4), 210–217.

Sloboda, J. and O'Neill, S. A. (2001). Emotions in everyday listening to music. In J. Sloboda and P. Juslin (Eds), *Music and Emotion. Theory and Research* (pp. 415–430). Hanover, NH: Wesleyan University Press.

Small, C. (1998). *Musicking: The Meanings of Performing and Listening*. Hanover, NH: Wesleyan University Press.

Snell, D. and Hodgetts, D. (2007). Heavy metal, identity and the social negotiation of a community of practice. *Journal of Community & Applied Social Psychology*, **17**(6), 430–445. doi:10.1002/casp.943.

Solli, H. P. (2015). Battling illness with wellness: A qualitative case study of a young rapper's experiences with music therapy. *Nordic Journal of Music Therapy*, **24**(3), 204–231.

Chapter 2

Group music therapy with adolescents referred for aggression

Andeline dos Santos

Introduction

I work as a music therapist in South Africa, one of the most aggressive countries in the world (Swartz, 2015). Increasing levels of aggression in schools here (Le Roux and Mokhele, 2011; Ncontsa and Shumba, 2013) reflect the violence and power imbalances that are prevalent in wider society (Ngqela and Lewis, 2012; Pahad and Graham, 2012). Poverty and the frustrations that flow from this form one of the crucial backdrops for understanding issues of youth aggression (Clark, 2012). In countries where economic inequality is greatest, so too are the levels of aggression (Wilkinson and Pickett, 2009).

Aggression takes many forms. It can be physical, verbal, non-verbal, or relational, as well as active or passive, direct or indirect. Aggression also serves various functions. It can be a response to perceived provocation (this is reactive and 'hot-blooded') or a proactive means to obtain a desired outcome (here it is planned and unemotional) (Vitaro et al., 2006). Aggression functions as part of complex social processes, for example, to stratify social systems, as observed in classroom bullying (Craig and Harel, 2004). Aggression can contribute to determining the dynamics of friendships (Wei and Jonson-Reid, 2011), and can serve as a means for obtaining power, control, status, popularity, and admiration within peer groups (Gini et al., 2011; Hawley, 2007; Jarvinen and Nicholls, 1996). When the adult-centric bias of much of the literature on youth at risk is questioned, 'problem behaviours' such as aggression can also be viewed as strategies used by adolescents to sustain health, resilience, and empowerment (Crombach and Elbert, 2014; Ungar, 2001; Ungar and Teram, 2000), identity and self-concept (Gooden, 1997), self-esteem (Copeland-Linder et al., 2012), status and belonging (Dahlberg and Potter, 2001; Gregson, 1994), and success (Hurrelmann and Engel, 1992).

Understanding aggression as a form of incompetence is rooted in models that construct a continuum where positive (prosocial) and negative (antisocial) behaviours reside on opposite ends (Hawley, 2007). In designing therapeutic processes, it is important to consider both how aggression can relate to deficits and damage, as well as how aggression can be an adaptive and functional response that is goal-directed and skilful in the context in which the adolescent finds themselves (Olthof et al., 2011).

Welcoming adolescents' multiplicity

Various theoretical approaches, including psychodynamic, developmental, and systemic, undergird how music therapy is considered and practised in relation to youth violence in schools. Katrina McFerran and Andreas Wölfl (2015) examine how each perspective is grounded in beliefs about the causes of violence and how music is used in everyday life. This directs the development of related programme aims, the selection of participants, and the use of techniques in music therapy sessions. My orientation is towards engaging with the multiple affordances of music and how individuals and groups actively appropriate these (Ansdell, 2014). As music is a dynamic, unfolding human process, rather than a static autonomous object (Small, 1998), so too can we regard adolescents in a way that is not limited to a perceived 'core identity'. When a person has been placed in a stable, unitary identity category such as 'aggressive adolescent' the tendency is for this to then override other more socially acceptable identities, such as 'loyal friend', 'dreamer', 'empathic sister', and so on. These go missing without further investigation (Kouri and Smith, 2013). Alternatively, it is possible to view adolescents as multiplicities and as lines of improvisational performance (Skott-Myre, 2008). I began to learn the value of this perspective from the outset of my work in the context of aggression. The following vignette illustrates my first encounter with the irreducibly multidimensional nature of young people at school who are referred to music therapy for being 'aggressive adolescents'.

After warmly welcoming the six members of my first group, and introducing them to the greeting song I suggest we start sessions with, I invite them into a djembe and vocal improvisation. The group members begin with some scepticism and cautious curiosity. Each member offers his or her own rhythm and vocal melody while listening carefully to how this blends with the music of the others in the group. As we are playing and singing together the energy level begins to rise from the tentative beginnings. Movements grow larger and facial expressions are open, engaged, and excited. The group is flowing synchronously. I begin to count in time with the beat, '1 ... 2 ... 3 ... 4 ... STOP!' Everyone stops with me instantaneously. I call: '... 2 ... 3 GO!', beginning again on the first beat of the new bar. They all join me precisely and boldly on this first beat. We are singing and playing the drums with strength, steadiness, and festivity. The group members' voices grow even louder in ascending whooping calls. Leihlani is now drumming as loudly as she possibly can. The others align their rhythm and dynamic level to hers. Some offer slight rhythmic variations, but overall it is her beat they match. She has created a current that pulls the groove. As the music climaxes Leihlani initiates a drum roll that builds explosively towards an ending. As she lifts her hands in the air after the last beat the rest of us do the same in a joint flourish with her. We laugh in a satisfied outburst that captures our joyfully playful musical connection.

Group music therapy can facilitate the range of expressions that emerge from adolescents-as-multiplicities and can contain and assist them in understanding and working with the multifaceted nature of their needs and strengths. These adolescents had the capacity to direct strength, force, and intensity towards harming others, as described in their reasons for referral and in their own descriptions of their social interactions. In this vignette it becomes apparent how they were also able to extend strength, force, and intensity towards generative synchrony. While low self-efficacy is a risk factor for aggression (Willemse et al., 2011), in group music therapy adolescents are afforded opportunities for leadership and competence. Although the members of this group were referred for rebellion against authority and resistance towards the structured tasks of the classroom, within musicking warmth, openness, and willingness to follow structure also became apparent. The structure that was offered was not rigid, though. It allowed for cohesion as well as flexibility, individuality, and autonomy to coexist. Some theorists suggest that the key task of middle adolescence is an increase in self-determination, agency, and autonomous control (Daddis, 2011; van Schalkwyk and Wissing, 2010). Growth in autonomy, however, does not negate the ongoing need for connectedness (Michiels et al., 2008). The capacity for 'autonomous-relatedness' (Oudekerk et al., 2015, p. 472) is vital for developing close relationships into adulthood and music therapy specifically offers opportunities to experience this.

Holding a non-judgemental space for the exploration of anger and self-control

Effortful control entails the ability to focus and shift attention, inhibit dominant responses, and initiate behaviour even in the absence of intrinsic motivation (White and Turner, 2014).

'The hardest thing at school is controlling my temper,' Shane says, 'because I do have a temper, a really bad one. It gets so bad that no-one can stop it'. I invite the group into a joint musical improvisation through which we can express the rise in anger intensity, explore the conditions within which this takes place, and reflect on what happens when we feel this way. We examine at what points along the anger and aggression trajectory Shane and the others in the group can still make alternative decisions to walk away rather than to explode, realistically acknowledging the complex demands of a social context where, according to group members, it is through aggression that one can construct the desired status of being 'the boss'.

The way that an adolescent interprets the cues of others can act as a risk factor for aggressive automaticity (Guo et al., 2016). Learning to take time to mentally critique an anger-evoking encounter before impulsively responding decreases aggressive behaviour (Heller et al., 2015). In group music therapy, adolescents can explore their perceptions of aggressive cues and I have often employed story creation techniques with recorded or improvised music. In a joint creative process the group develops multifaceted characters and situations. These stories can then be dramatized through role play with their musical soundtracks. As situations in the stories are worked with (and played with), aggressive cues can be interrogated. Alternative strategies can be explored and practised (such as breathing and altering one's experience of time through inwardly accessing musical flow).

Offering opportunities to practise generative negotiation

The ability to engage positively with conflict is essential to mutually satisfying relationships (Pedwell, 2014). This is addressed with adolescents who are referred to group music therapy for aggression by offering opportunities to negotiate and cooperate through songwriting, for example. A number of strategies for facilitating a group to generate lyrics and musical material are noted in the music therapy literature (Derrington, 2005; McFerran, 2010). I have found certain techniques useful, such as asking group members to select newspaper headlines that express an aspect of their life at present and then to collaboratively arrange them into a flow of verses and a chorus. I also invite group members to write poetry while listening to various evocative pieces of music and to then select lines from their individual poems and jointly arrange these as lyrics for their song. The melody and rhythm of the songs can be negotiated as well, and Philippa Derrington (2005) describes offering varying degrees of musical support when facilitating. I have experienced my task as also offering a fully engaged presence, asking questions when necessary to spark new directions of thought if there is an impasse, modelling accountability to group norms that have been developed by the group members (for example, listening to and respecting one another), and securely holding the group members' interactional navigation so that it remains a safe space for all involved. I have witnessed how interactions during songwriting processes include gentle friendliness, playful banter, bursting investment in personal contributions, and enthusiastic dissent. Disagreement forms part of the creative process; in fact it is necessary for the development of a musical product of which all group members are ultimately proud. Through this process group members gain experiences of negotiating generatively with others.

Voicing pain and holding the pain of others

The causes of aggression are complex, multifaceted, and reciprocal, including individual, relational, community, and societal dimensions (Anderson and Bushman, 2002; Barak, 2006; Potirniche and Enache, 2014; World Health Organization, 2002). In the groups I have worked with, adolescents referred for aggressive behaviour have shared stories of: being abused; being raped (multiple times); the death of parents (including parental suicide and resulting feelings of guilt that this could have been prevented, as well as violent deaths of parents who were gang members); parental abandonment and neglect; hunger; complex parental relationships including extramarital affairs with partners who treat the adolescents harshly, if acknowledging them at all; and experiences of parents being in prison.

Mark Berg et al. (2012) write of the 'victim-offender overlap' (p. 360). Increasing numbers of studies (for example by Lisa Broidy et al. (2006), Wesley Jennings et al. (2010), Janet Lauritsen and John Laub (2007), and Christopher Schreck et al. (2002)) have found that those who suffer from violence and those who perpetrate it are often the same people. They argue that 'although victimization and offending often are considered two separate domains, they are so intimately connected that perhaps it is not possible to understand them fully apart from one another' (p. 360). The adolescents in my groups have also shared experiences of peer rejection and being bullied, while simultaneously acknowledging their role in bullying others. The following vignette describes how this dynamic can be explored in group music therapy.

I have invited the group to listen to a gentle piece of music, to allow this to take them to a beautiful place in their minds, and then to draw this experience on their own piece of paper. Afterwards we discuss the images. Desiree explains that she has drawn a picture of herself and her child (who she gave birth to during our process of working together) beneath a tree in a beautiful park. She explains that the picture is very special to her. After each has shared about their drawing I ask them to exchange their page with someone else in the group and then … to destroy one another's picture. There are a range of responses, from gasps, to 'Uh!', to laughter. Once one begins the others follow. 'Eish, you are hurting me!' Marius says to Laetitia who is still cutting his picture into tiny pieces. Afterwards I ask how they experienced tearing one another's images as well as how they experienced having their own torn. We move into a discussion of when we have 'torn' others and when we have been 'torn'. Afterwards I invite them to create a new image out of all the torn pieces. Floyd notes, 'Even if you put it back together it's not the same anymore. Everything was torn before it was put back together. It's not the same.' I ask, 'Is it different in a good way or a bad way?' 'Both,' he answers. Desiree painstakingly finds all the small pieces of her picture and glues them together, exclaiming, 'I put myself and my child back together.' 'So even if someone tries to tear you apart you're going to put it back together?' I ask. 'Yes!' she states defiantly.

Difficulties in adjusting to life stressors is a risk factor for aggression in adolescence (Guo et al., 2016). This type of technique offers adolescents opportunities to share and explore difficult life experiences that they feel have damaged them. While other art-based processes are included, the music is central in the initial evocative experience. The music affords an emotive connection to a personally meaningful experience that is then visually represented. Without this emotional investment, the tearing of the drawings would not prompt the same depth of personal reflection. The technique also allows for an integrated exploration of experiences of being both a victim and a perpetrator of aggression. Crucially, this technique is facilitated when group members have established trust with one another and with the therapist over a period of time.

As members share difficult experiences, opportunities are provided for others in the group to grow in their capacity to show support. Empathy can be developed and expressed through both musical interactions and related verbal processing.

When Ammaarah explains that she is feeling heartbroken due to a break-up with her boyfriend, I suggest a group vocal improvisation to express care for her. Melissa tries to vocally improvise with the others, but stops, starts again, then stops and looks away. She tries once more, by smiling and singing 'We love you' awkwardly, in a slightly operatic voice. I suggest that we only sing sounds such as humming, instead of trying to find words. Later she begins to tap the djembe, but then stops again just as her rhythm begins to align with the others. It is difficult for Melissa to enter a shared affective musical space with Ammaarah and the rest of the group perhaps because she struggles to tolerate Ammaarah's pain, and/or her own. Although Melissa has been able to verbally express care and concern for the suffering of others, her music making reveals more about her pain-resilience as greater vulnerability is encountered in this experience. I gently say, 'Stay with it, Melissa. It's ok,' as I encourage her to build these capacities. 'Let's keep singing', Natalie responds, and with tears in her eyes she softly says, 'I hear it, I hear it.'

Musical improvisation within a contained therapeutic environment can allow for the ex-perience, expression, and reflection of emotion. Increasing awareness of one's own emo-tions is useful in developing the ability to respond empathically to others (Shechtman, 2003), as empathy is premised firstly upon an experience of self (Rodemeyer, 2006). Empathy can therefore be developed through opportunities to imaginatively live through the experiences of others. In music therapy, group members can practice other-directed presence (Rosan, 2012) by waiting, listening, and carefully paying attention to others. According to Stefan Koelsch (2013), empathy is enhanced when individuals listen to music together and experience congruous emotions. Through sharing within songwriting, receptive music techniques, or lyric analysis, for example, group members gain understanding of the experiences of others, frequently encountering similarities between the stories they hear and events in their own lives. In addition to placing them-selves 'in each other's shoes' and realising that often they have walked 'in the same shoes', musicking affords the creation of new, shared experiences. Interactional synchrony is created as bodies pulse together in a sustained period of coordinated 'groove' in group drumming, for example. As authors such as Tal-Chen Rabinowitch et al. (2013) have found, musical activities that encourage motor resonance, imitation, and entrainment promote empathy. People who are high in empathy are more able to tolerate and ac-commodate the views and feelings of others. This can assist in the inhibition of destruc-tive impulses and the selection of more constructive conflict-solving strategies (de Wied et al., 2007).

Conclusion

Actions, including aggression, gain meaning and legitimacy in the social context and interpersonal reciprocity in which they are used (Gergen, 2009). We engage in our be-haviours as participants of a confluence of relationships (an interdependent meaning-making system) within which these actions make sense. A music therapy group can offer adolescents a context within which the sense of aggression can be received, explored, and processed, but also where aggression becomes non-sense, and this can begin to offer young people new ways to interact within their social world. One group constructed ag-gression as a behaviour that makes sense as following from experiences of grief and sad-ness in a context where there is no one trustworthy to gain support from. In contrast, they spoke of our music therapy groups as a place where they could experience trust, share with others, and be supported. This then offers a confluence where aggression makes less sense. Members of another group described aggression towards their teachers and parents as being behaviour that makes sense as a breaking point of anger and frustration after being treated with dismissal, disregard, and disrespect. They explained that in music therapy they felt heard. Through various forms of musicking young people can experi-ence, explore, and share feelings of pain, loneliness, betrayal, difference, fear, and guilt in a relational context where they are concurrently experiencing the opposite: support, rela-tionship, trust, safety, containment, reliability, comfort, recognition, and validation—not only from the music therapist but, crucially, from each other. What legitimates aggression is undone as they interact in a new confluence.

This may not change their wider social environments, but for many this offers a rare interpersonal experience. The process provides a template for how warm and mutually respectful interactions with an adult and with their peers are possible. While significantly impacted by the harsh treatment they receive from others in their home and school environments, within music therapy they can also grow increasingly aware of how their own behaviour impacts the cycles of aggression that they are part of and how alternative behavioural strategies can elicit more generative responses from others. Importantly, they form a support system for one another that extends beyond the close of music therapy sessions.

Not only is music therapy a space to actively and creatively attempt different ways of being, it also offers a celebration of exactly who an adolescent is right now in generative ways: an 'abrasive attitude' is the spunky fuel of the lead rapping lyricist; shredding an image while experiencing confrontational music is an artistic statement that is valued, held, and understood; beating a drum with every ounce of force one can muster is a statement of presence and connection with others.

In the last session with one of the groups I ask about how the relational space that we have created between us has felt to them during our time together. Cherise answers by explaining that it was a space that she felt happy to be inside of, 'because we know each other better, Miss', to which Devon adds, 'without hurting each other'. 'Yes', I nod gently, 'without hurting each other'.

References

Anderson, C. and Bushman, B. (2002). Human aggression. *Annual Review of Psychology*, **53**, 27–51.

Ansdell, G. (2014). *How Music Helps in Music Therapy and Everyday Life*. Farnham: Ashgate Publishing.

Barak, G. (2006). A critical perspective on violence. In W. DeKeseredy and B. Perry (Eds), *Advancing Critical Criminology: Theory and Application* (pp. 133–154). Lanham, MD: Lexington Books.

Berg, M. T., Stewart, E. A., Schreck, C. J., and Simons, R. L. (2012). The victim–offender overlap in context: Examining the role of neighborhood street culture. *Criminology*, **50**(2), 359–390.

Broidy, L. M., Daday, J. K., Crandall, C. S., Sklar, D. P., and Jost, P. F. (2006). Exploring demographic, structural, and behavioral overlap among homicide offenders and victims. *Homicide Studies*, **10**, 155–180.

Clark, J. (2012). Youth violence in South Africa: the case for a restorative justice response. *Contemporary Justice Review*, **15**(1), 77–95.

Copeland-Linder, N., Johnson, S. B., Haynie, D. L., Chung, S., and Cheng, T. L. (2012). Retaliatory attitudes and violent behaviors among assault-injured youth. *Journal of Adolescent Health*, **50**, 215–220.

Craig, W. and Harel, Y. (2004). Bullying, physical fighting, and victimization. In C. Currie (Ed.) *Young People's Health in Context: International Report from the HBSC 2001/02 Survey* (pp. 133–144). Copenhagen: WHO Regional Office for Europe.

Crombach, A. and Elbert, T. (2014). The benefits of aggressive traits: A study with current and former street children in Burundi. *Child Abuse and Neglect*, **38**, 1041–1050.

Daddis, C. (2011). Desire for increased autonomy and adolescents' perceptions of peer autonomy: 'Everyone else can; why can't I?'. *Child Development*, **82**(4), 1310–1326.

Dahlberg, L. and Potter, L. (2001). Youth violence: Developmental pathways and prevention challenges. *American Journal of Preventative Medicine*, **20**, 3–14.

Derrington, P. (2005). Teenagers and songwriting: Supporting students in a mainstream secondary school. In F. Baker and T. Wigram (Eds), *Songwriting: Methods, Techniques and Clinical Applications for Music Therapy Clinicians, Educators and Students* (pp. 68–81). London: Jessica Kingsley.

de Wied, M., Branje, S. T., & Meeus, W. J. (2007). Empathy and conflict resolution in friendship relations among adolescents. *Aggressive Behavior*, **33**(1), 48–55.

Gergen, K. (2009). *Relational Being: Beyond Self and Community*. Oxford: Oxford University Press.

Gini, G., Pozzoli, T., and Hauser, M. (2011). Bullies have enhanced moral competence to judge relative to victims, but lack moral compassion. *Personality and Individual Differences*, **50**, 603–608.

Gooden, M. (1997). When juvenile delinquency enhances the self-concept: The role of race and academic performance. Unpublished doctoral dissertation, The Ohio State University.

Gregson, D. (1994). Normally very abnormal: A perspective on youth at risk. *Journal of Child and Youth Care*, **9**(2), 31–41.

Guo, X., Egan, V., and Zhang, J. (2016). Sense of control and adolescents' aggression: The role of aggressive cues. *PsyCH Journal*, **5**, 263–274.

Hawley, P. (2007). Social dominance in childhood and adolescence: Why social competence and aggression may go hand in hand. In P. Hawley, T. Little, and P. Rodkin (Eds), *Aggression and Adaptation: The Bright Side to Bad Behaviour* (pp. 1–30). London: Routledge.

Heller, S., Shah, A., Guryan, J., Ludwig, J., Mullainathan, S., and Pollack, H. (2015). Thinking, fast and slow? Some field experiments to reduce crime and dropout in Chicago. Institute for Policy Research, Northwestern University. Available at: http://home.uchicago.edu/ludwigj/papers/CBT%20paper%20thinking%20fast%20and%20slow%20NBER%20WP%20w21178.pdf (accessed 20 March 2017).

Hurrelmann, K. and Engel, U. (1992). Delinquency as a symptom of adolescents' orientation toward status and success. *Journal of Youth and Adolescence*, **21**(1), 119–138.

Jarvinen, D. W. and Nicholls, J. G. (1996). Adolescents' social goals, beliefs about the causes of social success, and satisfaction in peer relations. *Developmental Psychology*, **32**(3), 435–441.

Jennings, W. G., Higgins, G. E., Tewksbury, R., Gover, A. R., and Piquero, A. R. (2010). A longitudinal assessment of the victim-offender overlap. *Journal of Interpersonal Violence*, **25**(12), 2147–2174.

Koelsch, S. (2013). From social contact to social cohesion – The 7 Cs. *Music and Medicine*, **5**(4), 204–209.

Kouri, S. and Smith, J. (2013). What's under the dirt? Wondering as a transformation of self. *Relational Child and Youth Care Practice*, **26**(2), 42–46.

Lauritsen, J. L. and Laub, J. H. (2007). Understanding the link between victimization and offending: New reflections on an old idea. *Crime Prevention Studies*, **22**, 55.

Le Roux, C. and Mokhele, P. (2011). The persistence of violence in South Africa's schools: In search of solutions. *Africa Education Review*, **8**(2), 318–335.

McFerran, K. (2010). *Adolescents, Music and Music Therapy: Methods and Techniques for Clinicians, Educators and Students*. London: Jessica Kingsley.

McFerran, K. and Wolfl, A. (2015). Music, violence and music therapy with young people in schools: A position paper. *Voices: A World Forum for Music Therapy*, **15**(2). doi:10.15845/voices.v15i2.831.

Michiels, D., Grietens, H., Onghena, P., and Kuppens, S. (2008). Parent-child interactions and relational aggression in peer relationships. *Developmental Review*, **28**, 522–540.

Ncontsa, V. and Shumba, A. (2013). The nature, causes and effects of school violence in South African high schools. *South African Journal of Education*, **33**(3), 1–15.

Ngqela, N. and Lewis, A. (2012). Exploring adolescent learners' experiences of school violence in a township high school. *Child Abuse Research: A South African Journal*, **13**(1), 87–97.

Olthof, T., Goossens, F., Vermande, M., Aleva, E., and van der Meulen, M. (2011). Bullying as strategic behavior: Relations with desired and acquired dominance in the peer group. *Journal of School Psychology*, **49**, 339–359.

Oudekerk, B. A., Allen, J. P., Hessel, E. T., and Molloy, L. E. (2015). The cascading development of autonomy and relatedness from adolescence to adulthood. *Child Development*, **86**(2), 472–485.

Pahad, S. and Graham, T. (2012). Educators' perceptions of factors contributing to school violence in Alexandra. *African Safety Promotion Journal*, **10**(1), 3–15.

Pedwell, C. (2014). *Affective Relations: The Transnational Politics of Empathy*. New York: Palgrave MacMilllan.

Potirniche, N., and Enache, R. G. (2014). Social perception of aggression by high school students. *Procedia-Social and Behavioral Sciences*, **127**, 464–468.

Rabinowitch, T., Cross, I., and Burnard, P. (2012). Long-term musical group interaction has a positive influence on empathy in children. *Psychology of Music*, **41**(4), 484–498.

Rodemeyer, L. (2006). *Intersubjective Temporality: It's About Time*. Dordrecht: Springer.

Rosan, P. (2012). The poetics of intersubjective life: Empathy and the other. *The Humanistic Psychologist*, **40**, 115–135.

Schreck, C. J., Wright, R. A., and Miller, J. M. (2002). A study of individual and situational antecedents of violent victimization. *Justice Quarterly*, **19**, 159–180.

Shechtman, Z. (2003). Therapeutic factors in individual and group treatment for aggressive children: An outcome study. *Group Dynamics: Theory, Research, and Practice*, 7, 225–237.

Skott-Myhre, H. (2008). *Youth and Subculture as Creative Force: Creating New Spaces for Radical Youth Work*. Toronto: University of Toronto Press.

Small, C. (1998). *Musicking*. Middletown, CT: Wesleyan University Press.

Swartz, L. (2015). From Sharpeville to Marikana: The changing political landscape for mental health practice in a violent South Africa. In J. Lindert and I. Levav (Eds), *Violence and Mental Health: Its Manifold Faces* (pp. 381–390). Dordrecht: Springer.

Ungar, M. (2001). The social construction of resilience among 'problem' youth in out-of-home placement: A study of health-enhancing deviance. *Child and Youth Care Forum*, **30**(3), 137–153.

Ungar, M. and Teram, E. (2000). Drifting toward mental health: High-risk adolescents and the process of empowerment. *Youth and Society*, **32**(2), 228–252.

van Schalkwyk, I. and Wissing, M. P. (2010). Psychosocial well-being in a group of South African adolescents. *Journal of Psychology in Africa*, **20**(1), 53–60.

Vitaro, F., Brendgen, M., and Barker, E. (2006). Subtypes of aggressive behaviors: A developmental perspective. *International Journal of Behavioral Development*, **30**(1), 12–19.

Wei, H. and Jonson-Reid, M. (2011). Friends can hurt you: Examining the coexistence of friendship and bullying among early adolescents. *School Psychology International*, **32**(3), 244–262.

White, B. and Turner, K. (2014). Anger rumination and effortful control: Mediation effects on reactive but not proactive aggression. *Personality and Individual Differences*, **56**, 186–189.

Wilkinson, R. and Pickett, K. (2009). Income inequality and social dysfunction. *Annual Review of Sociology*, **35**, 493–511.

Willemse, M., Smith, M., and van Wyk, S. (2011). The relationship between self-efficacy and aggression in a group of adolescents in the peri-urban town of Worcester, South Africa: Implications for sport participation. *African Journal for Physical, Health Education, Recreation and Dance*, June, 90–102.

World Health Organization. (2002). *World Report on Violence and Health*. Geneva: WHO.

Chapter 3

Young people's uses of music for emotional immersion

Genevieve Dingle, Leah Sharman, and Joel Larwood

Development of emotion knowledge and regulation

Emotion regulation can be conceptualized as the ability to modify emotion in flexible and adaptive ways in response to the social context (Campos et al., 2011). Individuals with better emotion regulation skills are more socially competent, have better quality friendships, and show more prosocial behaviours than those with poor emotion regulation capacity (Eisenberg et al., 2007; Wranik et al., 2007). Adolescents commonly experience intense emotional states during puberty and the transition from childhood to adulthood (Casey and Caudle, 2013). At the same time, their full capacity to regulate emotions is still developing (Beauchaine, 2015; Hannesdottir and Ollendick, 2007). The development of these skills is important; failure to develop the capacity for emotion regulation is a trans-diagnostic risk factor for mental disorders in adolescents (McLaughlin et al., 2011).

So how are these emotion skills developed in children and young people, and how might music play a role? In everyday social interactions, emotions are conveyed through various cues including facial expression, body posture, vocal tone, and verbal message as well as context. The ability to correctly identify these emotion cues and integrate them into a meaningful whole occurs at different rates across the different cues, and research indicates that children can typically integrate information from multiple cues around the age of 8 years (Mondloch, 2012; Nelson and Mondloch, 2017; Nelson and Russell, 2012). However, some research suggests that the trajectory of development of emotion words (Baron-Cohen et al., 2010) and other emotion skills (Lawrence et al., 2015; McGivern et al., 2002; Thomas et al., 2007) slows down around the onset of puberty and early adolescence. This is a time of great physical, social, and emotional change, and the research summarized here suggests that adolescents may find the identification and regulation of emotions particularly challenging.

Music and emotion regulation in young people

Suvi Saarikallio and Jaakko Erkkila's (2007) study of eight young Finnish people revealed that musical activities helped to regulate the valence, intensity, and clarity of their emotions. In relation to valence, music strengthened positive feelings and helped the young people to move away from negative feelings. Music also regulated the intensity of the affect, typically increasing the intensity of emotional experiences. Adolescents reported that they frequently wanted to listen to music that was congruent with their current mood, and to become immersed with their feelings and sensations created by music. Music also affected the clarity of the experience by giving form to different feelings. The adolescents felt that sometimes music helped them to clarify their thoughts, and to make sense of their feelings.

Emotional immersion is a relatively new term in the field of music and emotion research. In the media technology field, emotional immersion is the type of immersion when the user feels emotionally aroused and absorbed by the narrative content of the story—such as in a video game or virtual reality experience (Zhang et al., 2017). We use a similar meaning in this chapter, where emotional immersion in music involves emotional arousal and absorption in the music—through sustaining an existing emotional state, or through intensifying it.

The functions of music to support wellbeing in young people were supported by the findings of a qualitative study using transcripts from three focus groups with participants aged 15–25 years (Papinczak et al., 2015). Four psychological mechanisms emerged from the transcripts to describe how music listening was related to wellbeing: relationship building, modifying cognitions, modifying emotions, and immersing in emotions (Fig. 3.1).

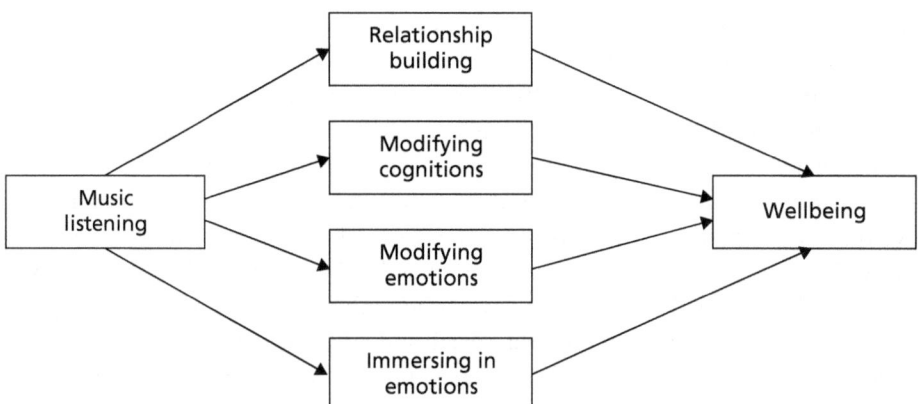

Fig. 3.1 Thematic map displaying commonly reported ways in which young people saw their music listening being linked with their wellbeing.

Reproduced with permission from: Zoe E. Papinczak, Genevieve A. Dingle, Stoyan R. Stoyanov, Leanne Hides, and Oksana Zelenko (2015) Young people's uses of music for well-being, *Journal of Youth Studies*, 18:9, 1119–1134, doi:10.1080/13676261.2015.1020935. © Copyright 2015 Taylor & Francis.

Here are some examples from Zoe Papinczak and colleagues' (2015) study of how young people used music to immerse in their emotions:

When something goes wrong you just kind of feel numb and you don't deal with it. And then you listen to something sad, it kind of triggers your reaction.

Immersing in the negative emotions through music helped some of these young people to experience them fully before feeling ready to move on. One young person said:

When you are in a certain mood and you listen to a song that matches that mood, it sort of amplifies those emotions more and you can sort of get over that emotion faster ... Instead of putting on a beat song and hiding under the rug, you listen to that sad song and really immerse yourself for a few minutes and then afterwards, I sort of feel better.

Some participants had created emotion-specific playlists or listened repeatedly to a particular song that reflected their feelings. Others allowed themselves some time to dwell on their negative feelings before moving onto happier, more positive music:

[when] I am sad, [I] can only listen to one song once and then after that, I have to move on, choose another song, finding something that is more encouraging. After that, I am happy.

To assess whether these theorized mechanisms linking music use with wellbeing were found in a larger sample of young people, the variables in the model (Fig. 3.1) were measured using self-report questionnaires which were administered to a second sample of 107 young people. Results showed that the pathways from music listening to the four psychological mechanisms were significantly supported, indicating that music was indeed being used by these young people for relationship building, cognitive change, emotional change, and emotional immersion. The pathways from the mechanisms to social wellbeing were also supported (Papinczak et al., 2015). This second study provided further evidence of how music use can lead to wellbeing via the four psychological mechanisms in a larger sample of young people, suggesting that emotional immersion can be an important function of music listening for young people. But is this unique to younger people, or do older adults use music for emotional immersion also?

Comparing younger and older people's music listening

To examine the nature and prevalence of music listening for emotional immersion further, we conducted an international online survey study of 372 adults aged 17–68 years (65% female) (Dingle and Sharman, unpublished). Respondents were asked to rate how often they listened to music to immerse in specific emotional states. The sample was subdivided into younger (17–25 years, $N = 103$) and older adults (26 years and older; $N = 241$), and

Table 3.1. Descriptive statistics and *t* tests on younger and older survey respondents on their use of music listening to immerse in positive and negative emotions

Listen to music to immerse in:	Response scale 1–5, mean (SD)		*t* test
	17–25 years	**26+ years**	
Happiness	4.24 (0.857)	4.17 (0.789)	0.805, ns
Sadness	3.68 (1.206)	3.27 (1.211)	2.850, *p* = 0.005
Anger	3.22 (1.35)	2.63 (1.231)	3.943, *p* < 0.001
Anxiety	2.17 (0.971)	2.15 (0.996)	0.170, ns
Love	4.02 (1.019)	3.83 (1.037)	1.561, ns
Wellbeing	4.47 (0.591)	4.44 (0.631)	0.302, ns

ns, not significant.

the two subgroups were compared on a number of variables related to music listening for emotion immersion. For instance, 'When I'm sad, I listen to music to fully experience my sadness' and 'When I'm happy, I listening to music to enhance my happiness'. Their responses were given on a five-point rating scale from 1 = strongly disagree to 5 = strongly agree. Results of bootstrapped *t* tests shown in Table 3.1 revealed that young people are significantly more likely to listen to music to immerse in feelings of sadness and anger than adults aged 26 years and over. Interestingly, there were no such age group differences in use of music to immerse in happiness, love, or to enhance feelings of wellbeing—which were highly endorsed by participants in both age categories. Perhaps unsurprisingly, participants of both age categories tended not to listen to music to immerse in feelings of anxiety (Dingle and Sharman, unpublished).

Correlational analyses were conducted on the full sample to determine if any relationships existed between the music for emotional immersion variables and participants' current depressed, anxious, or stressed mood (self-reported on single item ratings) or total score on the Difficulties in Emotion Regulation Scale (Gratz and Roemer, 2004). Results shown in Table 3.2 indicate that individuals who experience more difficulties in emotion regulation, and who are currently feeling depressed or anxious, endorse listening to music to immerse in sadness, anger, and anxiety to a greater extent.

These correlations do not tell us whether listening to music to immerse in negative emotions might make people feel more depressed and anxious, or whether pre-existing negative emotional states prompted individuals to listen to music in an attempt to experience and regulate their emotions, as suggested in the aforementioned studies by Papinczak et al. (2015) and Saarikallio and Errkila (2007). Further, in a critical interpretative analysis of 33 studies about music and mental health of young people, Katrina McFerran et al. (2016) concluded that there was a lack of experimental studies that might inform causative understandings. However, the authors added that a belief in a causal

Table 3.2. Bivariate correlations between the music for emotional immersion variables and participants' current mood and total scores on the Difficulties in Emotion Regulation Scale

Listen to music to immerse in emotional state:	Difficulties in Emotion Regulation Scale	Today I'm feeling depressed	Today I'm feeling anxious	Today I'm feeling stressed
Happiness	−0.092	−0.043	0.008	0.030
Sadness	0.205***	0.175***	0.121*	0.081
Anger	0.166**	0.110*	0.097	0.079
Anxiety	0.131*	0.133**	0.157**	0.086
Love	0.021	0.024	0.001	0.032
Wellbeing	−0.170**	−0.093	−0.025	−0.005

*, $p < 0.05$; **, $p < 0.01$; ***, $p < 0.001$.

link between music engagement and mental health was strongest in the voices of adolescent participants themselves, and qualitative analysis of interview data strongly attested to young people's faith in the positive benefits of music for health. To shed light on the issue of causation, laboratory studies where emotional states are evoked and music use is controlled, with emotions measured at multiple time points, are required.

Music to immerse in anger

Parents, religious groups, and policy makers have long been concerned about the potentially harmful effects of young people's music listening. Heavy rock, rap, and hip-hop have been sources of controversy for decades, with negative perceptions leading to censorship in many countries in an attempt to combat the supposed negative behavioural impact resulting from the music (Korpe, 2004; Negut and Sarbescu, 2013; Nuzum, 2001). Indeed, experimental research has found that young adults (unselected in terms of their musical preference) who listened to musically equivalent songs with and without violent lyrics showed increases in state hostility when they heard songs with violent lyrics (Anderson et al., 2003). Despite caveats such as the effect being short-lived among participants and dissipating quickly with intervening tasks, and the music not being chosen by the participants, this finding spoke to the mainstream perception of 'problem music'—a term coined by Adrian North and David Hargreaves (2006). That is, the perception that listening to some genres of music such as heavy metal, punk, alternative rock, hip-hop, and rap increases anger and aggressive behaviour.

In fact, research suggests that listeners' reactions to so-called problem music are largely determined by their musical preferences and beliefs about that music. In a study by Alexandra Negut and Paul Sârbescu (2013), participants were assigned to one of two conditions: the absence or presence of stereotype priming. In the primed group, participants were told 'Before you begin, we should mention that all the songs you will listen to contain, to a greater or lesser extent, obscene or violent lyrics. Also, some of these songs have been banned or censored by the NBC'. The priming absence group were not given this information. Both participant groups listened to a total of eight songs (three rock music tracks, four hip-hop music tracks, and one pop track, as a control song), after which they evaluated the lyrics in terms of different dimensions: violence, misogyny, alcohol or drugs consumption, sex, and satanism. Results showed that stereotype priming influenced participants' judgements and evaluations of the music lyrics in a more negative way, compared with those not exposed to priming (Negut and Sârbescu, 2013). Stereotyping about problem music may also affect mood states (e.g. hostility) when non-fans are asked to listen to problem music (Susino and Schubert, 2017).

In a naturalistic study, researchers found that after participants who listened to their own self-selected 'calming' music (of any genre) or to classical music chosen by the experimenter after experiencing stress or anger demonstrated significant reductions in anger and anxiety in both self-reported measures and physiological arousal (Labbé et al., 2007). Participants in another group (that was not selected for any particular music preference) showed an increase in anxiety levels after listening to heavy metal, a finding that underscores the importance of personal music preference in determining the emotional effect of music listening.

In an older study, William Gowensmith and Larry Bloom (1997) found that when selected heavy metal fans and non-fans listened to heavy metal or country music, heavy metal fans showed no differences in self-reported anger between their preferred or non-preferred music genre. Non-fans, on the other hand, showed an increase in self-reported anger to the heavy metal music compared to country music. It's unclear whether this was due to the nature of the music, listening to something they did not enjoy, or because it activated stereotypes about the type of music and associated behaviour (e.g. aggression, and hostility).

Other correlational research by Ehud Bodner and Moshe Bensimon (2015) involved two large samples of middle class university students, divided into those who were fans of the so-called problem music genres and non-fans of these genres. They compared the two groups in relation to various characteristics, including personality traits, self-esteem, and four subscales of the self-report delinquency questionnaire (body abuse, property damage, use of heavy drugs, and public disrespect). Across the two samples, they found no differences between fans of problem music and fans of other music genres in any measure except the one subscale of use of heavy drugs. Interestingly, problem music fans also reported more use of music to regulate mood states. The authors concluded that fans of problem music may be using music listening to regulate their mood and to alleviate (pre-existing) negative mood states. Although their correlational data could not substantiate this claim, this is congruent with our argument that some people listen to music to immerse themselves in negative emotions expressed by the music (such as anger), which may help to process and regulate their emotions.

Our own research on this topic built upon this idea in relation to the effects of heavy metal and other 'extreme' genres of music on anger (Sharman and Dingle, 2015). We recruited 39 participants (average age of 22 years, 72% males) who were fans of metal and extreme music and asked them to bring their music device along for an individual laboratory study. Each participant was made to feel angry using an anger interview procedure and then randomly assigned to either ten minutes of listening to extreme music from their own playlist or ten minutes of silence (the control condition). We found that average self-ratings of hostility, irritability, and stress increased during the anger induction, and then decreased after either listening to music or silence. Heart rate (a marker of angry arousal) increased during the anger induction and was sustained (not increased) in the music condition and decreased in the control condition. Ratings of positive emotions such as feeling 'active' and 'inspired' increased during music listening, an effect not seen in controls. Importantly, extreme music did not make these 39 participants angrier on average; rather, it appeared to match their physiological arousal and to result in more positive emotions at the end of 10 minutes. These results contradict the notion that extreme music makes angry people angrier and provides some small-scale evidence that listening to extreme music actually reduces levels of reported anger (hostility and irritability) among fans of extreme music genres (Sharman and Dingle, 2015).

Music to immerse in sadness

Just as music consumption increases in adolescence, so too does the frequency of sadness (Maughan et al., 2013). Indeed, the use of music to regulate mood is particularly prominent in the late stages of adolescence (Miranda and Claes, 2009; North et al., 2000) and over 10% of listeners in William Randall and colleagues' (2014) study reported using music to intensify a negatively valenced state. States of sadness have also been specifically related to an increased preference for sad music, which has been posited as potentially harmful for those at risk of depression (Garrido and Schubert, 2013, 2015a, 2015b). However, there are also counter findings that suggest that listening to mood-congruent sad music may be a healthy way to engage with one's experienced emotions (emotional immersion) (e.g. Papinczak et al., 2015; van den Tol and Edwards, 2013; van Goethem and Sloboda, 2011).

So, does listening to sad music pose a risk of harm to people experiencing depression? Interestingly there has been relatively little research conducted with samples experiencing clinical depression. Instead, proxy measures of depression risk have been used, such as participants' tendency towards rumination, which is characterized as attention to the causes and symptoms of distress without engaging in problem solving (Nolen-Hoeksema, 1991). Music with lyrics may have a particularly powerful influence on the mood of adolescents, who score more highly on a measure of ruminative thinking than adults (Sütterlin et al., 2012). Sandra Garrido and Emery Schubert (2013) found that high rumination was a predictor of habitual sad music listening (the proportion of music listened to that was sad) but not of overtly liking sad music. Extending this, Emily Carlson et al. (2015) found that using music for emotional discharge predicted diminished mental health in males.

Experimental studies also revealed that high ruminators were more susceptible to the emotional effects of music, showing a greater increase in sadness following sad music listening and a greater decrease in sadness following happy music listening (Garrido and Schubert, 2015a, 2015b). Suvi Saarikallio, Christian Gold, and Katrina McFerran (2015) have further proposed that there are healthy and unhealthy modes of engagement with music, with unhealthy ways including getting stuck in bad memories and struggling to disengage from musical cues of these memories. Their results revealed that unhealthy use of music was related to both increased psychological distress and decreased psychological wellbeing.

Although the use of music to purge sadness appears to be detrimental to mental health for some—perhaps especially for those at a higher risk of depression—the use of music in a way that promotes engagement with emotions has been related to positive mental health (Chin and Rickard, 2012, 2014), although decisions about research design, ways of assessing health, and the nature of musical engagement all influence this relationship and impact anticipated benefits (McFerran et al., 2016). Similar to Zoe Papinczak et al. (2015), Annamieke Van den Tol and Jane Edwards (2013) found that participants who select sad music to experience sadness also appear to gain a sense of empowerment. A follow-up study revealed that the use of sad music to engage with cognitions—to understand their feelings and thoughts—was perceived as helping to improve mood, as did listening to sad music for aesthetic pleasure (Van den Tol and Edwards, 2015). Consistent with the notion that sad music listening is beneficial for some people in the cognitive processing of sadness, Annamieke Van den Tol, Jane Edwards, and Nathan Heflick (2016) found sad music listening, but not happy music listening, was related to acceptance-based coping. A type of emotion-focused coping, acceptance-based coping has been described as 'coming to peace with' one's current situation, instead of trying to alter or deny the situation (Carver et al., 1989).

Joel Larwood's research on 128 young adults (mean age of 20 years, 40.6% males) indicated that using characteristically sad music in a sad state does not increase sadness, even among participants who scored highly on a measure of rumination (Larwood and Dingle, 2017). In our study, participants underwent a sadness induction (watching sad video clips) and were randomly assigned to one of three conditions: listening to experimenter-selected sad music (ESM), listening to self-selected music (SSM), or no music (control) for 5 minutes. Rumination was measured on the Rumination Reflection Scale (consistent with Garrido and colleagues' research). The experimenter-selected sad music was *You Don't Know What Love Is* performed by Chet Baker, which has a slow tempo, a minor mode, and sad lyrics, was used as a sad music stimulus in previous research (Ali and Peynircioglu, 2006) and was rated as the saddest of several music pieces pilot tested for this study. Participants in the self-selected music condition could select any music from their own device according to their preference so that we could examine ecologically valid music selection in an induced sad emotional state. Sadness was measured at baseline, post sadness induction, and post music or control using the Profile of Mood States depressed mood item. Results indicated that participants in the ESM condition demonstrated a

small decrease in sadness after listening, while both the control and the SSM participants demonstrated a substantial decrease in sadness, returning to their baseline (pre-
induction) levels of sadness (Fig. 3.2a). It is interesting that those in the control condition
scored similarly to the self-selected music participants, and noteworthy that only 28% of
participants in the SSM condition chose to listen to sad music (as indicated by their responses to the item 'The song I just listened to was sad'). An analysis of the influence of

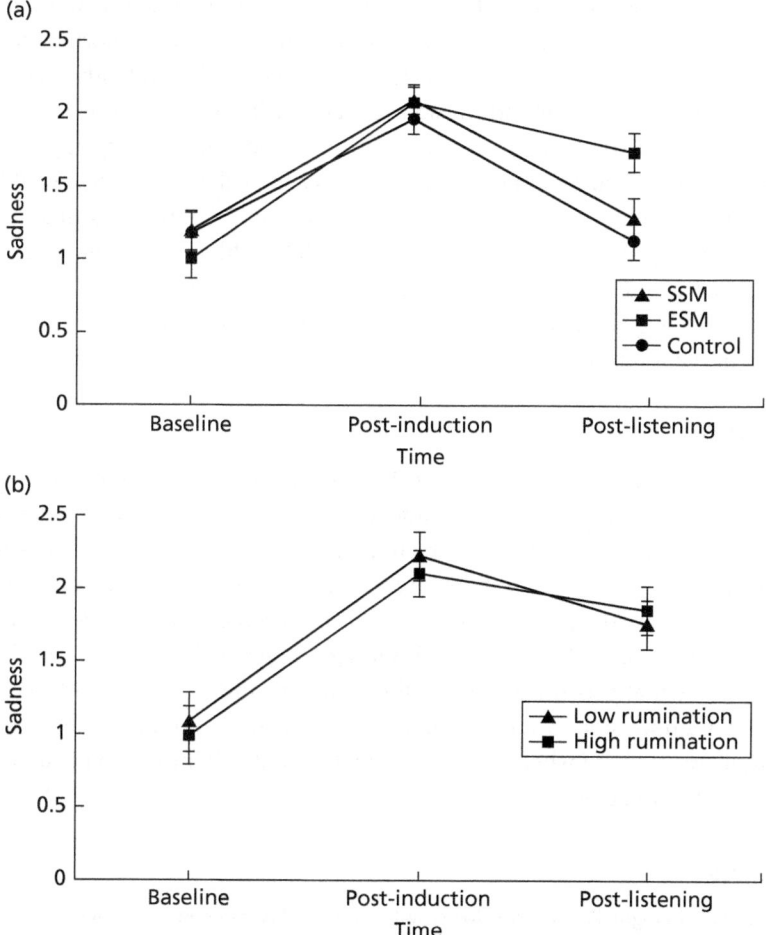

Fig. 3.2 (a) Profile of Mood States sadness scores at baseline, after sadness induction, and after
5 minutes listening to self-selected music (SSM, triangles), experimenter-selected sad music
(ESM, squares), or no music (control, circles). (b) Profile of Mood States sadness scores of the
ESM participants divided into high and low ruminators based on their scores on the Rumination
Reflection Scale.

From Larwood, J., & Dingle, G. A., 2017. I Get Knocked Down But I Get Up Again: The effects of listening
to music when sad. Poster presented at the Centre for Health Outcomes Innovation and Clinical Education
conference, Qld Brain Institute, University of QLD, 8 September 2017.

rumination on response to sad music (using only the participants in the ESM condition) revealed that listening to sad music did not make people feel sadder, even if they were high in rumination (see Fig. 3.2b).

Integrating the results from these studies indicates that sad musical and lyrical content alone do not worsen a sad state. The findings could be taken to support the position that it is selection and listening strategy that is pivotal in whether sad music worsens sadness, and not musical characteristics per se. There is currently evidence for both adaptive and maladaptive engagement with music in the context of mental health and affective outcomes. The field would benefit from more research with clinical samples experiencing depression as most of the studies summarized here have used normative samples in evoked sad states. Although there is evidence to suggest that individual factors such as rumination may affect how sad music is engaged with, there is no evidence to suggest that engagement styles are fixed. Thus, a growth and skill-building approach to the use of music for processing sadness should be pursued. Such an approach would be particularly inclusive of adolescents across the mental health spectrum as this population readily engages with music regardless of their mental health status. A growth and skill-building approach could both educate adolescents on what constitutes maladaptive music use, and actively engage them to practise adaptive engagement with their own preferred emotion-congruent music.

Conclusion

Taken together, the research presented in this chapter using diverse research methods shows preliminary support for our argument that young people may be immersing in music as a way of practising and understanding emotions—particularly negative emotions. More research is required to fully understand how music affects emotional states in young people who are diagnosed with mental health problems such as depression. Also, the potential effects of prolonged music listening and music listening in social contexts is largely unknown at this stage. Despite these caveats, the emerging evidence suggests that emotional immersion in music is not always harmful—it may also be helpful, and we need more research on when and under which conditions immersion is supportive of mental health and wellbeing.

References

Ali, S. O. and Peynircioğlu, Z. F. (2006). Songs and emotions: Are lyrics and melodies equal partners? *Psychology of Music*, **34**(4), 511–534.

Anderson, C. A., Carnagey, N. L., and Eubanks, J. (2003). Exposure to violent media: The effects of songs with violent lyrics on aggressive thoughts and feelings. *Journal of Personality and Social Psychology*, **84**(5), 960–971.

Baron-Cohen, S., Golan, O., Wheelwright, S., Granader, Y., and Hill, J. (2010). Emotion word comprehension from 4 to 16 years old: A developmental survey. *Frontiers in Evolutionary Neuroscience*, **2**, 109.

Beauchaine, T. P. (2015). Future directions in emotion dysregulation and youth psychopathology. *Journal of Clinical Child & Adolescent Psychology*, 44(5), 875–896.

Bodner, E. and Bensimon, M. (2015). Problem music and its different shades over its fans. *Psychology of Music*, 43(5), 641–660.

Campos, J. J., Walle, E. A., Dahl, A., and Main, A. (2011). Reconceptualizing emotion regulation. *Emotion Review*, 3(1), 26–35.

Carlson, E., Saarikallio, S., Toiviainen, P., Bogert, B., Kliuchko, M., and Brattico, E. (2015). Maladaptive and adaptive emotion regulation through music: A behavioral and neuroimaging study of males and females. *Frontiers in Human Neuroscience*, 9(August), 1–13.

Carver, C. S., Scheier, M. F., and Weintraub, J. K. (1989). Assessing coping strategies: A theoretically based approach. *Journal of Personality and Social Psychology*, 56(2), 267–283.

Casey, B. J. and Caudle, K. (2013). The teenage brain: Self control. *Current Directions in Psychological Science*, 22, 82–87.

Chin, T. and Rickard, N. S. (2012). The Music USE (MUSE) Questionnaire: An instrument to measure engagement in music. *Music Perception*, 29(4), 429–446.

Chin, T. and Rickard, N. S. (2014). Emotion regulation strategy mediates both positive and negative relationships between music uses and wellbeing. *Psychology of Music*, 42, 692–713.

Dingle, G. A. and Sharman, L. (unpublished). *Music and Your Mood survey*. University of Queensland.

Eisenberg, N., Hofer, C., and Vaughan, J. (2007). Effortful control and its socioemotional consequences. In J. J. Gross (Ed.), *Handbook of Emotion Regulation* (pp. 287–306). New York: Guilford Press.

Garrido, S. and Schubert, E. (2013). Adaptive and maladaptive attraction to negative emotions in music. *Musicae Scientiae*, 17(2), 147–166.

Garrido, S. and Schubert, E. (2015a). Moody melodies: Do they cheer us up? A study of the effect of sad music on mood. *Psychology of Music*, 43(2), 244–261.

Garrido, S. and Schubert, E. (2015b). Music and people with tendencies to depression. *Music Perception*, 32(4), 313–321.

Gowensmith, W. N. and Bloom, L. J. (1997). The effects of heavy metal music on arousal and anger. *Journal of Music Therapy*, 34(1), 33–45.

Gratz, K. L., and Roemer, L. (2004). Multidimensional assessment of emotion regulation and dysregulation: Development, factor structure, and initial validation of the Difficulties in Emotion Regulation Scale. *Journal of Psychopathology and Behavioral Assessment*, 26, 41–54.

Hannesdottir, D. K. and Ollendick, T. H. (2007). The role of emotion regulation in the treatment of child anxiety disorders. *Clinical Child and Family Psychology Review*, 10, 275–293.

Korpe, M. (2004). *Shoot the Singer!: Music Censorship Today*. London Zed Books.

Labbé, E., Schmidt, N., Babin, J., and Pharr, M. (2007). Coping with stress: The effectiveness of different types of music. *Applied Psychophysiology and Biofeedback*, 32(3–4), 163–168.

Larwood, J. and Dingle, G. A. (2017). I get knocked down but I get up again: The effects of listening to music when sad. *Poster presented at the Centre for Health Outcomes Innovation and Clinical Education conference*, Qld Brain Institute, University of QLD, 8 September 2017.

Lawrence, K., Campbell, R., and Skuse, D. (2015). Age, gender, and puberty influence the development of facial emotion recognition. *Frontiers in Psychology*, 6, 761.

McFerran, K. S., Garrido, S., and Saarikallio, S. (2016). A critical interpretive synthesis of the literature linking music and adolescent mental health. *Youth and Society*, 48(4), 521–528.

McGivern, R. F., Andersen, J., Byrd, D., Mutter, K. L., and Reilly, J. (2002). Cognitive efficiency on a match to sample task decreases at the onset of puberty in children. *Brain and Cognition*, 50, 73–89.

McLaughlin, K. A., Hatzenbuehler, M. L., Mennin, D. S., and Nolen-Hoeksema, S. (2011). Emotion dysregulation and adolescent psychopathology: A prospective study. *Behaviour Research and Therapy*, **49**(9), 544–554.

Maughan, B., Collishaw, S., and Stringaris, A. (2013). Depression in childhood and adolescence. *Journal of the Canadian Academy of Child & Adolescent Psychiatry*, **22**(1), 35–40.

Miranda, D. and Claes, M. (2009). Music listening, coping, peer affiliation and depression in adolescence. *Psychology of Music*, **37**(2), 215–233.

Mondloch, C. J. (2012). Sad or fearful? The influence of body posture on adults' and children's perception of facial displays of emotion. *Journal of Experimental Child Psychology*, **111**(2), 180–196.

Negut, A. and Sarbescu, P. (2013). Problem music or problem stereotypes? The dynamics of stereotype activation in rock and hip-hop music. *Musicae Scientiae*, **18**(1), 3–16.

Nelson, N. L. and Russell, J. A. (2012). Children's understanding of nonverbal expressions of pride. *Journal of Experimental Child Psychology*, **111**(3), 379–385.

Nelson, N. L., and Mondloch, C. J. (2017). Adults' and children's perception of facial expressions is influenced by cody postures even for dynamic stimuli. *Visual Cognition*, **25**(4–6), 563–574.

Nolen-Hoeksema, S. (1991). Responses to depression and their effects on the duration of depressive episodes. *Journal of Abnormal Psychology*, **100**(4), 569–582.

North, A. C., Hargreaves, D. J., and O'Neill, S. A. (2000). The importance of music to adolescents. *British Journal of Education Psychology*, **70**, 255–72.

North, A. C. and Hargreaves, D. J. (2006). Problem music and self-harming. *Suicide & Life-Threatening Behavior*, **36**(5), 582–590.

Nuzum, E. D. (2001). *Parental Advisory: Music Censorship in America*. New York: Perennial.

Papinczak, Z. E., Dingle, G. A., Stoyanov, S. R., Hides, L., and Zelenko, O. (2015). Young people's uses of music for wellbeing. *Journal of Youth Studies*, **18**(February), 1–16.

Randall, W. M., Rickard, N. S., and Vella-Brodrick, D. a. (2014). Emotional outcomes of regulation strategies used during personal music listening: A mobile experience sampling study. *Musicae Scientiae*, **18**(3), 275–291.

Saarikallio, S. and Erkkila, J. (2007). The role of music in adolescents' mood regulation. *Psychology of Music*, **35**(1), 88–109.

Saarikallio, S., Gold, C., and McFerran, K. (2015). Development and validation of the Healthy-Unhealthy Music Scale. *Child and Adolescent Mental Health*, **20**(4), 210–217.

Sharman, L. and Dingle, G. A. (2015). Extreme metal music and anger processing. *Frontiers in Human Neuroscience*, **9**(May), 272.

Susino, M. and Schubert, E. (2017). Cross-cultural anger communication in music: Towards a stereotype theory of emotion in music. *Musicae Scientiae*, **21**(1), 1–15.

Sütterlin, S., Paap, M. C. S., Babic, S., Kübler, A., and Vögele, C. (2012). Rumination and age: Some things get better. *Journal of Aging Research*, **10**, 267–327.

Thomas, L. A., De Bellis, M. D., Graham, R., and La Bar, K. S. (2007). Development of emotional facial recognition in late childhood and adolescence. *Developmental Science*, **10**, 547–558.

Van den Tol, A. J. M. and Edwards, J. (2013). Exploring a rationale for choosing to listen to sad music when feeling sad. *Psychology of Music*, **41**(4), 440–465.

Van den Tol, A. J. M. and Edwards, J. (2015). Listening to sad music in adverse situations: How music selection strategies relate to self-regulatory goals, listening effects, and mood enhancement. *Psychology of Music*, **43**(4), 473–494.

Van den Tol, A. J. M. Edwards, J., and Heflick, N. A. (2016). Sad music as a means for acceptance-based coping. *Musicae Scientiae*, **20**(1), 68–83.

van Goethem, A. and Sloboda, J. (2011). The functions of music for affect regulation. *Musicae Scientiae*, *15*(2), 208–228.

Wranik, T., Feldman-Barrett, L., and Salovey, P. (2007). Intelligent emotion regulation: Is knowledge power? In J. J. Gross (Ed.), *Handbook of Emotion Regulation* (pp. 393–407). New York: Guilford Press.

Zhang, C., Perkis, A., and Arndt, S. (2017). Spatial immersion versus emotional immersion, which is more immersive? 2017 Ninth International Conference on Quality of Multimedia Experience (QoMEX). Available at: http://ieeexplore.ieee.org/document/7965655/ (accessed 23 November 2018).

Chapter 4

Measuring adolescents' emotional responses to music: Approaches, challenges, and opportunities

Tan-Chyuan Chin

Introduction

Music listening increases substantially during adolescence (Roberts and Foehr, 2008) as music provides an ideal platform for young people to explore ways to manage mood (Saarikallio and Erkkilä, 2007), develop autonomy and identity (Marcia et al., 1993; North et al., 2000), as well as forming new experiences with music, affect, and contexts (Schubert et al., 2014). There is increasing evidence that many of the beneficial effects of music are mediated by a range of factors, such as the emotional impact that music has on an individual (Juslin and Sloboda, 2010), the ways in which music is used (Chin and Rickard, 2012; North and Hargreaves, 2008), the associated use of adaptive emotion regulation strategies (Chin and Rickard, 2014a, 2014b; Garrido and Schubert, 2013), and the individual's current state of wellbeing and context in which music is used (McFerran, 2016). Therefore, it is crucial to prioritize research that not only examines the broad range of adolescents' emotional responses to music, but also the contexts in which they occur.

Contemporary challenges facing researchers and practitioners in measuring and understanding the various components of emotional responses to music need to be balanced with informed, active participation from young people. For researchers, measurement can encompass both process and outcome indicators that provide the capacity to monitor change over time and examine the impact of music-based interventions on mental health and wellbeing. For practitioners, measurement forms a fundamental aspect of the needs analysis so that therapeutic sessions can be tailored to suit individuals' needs. The main aim of this chapter is to provide an overview of the various methods used for measuring emotional responses to music and to explore their utility, feasibility, and validity in research and practice with young people. The benefits and challenges of utilizing mixed-methods approaches will be considered. This chapter concludes that a blend of approaches will provide richer insight into research on the role of music in the lives of young people.

Emotions: concept and components

Emotions fall under the broader umbrella term of affect, and are generally described as a brief but intense affective reaction, which is focused on specific events and typically lasts for minutes to a few hours (Frijda, 2009; Juslin and Sloboda, 2010). Emotions are broadly defined as comprising several subcomponents: action tendencies, cognitive appraisal, expression (facial and vocal), physiological response, and subjective feeling (Juslin and Scherer, 2005; Scherer, 2005). Emotional experience of music can be further differentiated into felt (or induced) and perceived emotion (Evans and Schubert, 2008). Felt emotions are the actual emotions experienced in response to music. Perceived emotions refer to the recognition of emotions the composer is intending to convey through the music, without feeling it; for example, when an individual listens to a piece of sad music and recognizes that the intention of the music is to convey sadness, but does not personally feel sad when listening to the music. Felt and perceived emotions should not be viewed or treated as opposite extremes on a continuum (Zentner et al., 2008). Emotional responses of an individual can occur somewhere along the continuum from an emotion-free perception to intense emotional reactions. Apart from subjective feeling, a key differentiating factor between felt and perceived emotions is the association with physiological change, such as blood pressure, heart rate, skin conductance, and respiration (Krumhansl, 1997). Given the complex interplay between biochemical-neurophysiological, behavioural-expressive, and subjective-experiential components of emotions, I suggest that an accurate measurement of emotional responses to music should incorporate a mixed-methods approach, with convergent data from at least two components (Izard and Read, 1986).

Biochemical-neurophysiological component

The biochemical-neurophysiological component of emotions can be studied using techniques ranging from analyses of biochemical samples (such as saliva) to non-invasive methods such as electrocardiography (ECG), electroencephalography (EEG), functional magnetic resonance imaging (fMRI), or magnetoencephalography (MEG) (see Hodges (2010) for a comprehensive overview of psychophysiological measures). Emotion processing has been demonstrated to occur without conscious awareness (LeDoux, 1998; Tsuchiya and Adolphs, 2007), and therefore these methods are particularly useful for capturing individuals' unconscious responses to external stimuli such as music. Furthermore, a measure of this component of emotions when utilized in combination with subjective ratings of experienced feelings (felt emotions), can be used to distinguish between perceived and induced or felt emotions.

Behavioural-expressive component

The behavioural-expressive component can be studied using a coding system for participants' behavioural responses such as the number of blinks, body and facial movements, and level of alertness or disgust (Gross and Levenson, 1993). At least two independent coders with no knowledge of the experimental group assignment of the participants are required for objectivity and to establish interrater reliability of behaviour coding. The coding system from Gross and Levenson (1993) derives a score, on a six-point scale, for the duration, frequency, and intensity of each of the emotional response observed during a specified period of time.

Subjective-experiential component

The subjective-experiential component can be studied using methods such as self-report surveys, in-the-moment experience sampling, interviews, and diary methods. Self-report methods vary depending on the research questions and design, which then determine the timing requirements of the actual response task for participants. Continuous time-dependent responding provides the capacity to capture continuous emotional responses to music during an entire listening task (Schubert, 2010), whereas summative post-performance emotional responses are collected after the music piece has been played. Despite its ease and convenience of data collection and analyses, post-performance emotional response ratings are influenced by retrospective judgements of the music piece and have been found to be rated higher than averaged continuous response data (Rozin et al., 2004) and, even though correlated, their variances overlapped by only very little (Sloboda and Lehmann, 2001). This highlights the importance of selecting suitable indicators to adequately capture the construct of interest.

Mixed-methods approach

Each of the above-discussed three components captures a different aspect of an individual's emotional response. Therefore, having convergent data from at least two components will provide greater accuracy of the measurement. It is crucial, however, to balance the data collection with the burden and inconvenience placed on young participants. Burden on a participant can be broadly categorized in the following three aspects: invasiveness, intrusiveness, and time required. An overview of the estimated levels of burden on participant is presented in Table 4.1.

Apart from the effort and time required of participants, there are several other procedural factors for researchers and practitioners to consider. The majority of the biochemical-neurophysiological methods require not only specialized equipment or kits for data collection, but also additional technical and analytical knowledge and skills to process and interpret the collected data. Another consideration is the amount of time required to process and analyze the raw data. Indicators such as heart rate or temperature provide a sufficient reading at the time of data collection whereas raw data for measurement of muscular tension or skin conductance require additional time to process. Burden on researcher/practitioner can therefore also be broadly categorized in the following three aspects: specialized equipment to collect data, specialized training and/or knowledge to process and interpret data, and time required to process data for each participant. An overview of the estimated levels of commitment necessary from the researcher/practitioner, in terms of data collection and processing, is presented in Table 4.2.

Table 4.1. An overview of estimated burden on participant

	Estimated level of burden		
	Low	Moderate	High
Invasiveness of methods	No direct physical contact	Application of electrode and/or testing equipment	Drawing biological sample using syringe
Intrusiveness of methods	Minimal intrusion into daily activities	Multiple short responses (less than 10 minutes) required each day during data collection phase	Substantial responses (more than 10 minutes) required each day during data collection phase
Time required for each data collection	Less than 10 minutes	10–30 minutes	More than 30 minutes

The estimated levels of burden and commitment on participant and researcher/practitioner respectively are summarized alongside an overview of selected methods for each of the three components in Table 4.3. This summary table is not exhaustive but provides an indication of effort and time required to use the methods listed.

It is evident from Table 4.3 that most of the biochemical-neurophysiological indicators require moderate to high levels of time and effort from both participant and researcher/practitioner. There are, however, several indicators such as blood pressure, temperature, heart and pulse rate that require basic levels of time, effort, and procedure to set up, and which would suit contexts where immediate feedback is preferred. For instance, heart rate or temperature biofeedback can be used to help young people recognize their physiological responses to music. There is evidence that biofeedback training improves heart rate regulation, and the learned ability has further been demonstrated to transfer to emotional tasks or situations in the absence of feedback (Peira et al., 2013).

Table 4.2. An overview of estimated commitment from researcher/practitioner

	Estimated level of commitment		
	Low	Moderate	High
Specialized equipment	Basic and/or highly portable equipment	Portable equipment with basic software	Equipment and software set up in a laboratory
Specialized training and/or knowledge	Data are available with no further computation or processing required	Data need to be processed with basic software	Samples or data need to be processed externally or utilizing specialized software
Time required to process data for each participant	Less than 10 minutes	10–60 minutes	More than 60 minutes

Table 4.3. An overview of selected emotional response indicators and their estimated levels of participant burden and commitment from researchers

Type of emotional response	Indicator	Reference	Participant burden			Commitment from researchers		
			Invasiveness	Intrusiveness	Time	Specialist equipment	Specialist knowledge	Time
Biochemical-neurophysiological								
Biochemical responses	Blood glucose	Jing and Xudong (2008)	H	H	L	H	H	H
	Adrenaline/noradrenaline	Hirokawa and Ohira (2003)	H	H	M	H	H	H
	Salivary α-amylase (sAA)	Granger et al. (2007)	M	M	L	H	H	H
	Salivary cortisol (sCort)	Pressman and Cohen (2005)	M	H	L	H	H	H
	Salivary immunoglobulin A (s-IgA)	Hucklebridge et al. (2000)	M	M	L	H	H	H
Physiological responses	Blood pressure	Bernardi et al. (2006)	M	M	M	L	L	L
	Event-related potentials (ERPs) derived from electroencephalography (EEG)	Fox et al. (2005)	M	M	H	H	H	H
	Facial muscle activity using electromyography (EMG)	Khalfa et al. (2008)	M	M	H	H	H	H
	Heart and pulse rate	Blood and Zatorre (2001); Krumhansl (1997); Rickard (2004)	M	M	M	L	L	L
	Muscular tension	Rickard (2004)	M	M	M	H	H	H
	Pupillary responses	Gingras et al. (2015)	M	M	H	H	H	H
	Respiration	Krumhansl (1997)	M	M	M	M	M	M
	Skin conductance	Krumhansl (1997); Rickard (2004)	M	M	M	H	H	H
	Startle reflex	Mathieu et al. (2009)	M	M	H	H	H	H
	Temperature	Blood and Zatorre (2001); Rickard (2004)	M	M	M	L	L	L

(continued)

Table 4.3. Continued

Type of emotional response	Indicator	Reference	Participant burden			Commitment from researchers		
			Invasiveness	Intrusiveness	Time	Specialist equipment	Specialist knowledge	Time
Behavioural-expressive								
Behavioural responses	Number of blinks, body and facial movements	Gross and Levenson (1993)	M	M	M	M	M	H
Subjective-experiential								
Affect assessment along the dimensions of pleasure–displeasure and arousal–sleepiness	Affect Grid	Russell et al. (1989)	L	L	L	L	L	L
Basic emotions	Differential Emotion Scale (DES)	Izard et al. (1993)	L	L	L	L	L	L
Dimensions of emotional experience in response to music	Geneva Emotional Music Scales (GEMS)	Zentner et al. (2008)	L	L	L	L	L	L
Intensity of emotional experience	Affect Intensity Measure (AIM)	Larsen and Diener (1987)	L	L	L	L	L	L
Continuous emotional responses to music	Continuous-response method	Schubert (2010)	M	M	M	H	H	H

Description	Method	Reference						
Assessment of experiences in natural settings, in real time, and on repeated occasions	Experience Sampling Method (ESM)	Larson and Csikszentmihalyi (1983)	L	M	L	H	H	H
Emotional responses to music and contexts in which they occur	Experience Sampling Method (ESM)	Juslin et al. (2008)	L	M	L	H	H	H
Emotional responses and preferences to music	Experience Sampling Method (ESM)	Randall and Rickard (2013)	L	M	L	H	H	H
Daily emotion episodes	Diary studies	Bolger et al. (2003)	L	H	M–H	H	H	H
Study of musical emotions in everyday life	Diary studies	Sloboda and O'Neill (2001)	L	H	M–H	H	H	H

Note: L, low; M, moderate; H, high.

There are, however, concerns about the inconsistent findings with psychophysiological responses to music (Hodges and Sebald, 2011). These authors identified several important research-related issues ranging from not having standard research protocols or procedures, to there being no standards for selection of musical stimuli, variation of musical excerpts and experimental tasks across studies, to inconsistent reporting of participant individual variables such as gender, age, sociocultural factors, music training background, and preferences (Hodges and Sebald, 2011). Personality factors, such as extraversion and internal locus of control, may also mediate physiological response to music (Rickard, 2004). In future it is therefore important for researchers to consider including some of these individual variables, where relevant to the research question(s), and to clearly document procedures.

Indicators of the subjective-experiential component of emotional responses to music vary widely in terms of time and effort for both participant and researcher/practitioner. As these measures can be distributed online using web-based survey platforms, access and provision of measurements are more economical and scalable compared to biochemical-neurophysiological indicators. In contrast to standardized surveys (completed in one sitting), self-report methods that involve repeated sampling of momentary experiences in an individual's everyday life may pose moderate to high levels of interruption to the individual's regular routine. These methods also require greater amount of time for the researcher/practitioner to process and analyse collected data compared with standardized surveys. Despite these challenges, repeated sampling methods capture real-time feelings, thoughts, and actions in response to naturally occurring events, experiences, and situations, providing ecologically valid data, which can be used to construct individual profiles to assess intra- and interpersonal trends over time (Chin et al., 2016). Advancements in mobile technology provide greater capacity to capture real-time experiences and responses of young people, making mobile experience sampling a viable and complementary ecological approach for measuring emotional responses to music.

A mixed-methods approach to measuring emotional responses requires data to be collected from more than a single data source, as well as use of more than one type of analysis (Creswell and Plano Clark, 2007). Due to additional requirements of mixed-methods approaches, there are several factors for researchers/practitioners to consider when developing research design and planning data collection, processing, and analyses. Mixed-methods approaches require greater resources in terms of time, expertise, equipment, and funding and, as such, typically involve coordination of personnel with relevant knowledge and skills. However, these challenges are counterweighed by the strengths of the mixed-methods approach. Benefits include convergence of data, robustness of findings, overcoming limitations of single data source, increased capacity to address broader research questions, and the provision of important insights into understanding the nuances of emotional responses to music. Fig. 4.1 provides an illustration of the conceptual axes that may be useful for selecting and matching complementary indicators of emotional responses based on estimated burden on participants (y axis) and commitment from the researcher/practitioner (x axis).

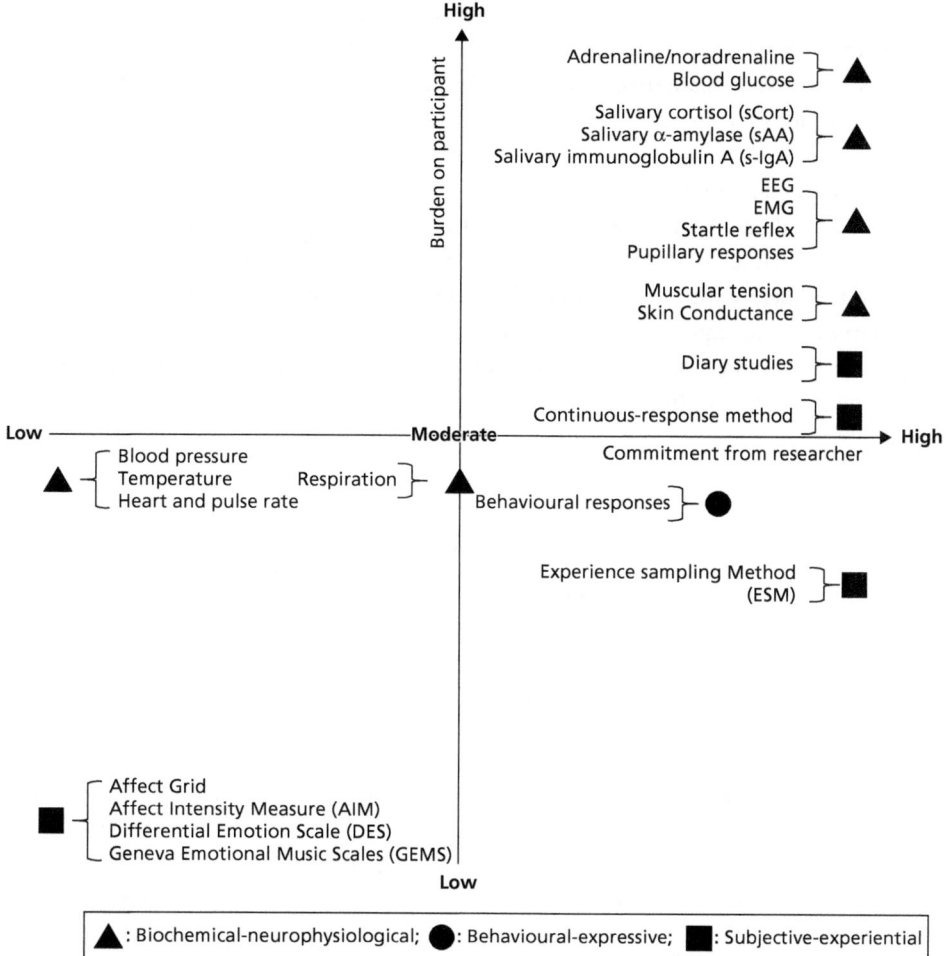

Fig. 4.1 Illustration of emotional response indicators classified on the conceptual axes of participant burden and level of commitment required of researchers/practitioners. EEG, electroencephalography; EMG, electromyography.

For instance, the indicators in the lower left quadrant in Fig. 4.1 will require low to moderate levels of commitment from the research/practitioner and impose low to moderate levels of burden or inconvenience to the participant. As for the indicators in the upper right quadrant, most of them require moderate to high levels of time and effort from both participants and researchers/practitioners. Perhaps, then, indicators in the two lower quadrants may be more suitable for research and work with younger participants.

Utility of the mixed-methods approach with young people

Mixed-methods approaches can be used across a variety of study designs, where decisions are guided by the reliance on each method and the timing of the use of the methods

(Creswell and Plano Clark, 2007). Mixed-methods approaches have been well utilized in research with young people and not only draw on strengths but also minimize the weaknesses of either qualitative or quantitative approaches. Methods are combined either concurrently or sequentially to address broader research questions more comprehensively (Creswell and Plano Clark, 2007). Some examples of adolescent studies using mixed methods are listed in Table 4.4.

Mixed-methods approaches are well suited for capturing the dynamic and complex range of emotional responses to music in young people and provide researchers with the capacity to validate multiple sources of data to obtain a comprehensive profile of emotional responses and experiences. It is, however, prudent for researchers and practitioners to regularly assess and monitor feasibility, adequacy, and efficiency of chosen methods to address the research question(s).

Table 4.4. Examples of adolescent studies utilizing mixed methods

Project aim	Method	Measure	Reference
To identify teacher behaviours that convey social support and the types of teacher support that were most strongly linked with subjective wellbeing	Quantitative	Self-report surveys	Suldo et al. (2009)
	Qualitative	Focus groups	
To explore the potential of music therapy for bereaved teenagers	Quantitative	Self-report surveys	McFerran et al. (2010)
	Qualitative	Focus groups	
To explore relationships between the cortisol awakening response (CAR), mental health, and wellbeing in a sample of healthy young adolescents	Biochemical-neurophysiological	Salivary cortisol	Rickard et al. (2016)
	Subjective-experiential	Self-report surveys	
To examine the feasibility of a newly developed mobile experience sampling app to study programme implementation in young people participating in wellbeing programmes	Subjective-experiential	Experience sampling method	Chin et al. (2016)
	Subjective-experiential	Self-report surveys	
To illustrate both the benefits and challenges associated with evaluation of positive education programme outcomes	Biochemical-neurophysiological	Salivary cortisol	Vella-Brodrick et al. (2017)
	Subjective-experiential	Experience sampling method	
	Subjective-experiential	Self-report surveys	
	Qualitative	Focus groups	

Conclusion

This chapter presents information about the types of methods and factors that need to be considered for the future work of measuring emotional responses to music in young people. Although not exhaustive, the benefits and challenges of using various indicators have been examined. Certain types of indicator appear to pose a lower burden to participants and can serve as complementary methods to capture adolescents' emotional responses to music. A considered, integrative approach of measurement will provide a rigorous evidence base for researchers and practitioners to obtain insights about contexts, applications, processes, and outcomes associated with adolescents' emotional responses to music. This in turn facilitates the design and development of relevant and helpful strategies or programmes that could be tailored to how a young person responds to music across various contexts and settings.

References

Bernardi, L., Porta, C., and Sleight, P. (2006). Cardiovascular, cerebrovascular, and respiratory changes induced by different types of music in musicians and non-musicians: The importance of silence. *Heart*, 92, 445–452.

Blood, A. J. and Zatorre, R. J. (2001). Intensely pleasurable responses to music correlate with activity in brain regions implicated in reward and emotion. *Proceedings of the National Academy of Sciences USA*, 98, 11818–11823.

Bolger, N., Davis, A., and Rafaeli, E. (2003). Diary methods: Capturing life as it is lived. *Annual Review of Psychology*, 54, 579–616.

Chin, T. C. and Rickard, N. S. (2012). The Music USE (MUSE) Questionnaire: An instrument to measure engagement in music. *Music Perception*, 29, 429–446.

Chin, T. C. and Rickard, N. S. (2014a). Emotion regulation strategy mediates both positive and negative relationship between music uses and well-being. *Psychology of Music*, 42, 692–713.

Chin, T. C. and Rickard, N. S. (2014b). Beyond positive and negative trait affect: Flourishing through music engagement. *Psychology of Well-Being*, 4, 25. doi:10.1186/s13612-014-0025-4.

Chin, T. C., Rickard, N. S., and Vella-Brodrick, D. A. (2016). Development and feasibility of a mobile experience sampling application for tracking program implementation in youth well-being programs. *Psychology of Well-Being*, 6, 1. doi:10.1186/s13612-016-0038-2.

Creswell, J. W. and Plano Clark, V. (2007). *Designing and Conducting Mixed Methods Approaches*. Thousand Oaks, CA: SAGE Publications.

Evans, P. and Schubert, E. (2008). Relationships between expressed and felt emotions in music. *Musicae Scientiae*, 12, 75–99.

Fox, N. A., Henderson, H. A., Marshall, P. J., Nichols, K. E., and Ghera, M. M. (2005). Behavioral inhibition: Linking biology and behavior within a developmental framework. *Annual Review of Psychology*, 56, 235–262. doi:10.1146/annurev.psych.55.090902.141532.

Frijda, N H. (2009). Emotion experience and its varieties. *Emotion Review*, 1, 264–271.

Garrido, S. and Schubert, E. (2013). Adaptive and maladaptive attraction to negative emotion in music. *Musicae Scientiae*, 17, 147–166.

Gingras, B., Marin, M., Puig-Waldmüller, E., and Fitch, W. T. (2015). The eye is listening: Music-induced arousal and individual differences predict pupillary responses. *Frontiers in Human Neuroscience*, 9, 619. doi:10.3389/fnhum.2015.00619.

Granger, D. A., Kivlighan, K. T., El-Sheikh, M., Gordis, E. B., and Stroud, L. R. (2007). Salivary α-amylase in biobehavioral research. *Annals of the New York Academy of Sciences*, **1098**, 122–144.

Gross, J. J. and Levenson, R. W. (1993). Emotional suppression: Physiology, self-report, and expressive behaviour. *Journal of Personality and Social Psychology*, **64**, 970–986.

Hirokawa, E. and Ohira, H. (2003). The effects of music listening after a stressful task on immune functions, neuroendocrine responses, and emotional states in college students. *Journal of Music Therapy*, **40**, 189–211.

Hodges, D. (2010). Psychophysiological measures. In P. N. Juslin and J. A. Sloboda (Eds), *Handbook of Music and Emotion: Theory, Research, Applications* (pp. 279–312). Oxford: Oxford University Press.

Hodges, D. and Sebald, D. (2011). *Music in the Human Experience: An Introduction to Music Psychology*. New York: Routledge.

Hucklebridge, F, Lambert, S., Clow, A., Warburton, D. M., Evans, P. D., and Sherwood, N. (2000). Modulation of secretory immunoglobulin a in saliva: Response to manipulation of mood. *Biological Psychology*, **53**, 25–35.

Izard, C. E., Libero, D., Putnam, P., and Haynes, O. (1993). Stability of emotion experiences and their relations to personality traits. *Journal of Personality and Social Psychology*, **64**, 847–860.

Izard, C. E. and Read, P. B. (1986). *Measuring Emotions in Infants and Children*. Cambridge: Cambridge University Press.

Jing, L. and Xudong, W. (2008). Evaluation on the effects of relaxing music on the recovery from aerobic exercise-induced fatigue. *Journal of Sports Medicine and Physical Fitness*, **48**, 102–106.

Juslin, P. N. and Scherer, K. R. (2005). Vocal expression of affect. In J. A. Harrigan, R. Rosenthal, and K. R. Scherer (Eds), *The New Handbook of Methods in Nonverbal Behavior Research* (pp. 65–135). New York: Oxford University Press.

Juslin, P. N., Liljeström, S., Västfjäll, D., Barradas, G., and Silva, A. (2008). An experience sampling study of emotional reactions to music: Listener, music, and situation. *Emotion*, **8**, 668–683.

Juslin, P. N. and Sloboda, J. A. (2010). *Handbook of Music and Emotion*. Oxford: Oxford University Press.

Khalfa, S., Roy, M., Rainville, P., Dalla Bella, S., and Peretz, I. (2008). Role of tempo entrainment in psychophysiological differentiation of happy and sad music? *International Journal of Psychophysiology*, **68**, 17–26.

Krumhansl, C L. (1997). An exploratory study of musical emotions and psychophysiology. *Canadian Journal of Experimental Psychology*, **51**, 336–353.

Larsen, R. J. and Diener, E. (1987). Affect intensity as an individual difference characteristic: A review. *Journal of Research in Personality*, **21**, 1–39.

Larson, R. and Csikszentmihalyi, M. (1983). The experience sampling method. *New Directions for Methodology of Social and Behavioural Science*, **15**, 41–56.

LeDoux, J. (1998). *The Emotional Brain: The Mysterious Underpinnings of Emotional Life*. New York: Touchstone.

Marcia, J. E., Waterman, A. S., Matteson, D. R., Archer, S. L., and Orlofsky, J. L. (1993). *Ego Identity: A Handbook for Psychosocial Research*. New York: Springer.

Mathieu, R., Mailhot, J., Gosselin, N., Paquette, S., and Peretz, I. (2009). Modulation of the startle reflex by pleasant and unpleasant music. *International Journal of Psychophysiology*, **71**, 37–42.

McFerran, K. S. (2016). Contextualising the relationship between music, emotions and the well-being of young people: A critical interpretive synthesis. *Musicae Scientiae*, **20**, 103–121.

McFerran, K. S., Roberts, M., and O'Grady. L. (2010). Music therapy with bereaved teenagers: A mixed methods perspective. *Death Studies*, **34**, 541–565.

North, A. C. and **Hargreaves, D. J.** (2008). *The Social and Applied Psychology of Music*. Oxford: Oxford University Press.

North, A. C., **Hargreaves, D. J.**, and **O'Neill, S. A.** (2000). The importance of music to adolescents. *British Journal of Education Psychology*, 70, 255–272.

Peira, N., Pourtois, G., and **Fredrikson, M.** (2013). Learned cardiac control with heart rate biofeedback transfers to emotional reactions. *PloS One*, 8(7), e70004.

Pressman, S. D. and **Cohen, S.** (2005). Does positive affect influence health? *Psychological Bulletin*, 131, 925–971.

Randall, W. M. and **Rickard, N. S.** (2013). Development and trial of a mobile experience sampling method (m-ESM) for personal music listening. *Music Perception*, 31, 157–170.

Rickard, N. S. (2004). Intense emotional responses to music: A test of the physiological arousal hypothesis. *Psychology of Music*, 32, 371–388.

Rickard, N. S., Chin, T. C., and **Vella-Brodrick, D. A.** (2016). Cortisol awakening response as an index of mental health and well-being in adolescents. *Journal of Happiness Studies*, 17, 2555–2568.

Roberts, D. F. and **Foehr, U. G.** (2008). Trends in media use. *The Future of Children*, 18, 11–37.

Rozin, A., Rozin, P., and **Goldberg, E.** (2004). The feeling of music past: How listeners remember musical affect. *Music Perception*, 22(1), 15–39.

Russell, J., Weiss, A., and **Mendelsohn, G.** (1989). Affect Grid: A single-item scale of pleasure and arousal. *Journal of Personality and Social Psychology*, 57, 493–502.

Saarikallio, S. and **Erkkilä, J.** (2007). The role of music in adolescents' mood regulation. *Psychology of Music*, 35, 88–109.

Scherer, K R. (2005). What are emotions? And how can they be measured? *Social Science Information*, 44, 695–729.

Schubert, E. (2010). Continuous self-report methods. In P. N. Juslin and J. A. Sloboda (Eds), *Handbook of Music and Emotion: Theory, Research, Applications* (pp. 223–253). Oxford: Oxford University Press.

Schubert, E., Hargreaves, D. J., and **North, A. C.** (2014). A dynamically minimalist cognitive explanation of musical preference: Is familiarity everything? *Frontiers in Psychology*, 5, 38. doi:10.3389/fpsyg.2014.00038.

Sloboda, J. A. and **Lehmann, A. C.** (2001). Tracking performance correlates of changes in perceived intensity of emotion during different interpretations of a Chopin piano prelude. *Music Perception*, 19, 87–120.

Sloboda, J. A. and **O'Neill, S. A.** (2001). Emotions in everyday listening to music. In P. N. Juslin and J. A. Sloboda (Eds), *Music and Emotion: Theory and Research* (pp. 415–430). Oxford: Oxford University Press.

Suldo, S. M., Friedrich, A. A., White, T., Farmer, J., Minch, D., and **Michalowski, J.** (2009). Teacher support and adolescents' subjective well-being: A mixed-methods investigation. *School Psychology Review*, 38, 67–85.

Tsuchiya, N. and **Adolphs, R.** (2007). Emotion and consciousness. *Trends in Cognitive Science*, 11, 158–167.

Vella-Brodrick, D. A., Rickard, N. S., and **Chin, T. C.** (2017). Evaluating positive education: A framework and case study. In N. J. L. Brown, T. Lomas, and F. J. Eiroa-Orosa (Eds), *The Routledge International Handbook of Critical Positive Psychology* (pp. 488–502). London: Routledge.

Zentner, M. R., Grandjean, D., and **Scherer, K. R.** (2008). Emotions evoked by the sound of music: Characterization, classification, and measurement. *Emotion*, 8, 494–521.

Chapter 5

Between down in the dumps and over the moon: Music therapy for young people with depression

Josephine Geipel

Introduction

Depression is among the most common psychiatric disorders in adolescents, with female adolescents being at higher risk for depression than male adolescents or children. It is characterized by a high rate of recurrence, which is especially striking as mood disorders in childhood and youth are strongly associated with the development of subsequent mental disorders in adulthood and suicidal ideation.

When working with depressive adolescents, symptoms such as depressed mood, loss of interest in activities they once found enjoyable, reduced energy, changed sleeping patterns or appetite, and feelings of guilt or low self-worth are apparent. For adolescents and children, depression often has derogatory effects including social withdrawal, poor school performance, and disturbances in family and peer relationships. In my clinical practice, these interpersonal problems are often the reason that patients seek professional help.

Treatment options for adolescent depression

Adolescents with depressive disorders are usually treated with pharmacotherapy or psychotherapy (particularly cognitive behavioural therapy) or a combination of both since these interventions have been amenable to outcome testing and therefore achieved positive results (Cheung et al., 2007). In addition to pharmacotherapy and well-established psychological interventions, there are a range of alternative and complementary treatment approaches available for adolescents with depression. Although there is a limited number of randomized controlled trials, experts frequently advocate for complementary approaches like exercise, relaxation/mindfulness, and creative arts therapies (Dolle and Schulte-Körne, 2014).

Music therapy for depressed young people

Many mental health institutions for young people employ music therapists because they experience music therapy as being beneficial for engaging and supporting adolescents in their programmes. In addition, research shows that music therapy is an effective intervention for adolescents with general psychopathology, showing medium (Gitman, 2010; Gold et al., 2004) to large effect sizes (Pesek, 2007). Until now, few scientists have researched the effects of music therapy on depressed adolescents. For adults, the positive impact of music therapy for decreasing depressive symptoms has been confirmed by evidence (Chan et al., 2011; Aalbers et al., 2017). Looking into research on music-based interventions with children and adolescents with internalizing symptoms, we also found evidence that music therapy may be beneficial for this special population (Geipel et al., 2018). The quantitative research evidence is nourished by qualitative studies, as well as supported by reports and case narratives from respected clinicians.

Music is of major importance in adolescents' identity formation, mood regulation, and peer-group-building processes (North et al., 2000). However, current research also associates music listening in depressed young people with both negative and positive outcomes, depending on the underlying coping strategies employed by the adolescent. Conversely, music making tends to mostly influence mood in a positive way (McFerran et al., 2016). According to Anna Maratos et al. (2011) the active doing of music making is characteristic of music therapy and a connotative way of dealing with typical symptoms in depression: music making fosters physical activity and interaction between musicians and gives pleasure.

Apart from some studies and chapters in collected editions, there is only a manageable amount of literature on music therapy with adolescents in general (McFerran, 2010). Until now, no music therapy guidelines for children or young people with depression have been explored. There are guidelines for adults with depression and/or anxiety (Jackson, 2013) and Catherine Carr and colleagues have an ongoing study to develop best practice guidelines in group music therapy for chronic depression (Carr et al., 2017). Some of the case studies and controlled studies with depressed young people also include descriptions of their approach, which can give guidance to clinicians and students (e.g. Hendricks, 2001; Hendricks and Bradley, 2005; Magnis, 2011; Porter et al., 2016).

Music therapy manual for depressed young people

The idea to develop a music therapy manual for depressive adolescents arose in the context of a research project in Heidelberg, Germany. When preparing for this project, I was torn between offering a standardized therapy treatment that met the requirements for validity and replicability of research and the need for a clinically meaningful and flexible therapeutic procedure that was tailored to the needs of the individual. I resolved to produce a music therapy manual that outlines certain principles and recommends interventions to achieve particular therapeutic aims. The manual intentionally avoids giving strict time cues, to give the music therapist the flexibility to react to the client's needs.

Table 5.1. Outline of the music therapy manual for young people with depression

Module	Goals	Intervention
Module 1: sensory modulation (sessions 1–12)	Introduction Relationship building	Exploration of expectations and wishes Exploration of the instruments
	Body-mind relaxation	Mindful listening to sounds/music
	Improved comprehension of impact of music on self	Receptive music therapy using client-preferred music
Module 2: emotion regulation (sessions 3–12)	Improved emotion recognition Improved perception of emotions Improved expression of emotions Improved comprehension of emotions and their impact on self Experience of feelings Modification of emotions Handling of emotional states and events	Referential improvisation of mood/emotions/emotional events Creating playlists Therapeutic songwriting
Module 3: interpersonal regulation (sessions 7–12)	Improved perception of one's own needs Exploring social roles Exploring diverse behaviours and their effect on one's self	Non-referential improvisation Musical role play
Sessions 11– 12	Conclusion and farewell	Recording of songs created Treatment evaluation

I used recent findings in music therapy/psychology research and current practical knowledge as the basis for developing the manual. This involved identifying general principles that define the therapists' stance. Single modules of the manual were then derived from research and these module-specific principles were outlined and interventions exemplified. Potential mechanisms are explained below.

Context

This manual is for short-term music therapy for adolescents between 13 and 17 years old who are experiencing a mild or moderate depressive episode. The young people are expected to participate in 12 individual sessions of music therapy inan outpatient setting. The particular interventions outlined in the manual were created as an adjunct therapy to psychotherapy and/or medical treatment provided by a qualified music therapist. Thus, it focuses on particular domains in the treatment of depression: sensory modulation, the improvement of emotion regulation, and interpersonal regulation. It contains methods that are in line with current music therapy practice and research. Table 5.1 shows the therapeutic aims and music therapy techniques used in the three phases of the music therapy manual for depressed adolescents.

General therapeutic principles

The general therapeutic principles highlighted in the manual can be understood as central for the whole therapeutic process as well as the therapist's attitude. They define a client-oriented approach.

The music therapist should:

◆ have a collaborative client–therapist stance

◆ offer acceptance and appraisal to the client

◆ offer feedback and interpretations

◆ listen, talk, and play adequately to the goal of the current process

◆ be authentic and provide therapeutic transparency

◆ build a trusting relationship

◆ provide positive experiences

◆ recognize the client's expertise of themselves

◆ respect the musical identity of the client.

Module 1: sensory modulation

Main focus of the module:

◆ build a trusting relationship

◆ introduce music therapy

◆ enable body-mind relaxation

◆ educate adolescents about influence of their preferred music on themselves.

The introductory module is focused on establishing a trusting relationship and to giving the client an idea of what to expect from the music therapy sessions. The therapist also uses the first two sessions to assess the client's music listening behaviour and to sensitize the adolescent to the impact music can have on their mood. It prepares them for the following module focusing on emotion regulation.

In my work, I include a technique to promote body-mind relaxation in the initial sessions with adolescents. This is because music has been suggested to have a stress-reducing effect that can induce relaxation that may be particularly beneficial for people with depression (Jorm et al., 2008). Relaxation can be induced through music on autonomic, endocrine, cognitive, and/or emotional levels and several underlying mechanisms may be relevant, depending on the environment and specific characteristics and experiences of a person. Rumination, difficulties in concentrating, and negative thoughts are symptoms that often affect depressive adolescents. To address these cognitive impairments, I suggest a shift of attention from internal to external events using mindful music listening practice.

Since a case history has been taken in advance, therapy starts in the first session with learning the expectations and wishes of the young person and introducing the concept of music therapy. An exploration of instruments establishes the basis for joint music making. The music therapist and the client play together on different instruments in the music therapy room. The music therapist notes which instruments the adolescent likes and how engaged and flexible they are in their playing. Depending on the age of the client the session can be conducted in a more playful or in a more structured way. Sometimes adolescents are shy or too cool in the beginning and need encouragement to engage. Some initial questions like 'What do you think is the loudest instrument?' or 'Which instruments you do not know?' can help getting them going. This should end up in a small, first improvisation, which gives the therapist the possibility to assess musical-emotional expression and flexibility.

Receptive music therapy with client-preferred music

There are many good reasons to listen to the preferred music of the adolescent client during the therapeutic process. First, it helps to open the dialogue and supports positive relationship building between client and therapist. Second, it can be a useful motivation for treatment, and third, it gives the depressed adolescent the possibility to engage with their composite feelings and to express them. A therapeutic dialogue around music listening can bring their intuitive music listening behaviour to consciousness. They can explore how they use music and what kind of coping strategies it serves.

Lucas (15) has a moderate depressive episode and a long history of being bullied in school. He is a big anime fan. Accordingly, he loves listening to the soundtracks of diverse anime films. He explains that while listening to music he would drift away in a fantasy world where he has super powers and self-confidence and where he can easily solve his negative everyday experiences in school. If he could see things more clearly afterwards this would be a helpful way of coping, but back in reality he still feels depressed. Even so, I validate Lucas's current feelings and behaviours and I chat with him about his music and what it makes him feel, with the intention of raising his consciousness about his music use.

Often adolescents are very competent in using their music for emotion regulation, but sometimes in a rather unconscious, non-intentional, and sometimes destructive way (McFerran and Saarikallio, 2014). Hence, the emphasis of listening to the client's preferred music is not necessarily for lyric analysis or to evolve a biographical narrative theme for discussion. Instead, the focus is on what and how they feel while listening to a particular piece of music and to assess what kind of coping strategy lies beyond listening to music.

Mindful music listening

An introduction to receptive music therapy can be used here with mindful listening to a single sound or a live improvisation with monochord and voice. The aim of this intervention is to help the adolescent focus and to practice maintaining their attention on listening. The music therapist leads the adolescent into the present moment by speaking gently and allowing time between statements. The adolescent is invited to sit as comfortably as possible and take some deep breaths. After a short body scan, which leads their attention through the different parts of their body, they are asked to redirect their attention to the sound in the room and then the music gently starts. If their mind wanders and gets stuck in thoughts, emotions, or other perceptions, they are reminded to simply notice where their mind is, and bring it back to the music as best they can.

This exercise is intended to reduce stress and can interrupt the tendency to ruminate. In the following sessions it also serves as a closing exercise as needed. If a session gets tough while concentrating on specific emotions, this can bring young people back down at the end of the session, so they feel safe to go home.

Module 2: emotion regulation

Main focus of the module:

- foster improvement of recognition, perception, expression, and comprehension of emotions and their impact on self
- foster experience of feeling
- empower adolescents to handle emotional states and events (with the help of music)
- validate current emotions
- reflect verbally and musically on emotional topics.

This manual has an emphasis on emotion regulation based on recent research supporting the hypothesis of depression mainly being a disorder of emotion regulation, involving severe mood disturbances (Campbell-Sills and Barlow, 2009). In the last 20 years diverse scientific disciplines have become interested in researching emotion regulation and music (Baltazar and Saarikallio, 2016). Neuroimaging studies have found strong associations between neural networks involved in music processing and those responsible for emotion regulation (Koelsch, 2014). Although there is an obvious connection between music and emotion regulation, it is not known exactly how the connection is best appropriated for wellbeing outcomes. Clarifying this connection does confirm that, when working on emotion regulation, music therapists should be aware that diverse mechanisms could elicit emotions in clients (Juslin and Västfjäll, 2008).

Creating playlists

Having raised awareness about music listening in Module 1, the music therapist then focuses on developing a playlist with the young person, aiming at the symptoms which seem most problematic to the adolescent. Regardless of whether depressed mood or a lack of energy is the biggest strain on the person, a playlist will be developed that aims to improve it with the preferred music of the adolescent. The concept of the iso principle (Altschuler, 2001) is introduced to the adolescent as a technique for mood management. The music therapist takes the role of a coach and honours the adolescent as the expert of their music and mood management. The therapist does not lose sight of musical and lyrical components of the playlist but also takes into account memories and feelings of the client towards single songs. It is recommended to use a music streaming service to develop the therapeutic playlist, as this makes sure both client and therapist have access to the playlist and ensures adherence to copyright laws. The playlist should be flexible and whenever the adolescent recognizes that one song does not work anymore or another one should be added the playlist can be revised. Success of this work has to be monitored by the therapist throughout the 12 sessions.

Angela (17) comes to music therapy with a moderate depressive episode. Apart from that she is dealing with bulimia and a borderline personality disorder. She has already had several stays in psychiatric hospitals because of suicidal ideation. She reports the biggest issue at the moment is her bad mood in the morning after she puts herself on the scales. As the bulimia is already a topic with her psychotherapist, we concentrate on the modulation of mood by creating a playlist. Angela choses to start with the song 'Believe in me' from Demi Lovato (Lovato, 2009), an artist who has bulimia herself and talks in this song about not losing courage. She imagines relating to this song when she is in her bad morning mood. It is a thoughtful quiet song compared to what Angela listens to in everyday life. When asked what kind of mood she wants to be in when she wakes up in the morning, she says she wants to feel balanced and self-confident. With the support of the therapist Angela finds 15 songs for her playlist, which ends with 'Without me' by Eminem (Eminem, 2002).

Referential improvisations of mood/emotions/emotional events

To support engagement in emotions, referential improvisations on single emotions like anxiety, sadness, joy, and anger, or on moods such as melancholy or optimism, will be played. Based on a therapeutic dialogue about a mood or an emotion, the patient chooses instruments which may be able to reflect this specific state and can give details concerning musical parameters fitting to the emotion or the mood. The therapist supports the client by grounding, holding, and containing the musical material that develops within the referential improvisation. The adolescent has the opportunity to express and experience emotions in a non-verbal way, and then the improvisation can act as a bridge to verbal communication. Referential improvisations of emotional events can be helpful to expand understanding of one's own emotions as well as the behaviour patterns relating to these emotions.

When Anna (16) starts music therapy she has mild depression, but cannot get herself out of bed to go to school in the mornings. She seems very controlled and describes how she absolutely does not understand why her situation is like that. She feels excellent. I introduce the basic emotions joy, anger, sadness, and anxiety to her. After being asked which feeling she wants to engage first, she decides on joy. She wants to play the piano and for me to support her at the drum kit. She starts playing a very slow melody in a minor key, and I hold her musically with a simple rhythm. Suddenly she stops and states that this is not joy but rather it is her current mood we were playing. We agree to go on with this improvisation to explore the mood a little more deeply. She is somewhat overwhelmed by her own feelings as she did not expect to be in a rather depressed mood until she expressed it. In the discussion afterwards Anna opens up for the first time and talks about her problems at home. At the end of the session she declares that she feels released.

Therapeutic singing/rapping

The voice is our primary instrument and therefore the most obvious source for emotional expression, as seen by groaning, sighing, and mumbling in everyday life. Using singing and rapping is therefore well matched and useful to provide the client with opportunities to express and experience emotions.

Laurien Hakvoort (2015) presents an interesting approach to therapeutic rapping, which can also be adjusted to therapeutic singing. The adolescent chooses the song to sing under the professional guidance of the music therapist. Then in the first step they focus on technical aspects of the song like intonation, articulation, and breathing. The therapist accompanies on the guitar or the piano. Depending on the song and the skills of the client, programmed rhythms can be added or the young person can also play guitar or piano while the therapist switches to the drum kit. In the second step the emphasis is on expression of emotions while singing, supported by the adherence to a good body posture and musical means, such as dynamics. The focus is now on the experience and expression of emotions and the improvement of self-confidence.

Nicole (15) has a mild depressive disorder and has been bullied ever since she can remember. She often shows a testiness when she comes home from school because she cannot understand why the other students in her class are giving her such a hard time. She keeps her head high by judging them as childish. We decide to sing a song which gives her the opportunity to express her feelings about this situation. In the following session she brings the German version of the song 'Let it go' from the Disney film Frozen (Buck and Lee, 2013). It is the song of a vulnerable and misunderstood girl who turns away from everybody, thinking she does not need anybody. While talking in the second step about how the singer may feel, she first states that she feels pride and after singing it another time she detects a loneliness which she can also connect to. Until Nicole came to music therapy she did not know she could sing, and encouraging her gave her an expanded sense of self. The therapeutic singing is finalized by the recording of the song. This serves as a witness and a resonator of her feelings.

Therapeutic songwriting

Songwriting can be a useful way to reflect verbally and musically on emotional topics in depth. The popularity of songs among adolescents and the structure songs provide make it easy for young people to relate to this idea. There are many approaches to therapeutic songwriting, including the work of Philippa Derrington (2005), that offer structure without becoming inflexible. In the first step, the therapist and adolescent talk about possible topics and ideas and then decide on one. As they have already worked on emotions and emotional events in earlier therapy sessions, there is material available for development through this new intervention. Different possibilities are available for writing lyrics which may use pre-composed lyrics or inventing them while playing and chatting. Sometimes adolescents bring prepared material based on poetry they have written at home or have created as schoolwork. Similarly, the music may be either based on melodies they already know or invented while improvising. The accompaniment is usually provided by the therapist, who follows the instructions of the adolescents concerning musical parameters. Depending on the quality of the therapeutic singing it may also be nice to document this intervention by recording it and/or writing it down.

Module 3: interpersonal regulation

Main focus of the module:

♦ improve perception of one's own needs

♦ explore different social roles

♦ explore diverse behaviours and their effect on one's self.

Depression occurs in an interpersonal context. Interpersonal strain may be the elicitor, the consequence, or the sustaining condition of depression; but in all these cases it should remain within the therapeutic focus. The main aim of this module is to explore experiences and develop flexible behaviours. This work may also target symptoms of low self-esteem, lack of self-confidence, and social withdrawal.

Musical role play

Musical role plays are helpful to explore interpersonal relationships, social situations, and aspects of self. Different instruments can be assigned to different persons as part of the improvised role play, minding that the characteristics of the instrument match with the characteristics of the person in the enacted situation. The client has the opportunity to realize relationship patterns and test diverse behaviours and their effect on others and themselves. By switching instruments between client and therapist, the client can gain insights into different roles and their needs.

Steven (17) came to music therapy after having a severe depressive episode. He already felt better when music therapy started, but had problems describing his own needs and expressing his feelings. After a referential improvisation on anger, I suggested we do a role play of a situation where he and two good friends were arguing about what to do during a trip to Munich. He described how he would stay calm on the outside but was very angry inside because he wanted to enjoy the time and not listen to them anymore. I played the two friends on the congas and Steven played himself on the djembe. After reviving the situation musically he felt the anger again. The congas were talking to each other very loudly and the djembe could not be heard at all. I encouraged him to try different patterns in the music, so he became more courageous and at the end of the session a quite long improvisation took place where the lead was changing between players in a way that felt more equal. In a therapeutic dialogue afterwards he could transfer the musical experience to situations in everyday life.

Treatment evaluation

By referring to the expectations and wishes they had at the beginning of therapy, young people can evaluate for themselves what has changed since they walked into music therapy for the first time. To make sure their growth and improvement will continue, it is also useful to discuss what remains to be changed by them or others and which of the things experienced in music therapy could help in promoting this.

Conclusion

Depression has been conceptualized as a disorder of emotion regulation and therefore music can be an excellent medium to support improvements in emotion regulation. Considering the in-between developmental state of adolescents, it is not appropriate to simply offer them interventions that were originally designed for children or adults, and it is critical to keep in mind that music is something crucial for identity formation, mood management, and peer-group formation. The therapy manual presented in this chapter offers many advantages in terms of its structure and its flexibility. It is valuable for a music therapist to have guidelines to follow without losing the possibility of integrating the own creativity and experience to reach therapeutic goals. The focus on the work with emotions makes sense since music therapists are experts in this field and taking this focus allows us to touch on other relevant topics such as self-esteem, loss of energy, and interpersonal problems. Everything is connected to difficulties in emotion processing. Adolescents regularly attended music therapy sessions based on this manual and this may have been partly because of the integration of their own music right from the beginning. They reported especially liking the playlist creation as this was something they could take home and use in between sessions.

There are a number of methods to address the therapeutic aims and follow the principles of this complementary music therapy manual for young people with depression. By using interventions derived from current practice and research I have provided suggestions about how qualified and trained music therapists might choose to treat young people with depression. The music therapist has the possibility of adapting interventions to the specific needs of the client using their own specific competences, gained through their professional training and clinical experience. This offers flexibility to the music therapist, as well as responsibility.

References

Aalbers, S., Fusar-Poli, L., Freeman, R. E., Spreen, M., Ket, J. C., Vink, A. C., et al. (2017). Music therapy for depression. *Cochrane Database of Systematic Reviews*, **11**, CD004517. doi:10.1002/14651858.CD004517.pub3.

Altschuler, I. (2001). A psychiatrist's experience with music as a therapeutic agent. *Nordic Journal of Music Therapy*, **10**, 69–76. doi:10.1080/08098130109478019.

Baltazar, M. and Saarikallio, S. (2016). Toward a better understanding and conceptualization of affect self-regulation through music: A critical, integrative literature review. *Psychology of Music*, **44**, 1500–1521. doi:10.1177/0305735616663313.

Buck, C. and Lee, J. (2013). *Frozen*. Walt Disney Studios Motion Pictures.

Campbell-Sills, L. and Barlow, D. (2009) Incorporation emotion regulation into conceptualizations and treatments of anxiety and mood disorders. In J.J. Gross (Ed.), *Handbook of Emotion Regulation* (pp. 542–559). New York: The Guilford Press.

Carr, C., O'Kelly, J., Sandford, S., and Priebe, S. (2017). Feasibility and acceptability of group music therapy vs wait-list control for treatment of patients with long-term depression (the SYNCHRONY trial): Study protocol for a randomised controlled trial. *Trials*, **18**, 149. doi:10.1186/s13063-017-1893-8.

Chan, M. F., Wong, Z. Y., and Thayala, N. V. (2011). The effectiveness of music listening in reducing depressive symptoms in adults: A systematic review. *Complementary Therapies in Medicine*, 19, 332–348. doi:10.1016/j.ctim.2011.08.003.

Cheung, A. H., Zuckerbrot, R. A., Jensen, P. S., Ghalib, K., Laraque, D., and Stein, R. E. K. (2007). Guidelines for Adolescent Depression in Primary Care (GLAD-PC): II. Treatment and ongoing management. *Pediatrics*, 120, e1313–e1326. doi:10.1542/peds.2006-1395.

Derrington, P. (2005). Teenagers and songwriting. Supporting students in a mainstream secondary school. In F. Baker and T. Wigram (Eds), *Songwriting: Methods, Techniques and Clinical Applications for Music Therapy Clinicians, Educators and Students* (pp. 68–81). London: Jessica Kingsley Publishers.

Dolle, K. and Schulte-Körne, G. (2014). Komplementäre Ansätze zur Behandlung von depressiven Störungen bei Kindern und Jugendlichen. *Praxis Kinderpsychologie Kinderpsychiatrie*, 63, 237–263.

Eminem (2002). *Without me, The* Eminem Show. Interscope Records, Santa Monica, CA.

Geipel, J., Koenig, J., Hillecke, T., Resch, F., and Kaess, M. (2018). Music-based interventions to reduce internalizing symptoms in children and adolescents: A meta-analysis. *Journal of Affective Disorders*, 225C, 647–656.

Gitman, K. (2010). The effects of music therapy on children and adolescents with mental or medical illness: A meta-analysis. PhD thesis. University at Buffalo, State University of New York.

Gold, C., Voracek, M., and Wigram, T. (2004). Effects of music therapy for children and adolescents with psychopathology: A meta-analysis. *Journal of Child Psychology and Psychiatry*, 45, 1054–1063. doi:10.1111/j.1469-7610.2004.t01-1-00298.x.

Hakvoort, L. (2015). Rap music therapy in forensic psychiatry: Emphasis on the musical approach to rap. *Music Therapy Perspectives*, 33, 184–192. doi:10.1093/mtp/miv003.

Hendricks, C. B. (2001). A study of the use of music therapy techniques in a group for the treatment of adolescent depression. PhD thesis. Texas Tech University.

Hendricks, C. B. and Bradley, L. J. (2005). Interpersonal theory and music techniques: A case study for a family with a depressed adolescent. *Family Journal*, 13, 400–405. doi:10.1177/1066480705278469.

Jackson, N. (2013). Adults with depression and/or anxiety. In L. Eyre (Ed.), *Guidelines for Music Therapy Practice in Mental Health* (pp. 339–377). Gilsum, NH: Barcelona Publishers.

Jorm, A. F., Morgan, A. J., and Hetrick, S. E. (2008). Relaxation for depression. *Cochrane Database of Systematic Reviews*, 4, CD007142. doi:10.1002/14651858.CD007142.pub2.

Juslin, P. N. and Västfjäll, D. (2008). Emotional responses to music: The need to consider underlying mechanisms. *Behavioral and Brain Sciences*, 31, 559–575. doi:10.1017/S0140525X08005293.

Koelsch, S. (2014). Brain correlates of music-evoked emotions. *Nature Reviews Neuroscience*, 15, 170–180. doi:10.1038/nrn3666.

Lovato, D., 2009. *Believe in me, don't forget*. Hollywood Records, Burbank, CA.

Magnis, E. S. (2011). Finding a vocal path through depression. PhD thesis. Pacifica Graduate Institute.

Maratos, A., Crawford, M. J., and Procter, S. (2011). Music therapy for depression: It seems to work, but how? *British Journal of Psychiatry*, 199, 92–93. doi:10.1192/bjp.bp.110.087494.

McFerran, K. S. (2010). *Adolescents, Music and Music Therapy*. Philadelphia, PA: Jessica Kingsley.

McFerran, K. S., Garrido, S., and Saarikallio, S. (2016). A critical interpretive synthesis of the literature linking music and adolescent mental health. *Youth & Society*, 48, 521–538. doi:10.1177/0044118X13501343.

McFerran, K. S. and Saarikallio, S. (2014). Depending on music to feel better: Being conscious of responsibility when appropriating the power of music. *Arts in Psychotherapy*, 41, 89–97. doi:10.1016/j.aip.2013.11.007.

North, A. C., Hargreaves, D. J., and O'Neill, S. A. (2000). The importance of music to adolescents. *British Journal of Educational Psychology*, **70**, 255–272. doi:10.1348/000709900158083.

Pesek, U. (2007). Musiktherapiewirkung—eine Meta-Analyse. *Musiktherapeutische Umschau*, **28**, 110–135. doi:10.13109/muum.2007.28.2.110.

Porter, S., McConnell, T., McLaughlin, K., Lynn, F., Cardwell, C., Braiden, H.-J., Boylan, J., Holmes, V., and the Music in Mind Study Group (2016). Music therapy for children and adolescents with behavioural and emotional problems: A randomised controlled trial. *Journal of Child Psychology and Psychiatry*, **58**, 586–594. doi:10.1111/jcpp.12656.

Chapter 6

Musical affect regulation in adolescents: A conceptual model

Margarida Baltazar

Introduction

The ubiquity of music in adolescents' lives has conferred it an immense responsibility and incomparable power: the one of lifting shattered emotions, blowing the blues away, keeping it low, or changing the key. But what exactly is the role of music and how can we study it? Is there something special about music? This chapter will explore how adolescents use music to self-regulate their affect. A conceptual model of affect regulation through music will be presented, drawing support from both psychology and music research.

Affect and affect regulation

When talking about their relationship with music, adolescents often report the regulation of different affect dimensions simultaneously (e.g. 'I received emotions of joy and happiness and emotional sensations. I got into a good mood and I started feeling ample [*sic*] and happy. I started to feel like dancing', Saarikallio et al., 2017). Given this overlap in daily life experience, this chapter follows the suggestion of Baltazar and Saarikallio (2016) and adapts the umbrella term affect in order to include the states related to the positive/negative evaluation of external and internal stimuli. This term allows us to gather together states such as emotions, moods, motivational impulses, stress responses, and arousal (Juslin and Sloboda, 2010; Scherer, 2005). Affect regulation is then taken to mean all the attempts made by the young person at creating, changing, or maintaining any of these affective states. Only the regulation of one's own affective states (i.e. self-regulation) will be addressed in this chapter.

Affect is highly informative: through our feelings, we get valuable cues about what is happening around us and its meaning (Damasio, 2000). However, affect cannot flow freely in a constant stream of strong emotions, moving moods, and varying levels of arousal. It requires regulation and this is a constant process where the person strives for a better balance between personal goals, emotions, and context (Tamir and Ford, 2012; Aldao and Nolen-Hoeksema, 2012; Tamir, 2016).

Adolescence is a special developmental stage because major changes occur at several levels—be it affective, biological, cognitive, social, and identity levels (for a review, see Gowers, 2005). During these changes, emotional experiences can be more intense and unstable and social or external regulation may be decreased (Yap et al., 2007). Due to the developmental challenges faced, adolescence and early adulthood are critical points of vulnerability (Steinberg, 2005). If the adolescent is lacking self-regulation skills, there is an increased risk of social difficulties, lower psychological and emotional adjustment, and internalization and externalization symptoms (Garnefski et al., 2005).

Model of affect self-regulation through music: putting the pieces together

The model depicted in Fig. 6.1 combines several components of musical affect regulation that have been identified in recent literature (Van Goethem and Sloboda, 2011; Baltazar and Saarikallio, 2016, 2017a). In this model, affect regulation is one among many functions of music. The affective goals influence the choice of musical activities, regulatory strategies, and musical mechanisms. Regulation strategies and musical mechanisms form specific associations represented in the triangle of cognition, feelings, and body. The process of regulation results in changes that, in the long term, are related to the adolescents' wellbeing. Affect regulation is a continuous process, embedded in an intricate pattern of contextual and individual factors.

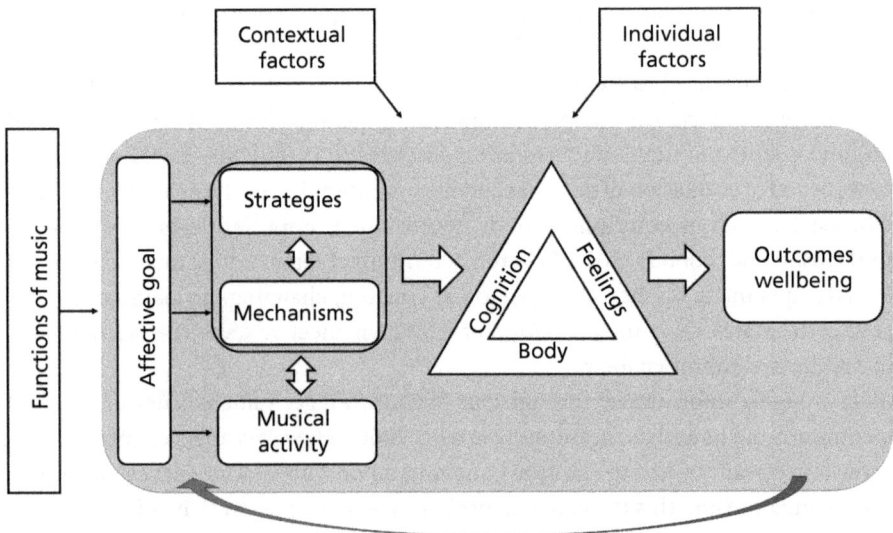

Fig. 6.1 Integrative model of affect self-regulation through music.
Baltazar, M. and Saarikallio, S. (2017a). Conceptual model of musical affect regulation. *Figshare*. https://figshare.com/articles/Conceptual_model_of_musical_affect_self-regulation/5350105/3 (accessed 27 November 2018).

The act of regulation is considered to be driven by an affective goal, even if unconsciously (Koole and Rothermund, 2011; Tamir, 2016). In a healthy individual, affect regulation is flexible (Marik and Stegemann, 2016) and the behaviour, regulation strategies, and interaction with available resources in the environment adjust to better fit the affective goal. Similarly, in the context of music use, the affective goal guides the adolescent's decisions regarding the musical activity to engage in, the strategy to apply, and the musical mechanisms on which to focus.

Adolescents might use music to achieve several affective goals, such as decreasing negative affect, increasing or maintaining positive affect, and intensifying negative states (Papinczak et al., 2015; Saarikallio and Erkkilä, 2007; Tarrant et al., 2000). In psychology studies, adolescents have been found to be more prone than adults to engage in negative states or to dampen positive affect (Riediger et al., 2009) and this pattern has also been found in music listening (Cohrdes et al., 2017). Nevertheless, the goals pursued and their outcomes are heavily influenced by the adolescents' mental wellbeing and individual factors (Miranda and Gaudreau, 2011; Schwartz and Fouts, 2003). Of particular interest is that an increased use of music to cope with negative states has been correlated with higher levels of depression symptoms (Miranda and Claes, 2009).

Musical activities

Adolescents engage in music through several types of activities—listening attentively or in the background, dancing, singing, watching music videos, composing songs, and writing lyrics, among others (Saarikallio and Erkkilä, 2007; Van Goethem, 2010). One way of seeing these musical activities can be the concretization of an affective need and goal (Van Goethem and Sloboda, 2011); they give the adolescent the resources for action and put into practice the desired strategies. An ecological approach to music suggests that musical situations convey affordances; i.e. possibilities of action belonging to an object or environment in relation to an organism (Gibson, 1977). It has been argued that each musical activity has different affordances (Krueger, 2014; DeNora, 2000), thus supporting different regulatory actions.

Empirical results seem to support this claim. Adolescents interact with different musical activities with different purposes and strategies. In Saarikallio and Erkkilä's (2007) study, even though music listening was the most common activity for self-regulation, interesting patterns concerning other musical activities emerged. For example, singing was used for reviving, relaxing, and re-energizing through the strategy revival and forgetting about current negative mood through diversion. Writing songs, in turn, while having in common the support of relaxation and revival, was also associated with achieving new insights and understandings about the situation/feeling through mental work. These associations point to the interdependence between music, its features, and the strategic possibilities offered. For this reason, there is a bidirectional arrow between musical activity and the group of strategies and mechanisms in Fig. 6.1.

Regulation strategies and musical mechanisms: at the interface between the adolescent and music

There is something fascinating in studying how the characteristics of music support its affective uses. Micro-level examination may deepen our understanding of why music is so efficient and engaging. We recently conducted a study that provides useful insights into the internal organization of strategies and mechanisms and the associations between them. Data was collected through an online questionnaire from adolescents and young adults concerning their most recent episode of affect regulation through music (more details in Baltazar and Saarikallio, 2017b). Participants were asked about the reason they chose music over other activities (e.g. talking to a friend, exercising). Four options were provided, each one representing the intention to focus on one of the four levels of musical affect regulation suggested by Van Goethem (2010): goals ('I wanted to be in a certain affective state'), strategies ('I wanted to use music as a "tool" that could help me'), musical activities (tactics in Van Goethem, 2010; 'I wanted to engage in music by, for example, listening, playing, or dancing to it'), and mechanisms ('I wanted to feel music's impact on me'). The answers were unequally distributed ($\chi^2(3) = 36.98$, $p < 0.001$). The participants selected the options relative to strategies and mechanisms equally often, both with a proportion significantly higher than the expected mean ($z = 3.38$, $p < 0.001$). According to these young informants, the strategies that they can use through music and music's emotional impact on them are the main motivators for engaging in music. Based on this, we identified regulatory strategies and musical mechanisms as the core elements for the adolescents' experience (Fig. 6.1) and considered that their associations deserve further exploration.

Strategies

In a musical context, we consider strategies to be the behavioural and cognitive tools employed while performing a certain musical activity to achieve an affective goal. Regulation strategies are inherent to any human behaviour and have been widely studied in psychology (for a review, see Gross, 2015). However, general models from psychology do not necessarily transpose directly to the case of musical self-regulation (Randall et al., 2014). Consequently, music researchers have been devoted to the identification and analysis of the strategies involved in musical uses. Saarikallio and Erkkilä (2007) identified the following strategies used by the adolescent participants in their study: entertainment (creating a fun environment and seeking amusement), revival (relaxing, energizing, and revitalizing), strong sensation (seeking powerful feelings of pleasure, enjoyment, and excitement), diversion (detaching from undesired thoughts or feelings), discharge (expressing, releasing, or venting emotions), mental work (reflecting on and reappraising situations and reactions), and solace (seeking comforting, connecting, and meaningful experiences).

In the survey study, we presented a set of strategies for the participants to identify which ones they had used in the musical episode they were reporting (the list of strategies was based on a literature review by Baltazar and Saarikallio, 2016). Three dimensions emerged from the analysis, representing distinct components underlying affect regulation: cognition, feelings, and bodily reactions (Fig. 6.2). The poles of each dimension mean a higher or lower involvement of the corresponding component.

As seen in Fig. 6.2, the higher and lower focus on cognition, feelings, and bodily reactions while self-regulating through music creates six major groups of strategies: cognitive work (reappraisal, perspective taking, reflection, acceptance), entertainment (seek pleasurable feelings through fun), affective work (modulation of feelings, induction of strong sensations), distraction (turn the attention away from thoughts, feelings, or surroundings), revival (relaxation, energizing, increasing flow and endurance), and focus on situation (direct the attention to the surroundings, task in hand, or situation).

Interestingly, these groups of strategies can be further categorized in two: analytical and change-oriented strategies versus repairing and pleasure-oriented strategies. The left side of Fig. 6.2 is thus characterized by an active, contemplative, and cognition-loaded regulation, while the right side is characterized by a more passive, pleasure-oriented, and body-focused regulation.

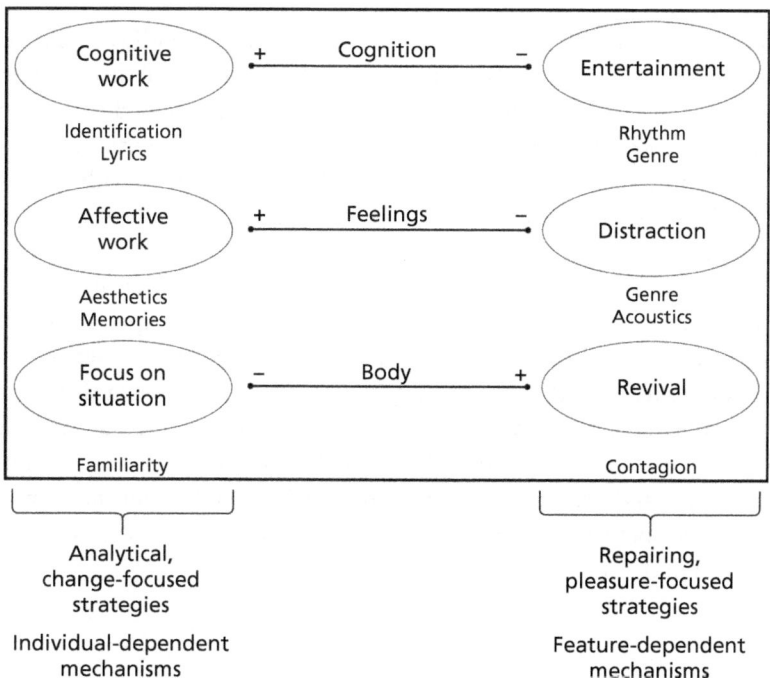

Fig. 6.2 Associations between strategies and mechanisms across three dimensions (cognition, feelings, body).

Note: the plus/minus signs indicate the higher/lower use of that dimension's component (e.g. cognition). Adapted from Baltazar and Saarikallio (2017b), Musicae Scientiae (advance online publication). Copyright ® 2017 (Baltazar and Saarikallio). doi: 10.1177/1029864917715061. Adapted by permission of SAGE publications.

Musical mechanisms

Studies on adolescents' musical regulation often report statements such as 'First I am captivated by the lyrics, and then I pay attention to the melody, sonorities, and all that' or 'Someone is singing, then the music's rhythm .... It reaches inside me and makes me relax' (Baltazar, 2009). These testimonies imply that there are qualities in the music itself or in the dyad 'individual-music' that facilitate affective change. In this chapter, musical mechanisms refer to the aspects linked to music that can induce affect and support affective change.

Initial explorations of this topic have been supporting the link between musical qualities and self-regulation. Saarikallio et al. (2017) examined the interplay between strategies and mechanisms in adolescents' relaxation through music and observed that two major groups of mechanisms were used: musical (including acoustic features and emotional character of the song) and mental (including imagery and memories). Additionally, studies with adults have overall identified a large list of mechanisms that adolescents might potentially use as well (lyrics, rhythm, memories, genre, acoustic features, identification with the artist or song, aesthetics, preferences, associations, familiarity with the music, contagion, and imagery; see review in Baltazar and Saarikallio, 2016).

Based on these findings, the survey asked the participants to identify the relevant mechanisms for the reported episode. The following mechanisms contributed significantly to the model in Fig. 6.2: identification with the artist or song, lyrics, rhythm, genre, aesthetics, memories, acoustics, contagion, and familiarity with the music. The young participants tended to get support from each mechanism in association with certain groups of strategies; these associations are illustrated in Fig. 6.2 by placing the mechanism under the respective major strategy.

These mechanisms cover a wide range of features one can identify in relation to music. The results suggest that musical mechanisms can be grouped into individual-dependent mechanisms (left side of Fig. 6.2: identification, lyrics, aesthetics, memories, and familiarity with the music) and feature-dependent mechanisms (right side of Fig. 6.2: contagion[1], genre, acoustics, and rhythm). The feature-dependent mechanisms are related to more universal characteristics of music regarding sound, style, expressed arousal, and valence, while the individual-dependent mechanisms reflect a unique experience between the person and music and are linked to associations, significations, and preferences.

---

[1] Even though the term *contagion* might suggest an individual association, it refers to the expressed emotions of the music, which then are 'mimicked' by the individual (Juslin and Västfjäll, 2008). Similarly, *rhythm* can induce affect through entrainment. All perception is, at some level, subjective and individual and even the feature-dependent mechanisms are imbued with this subjectivity.

Regulation strategies and musical mechanisms: underlying associations

There is an interesting pattern visible in Fig. 6.2 that sheds some light on how musical mechanisms support the affective needs of young people. Individual-dependent mechanisms (e.g. memories) are associated with analytical and change-oriented strategies (e.g. affective work). Feature-dependent mechanisms (e.g. rhythm) are, in contrast, associated with repairing and pleasure-oriented strategies (e.g. entertainment). One might conclude that personally meaningful aspects of music have a stronger impact on affect regulation that requires larger efforts in terms of cognitive, affective, and attention processing (left side of the Fig. 6.2), while regulation processes that disengage from the situation and internal processes (such as the ones on the right side of Fig. 6.2) benefit from mechanisms intrinsic to music.

Affective outcomes and wellbeing

One of the driving factors for the growth of research on strategies underlying music use is their strong connection to health and affective outcomes. More and more, research has been showing that regulation strategies are a mediating variable between music uses, genre preferences, and mental health (e.g. Chin and Rickard, 2014; Thomson et al., 2014). The development of adaptive and flexible regulation tools during adolescence is crucial for youth's wellbeing and mental health. Depending on the strategies used, music can be a risk or protective factor (Miranda, 2013; McFerran, 2016). The affective outcomes and wellbeing implications are not explored in this chapter; however, it is worth noting that, according to this model, affective musical regulation impacts—positively or negatively—the adolescent's wellbeing through the cumulative process of affective outcomes.

Individual and contextual factors

Self-regulation is deeply influenced by individual and contextual factors. These two factors have reciprocal relationships, as children and adolescents are raised in a sociocultural environment that undoubtedly shapes their biopsychological development (Raver, 2004).

Just as there are several types of music, there are different listeners (Ter Bogt et al., 2011). The relationship with music is rather personal, and individual traits play an important role in how adolescents use music to self-regulate. The number of hours adolescents spend listening to music, their preferred style of affect regulation, the most relevant function of music and, even, the affective outcomes of music engagement have all been traced back to individual factors such as emotional reactivity (e.g. Roberts et al., 1998), symptomatology (e.g. McFerran et al., 2015), developmental stage (e.g. Leipold and Loepthien, 2015), and level of engagement with music (e.g. Ter Bogt et al., 2011).

As for contextual factors, one should bear in mind that the sociocultural context is a powerful shaping force that influences musical behaviour on several levels. These influences can be observed on, for example, the adolescents' musical preferences or on their use of music to express their cultural identity (for a review, see Miranda et al., 2015). Importantly, given the culture-dependent function and meaning of emotions (Ratner, 2000), adolescents need to adhere to sociocultural rules regarding their self-regulation (Eisenberg and Zhou, 2000). Lastly, the specific situation surrounding the adolescent at the moment of regulation greatly dictates what are the needs, possible actions, available strategies, and desired outcomes of affect regulation (e.g. Boekaerts, 2002).

Conclusion

Adolescents have incorporated music in their lives and entrusted it with an important function: to help them regulate emotions, moods, and energy levels. Affect regulation is one of the many functions played by music, but it is one of the most relevant for youth's wellbeing and development.

According to the conceptual model presented in this chapter, regulatory strategies and musical mechanisms are at the core of musical regulation. Through the interaction between these two components, adolescents pursue their affective goals across the levels of cognitive, affective, and sensorial functioning. This is a dynamic process, constantly influenced by internal and external factors. The aim of this model is to provide researchers with a solid conceptual background for future studies. Prevention and intervention programmes might likewise benefit from this conceptual endeavour due to the identification of key elements underlying the adolescents' musical self-regulation and contributing to their wellbeing. However, more research is needed to better understand the interconnections between each of the dimensions identified. The model can, therefore, be seen as eternally 'under construction'.

References

Aldao, A. and Nolen-Hoeksema, S. (2012). The influence of context on the implementation of adaptive emotion regulation strategies. *Behaviour Research and Therapy*, **50**(7–8), 493–501.

Baltazar, M. (2009). All you need is music: Caracterização da regulação emocional dos jovens através da música. Master's Thesis. University of Lisbon.

Baltazar, M. and Saarikallio, S. (2016). Toward a better understanding and conceptualization of affect self-regulation through music: A critical, integrative literature review. *Psychology of Music*, **44**(6), 1500–1521.

Baltazar, M. and Saarikallio, S. (2017a). Conceptual model of musical affect regulation. *Figshare*. https://figshare.com/articles/Conceptual_model_of_musical_affect_self-regulation/5350105/3 (accessed 27 November 2018).

Baltazar, M. and Saarikallio, S. (2017b). Strategies and mechanisms in musical affect self-regulation: A new model. *Musicae Scientiae*, advance online publication. doi:10.1177/1029864917715061.

Boekaerts, M. (2002). Intensity of emotions, emotional regulation, and goal framing: How are they related to adolescents' choice of coping strategies? *Anxiety, Stress & Coping*, **15**(4), 401–412.

Chin, T. and Rickard, N. S. (2014). Emotion regulation strategy mediates both positive and negative relationships between music uses and well-being. *Psychology of Music*, **42**(5), 692–713.

Cohrdes, C., Wrzus, C., Frisch, S., and Riediger, M. (2017). Tune yourself in: Valence and arousal preferences in music-listening choices from adolescence to old age. *Developmental Psychology*, **53**(9), 1777–1794.

Damasio, A. (2000). A second chance for emotions. In R. D. Lane and L. Nadel (Eds), *Cognitive Neuroscience of Emotion* (pp. 12–23). New York: Oxford University Press.

DeNora, T. (2000). *Music in Everyday Life*. Cambridge: Cambridge University Press.

Eisenberg, N. and Zhou, Q. (2000). Regulation from a developmental perspective. *Psychological Inquiry*, **11**(3), 166–171.

Garnefski, N., Kraaij, V., and van Etten, M. (2005). Specificity of relations between adolescents' cognitive emotion regulation strategies and internalizing and externalizing psychopathology. *Journal of Adolescence*, **28**(5), 619–631.

Gibson, J. J. (1977). The theory of affordances. In R. Shaw and J. D. Bransford (Eds) *Perceiving, Acting, and Knowing: Toward an Ecological Psychology* (pp. 67–82). Hillsdale, NJ: Lawrence Erlbaum Associates.

Gowers, S. (2005). Development in adolescence. *Psychiatry*, **4**(6), 6–9.

Gross, J. J. (2015). Emotion regulation: Current status and future prospects. *Psychological Inquiry*, **26**(1), 1–26.

Juslin, P. N. and Sloboda, J. A. (2010). Introduction: Aims, organization, and terminology. In P. N. Juslin and J. Sloboda (Eds), *Handbook of Music and Emotion: Theory, Research, Applications* (pp. 3–12). New York: Oxford University Press.

Juslin, P. N. and Västfjäll, D. (2008). Emotional responses to music: The need to consider underlying mechanisms. *Behavioral and Brain Sciences*, **31**(5), 559–621.

Koole, S. L. and Rothermund, K. (2011). "I feel better but I don't know why": The psychology of implicit emotion regulation. *Cognition & Emotion*, **25**(3), 389–399.

Krueger, J. W. (2014). Affordances and the musically extended mind. *Frontiers in Psychology*, **4**, 1003–1015.

Leipold, B. and Loepthien, T. (2015). Music reception and emotional regulation in adolescence and adulthood. *Musicae Scientiae*, **19**(1), 111–128.

Marik, M. and Stegemann, T. (2016). Introducing a new model of emotion dysregulation with implications for everyday use of music and music therapy. *Musicae Scientiae*, **20**(1), 53–67.

McFerran, K. S. (2016). Contextualising the relationship between music, emotions and the well-being of young people: A critical interpretive synthesis. *Musicae Scientiae*, **20**(1), 103–121.

McFerran, K. S., Garrido, S., O'Grady, L., Grocke, D., and Sawyer, S. M. (2015). Examining the relationship between self-reported mood management and music preferences of Australian teenagers. *Nordic Journal of Music Therapy*, **24**(3), 187–203.

Miranda, D. (2013). The role of music in adolescent development: Much more than the same old song. *International Journal of Adolescence and Youth*, **18**(1), 5–22.

Miranda, D. and Claes, M. (2009). Music listening, coping, peer affiliation and depression in adolescence. *Psychology of Music*, **37**(2), 215–233.

Miranda, D. and Gaudreau, P. (2011). Music listening and emotional well-being in adolescence: A person- and variable-oriented study. *Revue Européenne de Psychologie Appliquée/European Review of Applied Psychology*, **61**(1), 1–11.

Miranda, D., Blais-Rochette, C., Vaugon, K., Osman, M., and Arias-Valenzuela, M. (2015). Towards a cultural-developmental psychology of music in adolescence. *Psychology of Music*, **43**(2), 197–218.

Papinczak, Z. E., Dingle, G. A., Stoyanov, S. R., Hides, L., and Zelenko, O. (2015). Young people's uses of music for well-being. *Journal of Youth Studies*, **18**(9), 1119–1134.

Randall, W. M., Rickard, N. S., and Vella-Brodrick, D. A. (2014) Emotional outcomes of regulation strategies used during personal music listening: A mobile experience sampling study. *Musicae Scientiae*, **18**(3), 275–291.

Ratner, C. (2000). A cultural-psychological analysis of emotions. *Culture & Psychology*, **6**(1), 5–39.

Raver, C. C. (2004) Placing emotional self-regulation in sociocultural and socioeconomic contexts. *Child Development*, **75**(2), 346–353.

Riediger, M., Schmiedek, F., Wagner, G. G., and Lindenberger, U. (2009). Seeking pleasure and seeking pain: Differences in prohedonic and contra-hedonic motivation from adolescence to old age. *Psychological Science*, **20**(12), 1529–1535.

Roberts, K. R., Dimsdale, J., East, P., and Friedman, L. (1998). Adolescent emotional response to music and its relationship to risk-taking behaviors. *Journal of Adolescent Health*, **23**(1), 49–54.

Saarikallio, S. and Erkkilä, J. (2007). The role of music in adolescents' mood regulation. *Psychology of Music*, **35**(1), 88–109.

Saarikallio, S., Baltazar, M., and Västfjäll, D. (2017). Adolescents' musical relaxation: Understanding the related affective processing. *Nordic Journal of Music Therapy*, **26**(4), 376–389.

Scherer, K. R. (2005). What are emotions? And how can they be measured? *Social Science Information*, **44**(4), 695–729.

Schwartz, K. D. and Fouts, G. T. (2003). Music preferences, personality style, and developmental issues of adolescents. *Journal of Youth and Adolescence*, **32**(3), 205–213.

Steinberg, L. (2005). Cognitive and affective development in adolescence. *Trends in Cognitive Sciences*, **9**(2), 69–74.

Tamir, M. (2016). Why do people regulate their emotions? A taxonomy of motives in emotion regulation. *Personality and Social Psychology Review*, **20**(3), 199–222.

Tamir, M. and Ford, B. Q. (2012). Should people pursue feelings that feel good or feelings that do good? Emotional preferences and well-being. *Emotion*, **12**(5), 1061–1070.

Tarrant, M., North, A. C., and Hargreaves, D. J. (2000). English and American adolescents' reasons for listening to music. *Psychology of Music*, **28**(2), 166–173.

Ter Bogt, T. F. M., Mulder, J., Raaijmakers, Q. A. W., and Gabhainn, S. N. (2011). Moved by music: A typology of music listeners. *Psychology of Music*, **39**(2), 147–163.

Thomson, C., Reece, J., and Di Benedetto, M. (2014). The relationship between music-related mood regulation and psychopathology in young people. *Musicae Scientiae*, **18**(2), 150–165.

Van Goethem, A. (2010). Affect regulation in everyday life: Strategies, tactics and the role of music. PhD Thesis. Keele University.

Van Goethem, A. and Sloboda, J. A. (2011). The functions of music for affect regulation. *Musicae Scientiae*, **15**(2), 208–228.

Yap, M. B., Allen, N., and Sheeber, L. (2007). Using an emotion regulation framework to understand the role of temperament and family processes in risk for adolescent depressive disorders. *Clinical Child and Family Psychology Review*, **10**(2), 180–196.

Chapter 7

Music and violence: Working with youth to prevent violence

Andreas Wölfl

Introduction

Music as a space of experience fulfils an important function in the confrontation, the learning, and the regulation of one's own feelings, as well as for the development of one's own identity. It is also relevant for dealing with aggressive feelings. In discussions with young people about the relationship between music and violence, three categories can be discerned. First, music can be used for regulating affect by calming down and distracting. Second, aggressive music can reflect aggressive feelings and give an emotional space of understanding for one's own moods such as disappointment, anger, and rage. A third possibility is that stimulating music can intensify aggressive feelings and increase preparedness for violent behaviour (Wölfl, 2017). This leads to the question of how music and music therapy approaches can be used in working with young people to prevent violence.

Youth violence

Violence is a complex phenomenon that seems to lack a general definition, as individual and cultural understandings are required that vary and change in different countries, regions, and groups and occur in the context of local current events. For example, beatings are accepted as a means of education in some cultures whereas they are seen as a form of violence and forbidden in other countries. In an effort to achieve an internationally recognizable definition, the World Health Organization describes violence as 'the intentional use of physical force or power, threatened or actual, against oneself, another person, or against a group or community, that either results in or has a high likelihood of resulting in injury, death, psychological harm, maldevelopment or deprivation' (World Health Organization, 2002). This definition includes not only interpersonal violence but also suicidal behaviour and armed conflicts. It encompasses the most diverse of actions and extends beyond concrete physical action to also include threats and intimidation.

Youth violence is associated with an increase in aggressive potential (moods, feelings, behaviours) at an individual level, which usually decreases again in the adult age. Developmental psychology studies have linked this phenomenon to neurobiological

Table 7.1. Important risk factors on different levels

Individual (Biological disposition and personal history factors)	Relationship (Close relationships: family, friends, intimate partners, and peers)	Community/society (Contexts in which social relationships and broad societal factors exist)
Affect control: ◆ lack of impulse control ◆ lack of frustration tolerance in rejection ◆ persisting phases of loneliness (isolation) ◆ depression.	Experiences of: ◆ domestic violence ◆ strict physical penalties ◆ trauma ◆ neglect ◆ exclusion and isolation ◆ benefiting from violence through enhanced prestige, group membership, etc.	Experiences of: ◆ exclusion ◆ isolation ◆ disadvantage ◆ distributional injustices ◆ aggressive social. Interaction: ◆ benefiting from violence through enhanced prestige, group membership, etc. ◆ violence in the media.
Value and norm orientation: ◆ lack of normative assessment criteria and values ◆ lack of empathy ◆ normative agreement with aggressive behaviour.	Lack of guidance by the parents Affiliation with violent peer groups Inability to distance oneself from other persons or violent group dynamics	Availability of weapons Environment of high crime and poverty rates Culture of violence Periods of social and political changes and armed conflicts

changes and rebuilding processes as well as to psychosocial developments and challenges (World Health Organization, 2002).

Risk factors

The World Health Organization uses an ecological model for explaining violence that encapsulates individual, relationship, community, and societal factors. There are multiple risk factors that increase the prevalence of violence during adolescence and encourage the continuation of aggressive behaviour into adulthood. These risk factors are lack of affective regulation, aggressive attitudes, and lack of empathy, values, and norms, as well as failure at school and lack of education and social success (World Health Organization, 2002). The risk factors listed in Table 7.1 are mentioned as particularly important by a range of experts (World Health Organization, 2002; Cierpka, 2008; Wahl, 2009; Gugel, 2010; Bauer, 2011).

Violence prevention

Efforts to prevent violence usually include a range of measures which, in the best case, cover all four levels of individual, relationship, community, and society. Within the field of prevention, a distinction is often made between primary, secondary, and tertiary prevention. The task of primary prevention is to identify stress factors and developmental risks at an early stage and to influence the development of constructive patterns of action and conflict resolution in the build up to violence and to prevent the use of violence (World Health Organization, 2002; Gugel, 2010).

Music and youth violence

As a universal language of emotion, music can be used by persons in all cultures to calm, distract from, and deal with aggressive emotions as well as to stimulate aggressive moods and violence. A number of non-specific preventative effects of music can be identified under certain conditions and an analysis of protective factors for dealing with aggressive/ violence-glorifying music includes the following (Wölfl, 2017):

- aspects intrinsic to music such as change and positive resolution of aggressive dynamics in a piece of music or obvious and subtle possibilities for distancing oneself by alienation and exaggeration of violence
- social aspects, such as critical discussion with friends and parents
- individual change processes, such as the management of mental crises and the development of new perspectives and options for action.

Risk factors associated with music include a lack of affective regulation and the inability to tolerate others' musical listening choices, an increasing a sense of isolation due to unpopular music preferences, the idealization of a strong, aggressive self-image, and overidentification with a violent group (Wölfl, 2017). It is possible to observe the ways that youth consciously use music in groups and communities for self-regulating as well as stimulating aggression through listening to music (Wölfl, 2017). For example, at peace concerts, songs that calm aggressive moods, strengthen the community, and emphasize a tolerant, peaceful attitude are common. In violent contexts, the emphasis may be more on rhythm and intensity, in order to build a sense of unity and energy.

A significant step towards reinforcing preventive factors could be to engage people in active music making rather than receptive music listening. Joint active music making has been shown in a number of different investigations to have a number of non-specific effects that may prevent aggressive behaviour (Bastian, 2000). The criminologist Christian Pfeiffer (Neumann, 2008) has shown through survey data that the likelihood of violent behaviour in children who actively play music is significantly lower than in other comparison groups. However, in the case of shared music making, aggressive impulses can also be intensified, for example in the joint singing and drumming of combatants during violent episodes of hooliganism (Liell, 2001).

Music as a therapeutic instrument for the prevention of violence

Music therapy for the prevention of violence takes a particular, interpersonal focus in regards to the effects of music. Although music may not lead to fundamental changes in the rate of crime or poverty at a societal level, it can be used to promote positive social impulses and prosocial atmospheres and to strengthen the sense of community at a micro level. In addition, at the level of psychotherapeutic prevention, it can offer new and corrective relationship experiences at the relationship level and promote the regulation of aggressive impulses and dealing with difficult feelings at the individual level.

In practice, music therapists have developed a range of approaches to the prevention of violence, but only a few case studies, theoretical works, and scientific evaluations are published (McFerran and Wölfl, 2015). Three publications are available in the English language about individual work with aggressive adolescents (Castellano and Wilson, 1970; Kivland, 1986; Strange, 2012) and two others describe work with teenagers who have experienced childhood trauma (Derrington, 2012; Viega, 2013). In addition, both unspecific and specific music therapy group formats for the prevention of violence have been reported (Nöcker-Ribaupierre and Wölfl, 2010; McFerran, 2014; Wölfl, 2014, 2016). Finally, community music therapy programmes in school systems, which foster respectful and self-responsible relationships, may prompt behaviours that prevent violence (Elefant, 2010; Baines, 2013; Rickson and McFerran, 2014; Krüger and Stige, 2015).

The position paper 'Music, violence and music therapy with young people in schools' (McFerran and Wölfl, 2015) describes psychodynamic, social learning, and systemic models for understanding the emergence and avoidance of violence (Cierpka, 2008; Bandura, 1978; Stige and Aarø, 2012). The paper differentiates systemic, group-specific, and individual formats into a systematic framework.

In accordance with the ecological model proposed by the World Health Organization to explain the emergence of violence (World Health Organization, 2002), it seems to be useful and effective to offer music therapy approaches that aim to prevent violence at different levels (community, group, individual) and which are able to take account of the interactions between the different levels. Table 7.2 lists the different types of programme that address violence.

Community-focused programmes

Community-focused formats emphasize change processes within larger systems. They aim at atmospheric and structural changes in the community and society in order to promote the (further) development of respectful humanist and democratic cultures that enable members of the community to live equitably and to use and benefit from these advantages independently. Programmes that target community change strive to impact processes at the macro and meso levels. These processes cause changes in the formation of relationships and in the attitudes of individuals. In the context of youth work, these programmes might aim to reduce bullying and exclusion at school and to increase wellbeing and bonding through positive experiences such as collaborative music productions and music participation programmes. Ideally, entire school systems are involved in these programmes over a sustained period of time. In working at this level, strategies are imbedded that impact how the music culture can be independently pursued after the music therapist's involvement has ended (McFerran, 2014; Rickson and McFerran, 2014).

Table 7.2. Different types of programme addressing violence

Most relevant theoretical orientation	Beliefs about causation	Uses of music	Programme aims	Participants	Format
Psychodynamic	Traumatic early childhood experiences	Priming	To provide positive experiences of relationship that mediate the effects of stressors	At-risk youth with challenging behaviours	Process-oriented and Individual
Developmental	Modelling of violent behaviours in different life-contexts (family, peers, institutions)	Non-verbal Expression of feelings, Building Relationship in the group, space for experimental development of solutions to conflict and violent situations	To understand aggressive emotions, and to develop constructive strategies for conflict resolution	Mixed groups made up of whole school-classes with some students, who show propensity to aggressive and violent behaviour	Short or medium term semi-structured and process-oriented group programme
Systemic	Societal expectations about power	Represents societal attitudes	To critically examine attitudes towards men and women	Mixed groups with sustained participant engagement	Process in working with system, consultation to support sustainable uses in future

McFerran, Katrina Skewes; Wölfl, Andreas. *Music, Violence and Music Therapy with Young People in Schools: A Position Paper. Voices: A World Forum for Music Therapy*, [S.l.], v. 15, n. 2, jun. 2015. ISSN 1504-1611. Available at: <https://voices.no/index.php/voices/article/view/831/689>. Date accessed: 29 Aug. 2018. doi:10.15845/voices.v15i2.831.

Uses of music

A music therapy programme will often take the musical preferences of the different groups of young participants into account. Programmes frequently utilize popular music that participants relate to, as well as utilizing instruments that individuals are interested in exploring. During these programmes, the facilitator is sensitive to openly recognizing and acknowledging open and subtle forms of xenophobia, glorification of violence, and destructiveness in the discussion of preferred music. Facilitators may challenge content as well as tolerate and explore examples of lyrics and music that highlight sexism, racism, homophobia, entitlement, and binary constructions of identity (Scrine, 2016). While younger children often enjoy the opportunity to participate in musical improvisations and role playing, teenagers mostly prefer to utilize their own musical preferences, such as rap music, rock, beats, and other contemporary genres. The theory of community music therapy or systemic theories have been influential in the design of these types of programme (Stige et al., 2010; McFerran, 2014; Rickson and McFerran, 2014).

Benefits

The potential for community-focused music therapy programmes is the development of a shared music culture that aims at the wellbeing of all in the community and supports respectful and constructive forms of communication that counteract destructive behaviour. In these processes, everyone is involved and can experience themselves as part of the community. Young people have the opportunity to participate actively, to question critical behaviour, and to take responsibility for shared wellbeing in creative activities.

Within the MusicMatters programme in Australia, it is common to work with whole class groups to use music for learning about aspects of the wellbeing curriculum. In one school this involved three different class groups changing the lyrics to known songs to address the topic of bullying. Each class chose their own song and approached the project quite differently. One class created a rap music video that illustrated how a bully should be called out and asked to be more respectful of the rights of others. Another class wrote and sang a song about love and the many benefits of being kind to one another. A third class created a three-verse song where different groups danced, sang, and played instruments for their own verse, reciting simple lyrics about being nice and having fun. This highlighted the different levels of understanding within the classes, and the function of music making was to make the material accessible to diverse students. Following this activity, the class teachers used lyric substitution for the subsequent curriculum unit, and reported that student engagement in difficult topics such as respectful relationships and gender-based violence conversations was higher than in their previous attempts at that material.

Group programmes

Music therapy programmes that target violence prevention often utilize a semi-structured approach for whole class groups which can involve short intensive programmes or medium-term half-year and yearly projects. These types of programme explicitly discuss bullying and violence and promote the construction of respectful group interactions. Group drumming and music improvisation have been used to foster positive interactions between group members and to generate a range of constructive solutions for dealing with aggressive situations (McFerran and Wölfl, 2015). One specific group programme developed to prevent violence (Wölfl, 2016) encompasses a variety of music therapy techniques that are flexibly applied to a wide range of target groups, issues, and thematic areas, as well as being responsive to the interests of young people. The aim is to strengthen the affective regulation of the individual young people and to promote a group-oriented value orientation which seeks respectful and constructive solutions to conflicts and prevents aggression and violence. Other objectives are the integration of all young people into the class community and the promotion of well-grounded social competence. Possible developmental problems or disorders due to trauma and neglect are countered by the mediation of non-verbal and verbal basic competences and, if necessary, supplemented by individual support measures and sessions (Nöcker-Ribaupierre and Wölfl, 2010; Wölfl, 2014, 2016).

Uses of music

The basis of the musical approach is often structured music improvisation on easy-to-play instruments, which gives all children and young people the opportunity to make music regardless of their musical preferences or musical background. For example, in the DrumPower programme (Wölfl, 2016), rhythmic work with drums provides a foundation which is generally accessible to all children and teenagers. This is supplemented with improvised music on easy-to-play sound instruments, voice work, and musical role playing. Skills are developed in the improvisations as students come into contact with one another in ways that are playfully experienced and can be practised over a number of experiences. Affect regulation is mediated through dynamic improvisations, and stop-exercises support development of the ability for delimitation and self-control as the acceptance of limits is rehearsed. In thematic improvisations about conflict, bullying situations, and violence, young people propose consensual values and develop constructive behaviours.

Through the use of improvised music, the musical space is opened to all participants regardless of musical preferences and skills. The use of improvisation reveals implicit and explicit resources and potential of the young people, as well as uncertainties and deficits. For example, well-trained therapists can make professional assessments through musical attunement processes, knowing that disturbances in affective regulation are likely to relate to individual development. The use of structure is intentionally employed to scaffold individual's resources and to balance possible uncertainties and deficits with new experiences and skills. The theoretical background for these programmes is based on integrative conceptualizations that involve developmental psychological and/or psychodynamic comprehension models (Nöcker-Ribaupierre and Wölfl, 2010; Wölfl, 2014, 2016).

Benefits

The opportunity for group programmes to address the prevention of violence largely results from the fact that working with the entire class also naturally involves young people from high-risk groups who often escape social therapeutic efforts. By working with improvised music, uncertainties in coordination and regulatory processes can be quickly revealed and playfully engaged, while competencies can also be conveyed and celebrated. Focusing on the topics of bullying and violence can lead to conscious debate within the whole group allowing the therapist to promote values congruent with social cohesion and avoiding violence as a means of conflict resolution.

One technique of the German DrumPower programme is to use stop-exercises where the group drums more and more loudly until they are interrupted by a student with a clear stop sign. In one group, a boy explained how he never wanted to use violent behaviour, but that he simply punched anyone who made offensive remarks about his parents. Through group discussion and short role plays it became very clear that his adversaries never really noticed how deeply they hurt him with their statements and, to them, he appeared to blow up very abruptly, as though without warning. He was asked by the others to use the stop sign before that moment and to show his limits clearly. He took this technique back in to his school life and the aggressive interactions decreased markedly.

Individual programmes

Music therapy work with individuals mostly takes place when young people have become so resistant that they demonstrate aggressive behaviour that can no longer be tolerated in regular schools or in the family environment. These are often found in Western indus-trialized countries in the fields of youth welfare, clinical treatment, and juvenile justice. In addition, music therapists working with traumatized adolescents in crisis areas or in refugee institutions often utilize an individual format.

Individual preventive music therapy approaches prior to the eruption of aggressive be-haviour is usually not funded by national health systems (McFerran, 2017) and is usually addressed by educational social workers or welfare systems. In addition, offers to par-ticipate in preventive programmes are frequently refused by the young people and their families, since no subjective necessity is perceived. In collective societies, the handling of aggressive phenomena is regulated within the family and the social or religious commu-nity, without the inclusion of outsiders (Bauer, 2011).

Uses of music

Individual music therapy sessions focus on the development of a relationship through engaging in musical possibilities that foster establishment of a therapeutic relationship. A wide range of music therapy methods might be included, from listening to music, playing music, and singing songs to improvisation. The development of sustained mo-tivation, a secure space, and a sustainable therapeutic relationship (Lutz Hochreutener, 2009), which allows for the expression of critical comments and may promote a change in impulses within the context of a corrective therapeutic relationship, is crucial. In the therapeutic process, it is important to understand the subjective importance of aggres-sive behaviour, to recognize interactions, and then to suggest constructive coping pro-cesses with the young people. For example, aggressive behaviour as an expression of self-assertion may require the differentiation between powerful action and damaging destruction. Aggressive behaviour in conflict situations requires affective regulation and the ability to constructively resolve conflicts, respecting the position and opinion of others.

Music as a third element in therapy can be an additional motivation to remain com-mitted to such relationships and sustain contact. The wide spectrum of musical possibil-ities increases the likelihood that the musical wishes of the young people will be honoured. This should include listening, singing, and playing preferred music as well as songwriting, various forms of dancing, movement, and musical role plays in addition to the traditional approaches of music listening and music improvisation. When listening to and playing aggressive music, a shared reality in the musical experience can allow non-verbal under-standing of moods and feelings. Discussions about the musical experience can then in-spire mental comprehension processes (Smetana, 2017).

Besides the expression of aggressive feelings, the music may offer many possibilities to regulate destructive impulses and soothe and change aggressive moods. These might involve listening to soothing music, being distracted through shared music making, or participating in tuning-in exercises with improvised music. Improvisation can open up a free space to express feelings and can bring the young people into contact with emo-tions behind their aggression, like loneliness and frustration, or with their challenges in regulative interaction, which they may not have learned in their childhood. The young people can experience different emotional qualities while making music and learn to use them for calming and for activating control over aggressive impulses. With an increase in action and control competencies, ideas for alternative behaviours can be developed and practised in musical trials. In this way, basic beliefs can be changed and new prosocial values can be developed.

Benefits

The opportunity for individual music therapy work is based on the interests and concerns of the respective young people, so that their motivation is taken into account and they are individually acknowledged and understood. The treatment of the aggressive subject can lead to a deeper self-understanding and extend the mental apprehension of their ag-gressive behaviour and connect it with basic experiences in their development. In the therapeutic process, it can also lead to a new corrective relationship experience, which mediates affective-regulating experiences and value-oriented evaluation criteria. As a protective, motivating, and mediating factor, music can offer a creative and positively oc-cupied space for working with the respective topics in the foreground.

In her music therapy practice in the UK, Philippa Derrington (2012) offered young people opportunities to express their feelings in longer-term music therapy. This included listening and playing along to songs of their choice, improvising together or writing lyrics. One student, for example, learned to develop a language for his feelings by rapping improvised lyrics to a beat that was set up from his phone through speakers. His ag-gression was channelled into this activity which was also performed to a video camera and witnessed by the therapist. This process happened each week for 6 months, which began to generate feelings of acceptance in the student, and he appeared to feel more and more understood. Through this ongoing therapeutic relation-ship, the student recognized that his feelings were understandable and digestible but that did not mean that he had a right to act aggressively. The more he developed an expression of his emotions in music therapy, the less his aggressive outbursts in everyday life occurred and he became more capable of dealing with his feelings.

Conclusion

Within each of these programmes, music therapy has finely graded procedures which can be applied variably and precisely to the prevention of violence and destructiveness, depending on the particular problem and the context. This ranges from the perception and the handling of feelings when listening to music through to the creative shaping of coordination and cooperation processes in music making, and the discussion of aggressive content from lyrics to the practice of affective regulation and the working through of personal, traumatic experiences of violence. Music therapists use direct and indirect interventions in individual work, in groups, and in the community to strengthen individuals for constructively dealing with aggressive situations and practising delineation of malignant influences of aggressive groups.

For violence prevention, the special importance of the approaches presented lies in the power of the music to touch people emotionally and to motivate young people to take part in projects, to inspire themselves, to take responsibility, and to overcome motivational challenges in the process. In both group and individual settings music can release and sustain high motivation, especially when the musical interests of young people are utilized, so that everyone can find a way of participating in the preventive work. Music preferences can be used to communicate essential aspects of violence prevention such as affective regulation, value development, demarcation, difference formation (priming), and constructive competencies, in the build-up to violent behaviour, and are altered with the power of the intrinsic motivation of young people. The future challenge for music therapy will be to build bridges and combine the described programmes into dominant concepts in order to provide work with young people to prevent violence, which could be widely accepted in different places and contexts.

References

Baines, S. (2013). Music therapy as an anti-oppressive practice. *The Arts in Psychotherapy*, **40**, 1–5. doi:10.1016/j.aip.2012.09.003.

Bandura, A. (1978). Social learning theory of aggression. *Journal of Communication*, **28**(3), 12–29. doi:10.1111/j.1460-2466.1978.tb01621.x.

Bastian, H. G. (2000): *Musik (erziehung) und ihre Wirkung. Eine Langzeitstudie an Berliner Grundschulen*. [Music (Education) and Its Effect. A Long-Term Study at Primary Schools in Berlin]. Mainz: Schott Musik International.

Bauer, J. (2011): *Schmerzgrenze. Vom Ursprung alltäglicher und globaler Gewalt*. [Threshold of Pain. From the Origin of Everyday and Global Violence]. Munich: Karl Blessing.

Castellano, J. A. and Wilson, B. L. (1970). The generalization of institute therapy to classroom behaviour of an electively mute adolescent. *Journal of Music Therapy*, **7**, 139–143. doi:10.1093/jmt/7.4.139.

Cierpka, M. (Ed.) (2008). *Möglichkeiten der Gewaltprävention*. [Possibilities for Prevention of Violence]. (2nd edn). Göttingen: Vandenhoeck & Ruprecht. doi:10.13109/9783666462092.

Derrington, P. (2012). Music therapy for youth at risk: An exploration of clinical practice through research. Unpublished doctoral thesis. Anglia Ruskin University.

Elefant, C. (2010). Giving voice: Participatory action research with a marginalized group. In B. Stige, G. Ansdell, C. Elefant, and M. Pavlicevic (Eds), *Where Music Helps: Community Music Therapy in Action and Reflection* (pp. 132–142). Surrey: Ashgate.

Gugel, G. (2010): *Handbuch Gewaltprävention II. Für die Sekundarstufen und die Arbeit mit Jugendlichen. Grundlagen–Lernfelder–Handlungsmöglichkeiten*. [Handbook on Prevention of

Violence II. For Secondary Level and Working with Young People. Basics-Learning Fields – Possibilities of Action]. Tübingen: Institut für Friedenspädagogik.

Kivland, M. J. (1986). The use of music to increase self-esteem in a conduct disordered adolescent. *Journal of Music Therapy*, **23**, 25–29.

Krüger, V. and Stige, B. (2015). Between rights and realities–music as a structuring resource in child welfare everyday life: a qualitative study. *Nordic Journal of Music Therapy*, **24**, 99–122. doi:10.1080/08098131.2014.890242.

Liell, Chr. (2001). *Die Rezeption von Musik und deren "Wirkung" auf das Gewalthandeln Jugendlicher* [Reception of Music and Its Impact on Violent Behaviour of Adolescents]. Available at: www.db-thueringen.de/servlets/MCRFileNodeServlet/dbt_derivate_00001317/liell.html (accessed 24 March 2018).

Lutz Hochreutener, S. (2009): *Spiel—Musik—Therapie*. [Game—Music—Therapy]. Göttingen: Hogrefe.

McFerran, K. S. (2014). Music therapy in the schools. In B. Wheeler (Ed.), *Music Therapy Handbook* (pp. 328–338). New York: Guildford Press.

McFerran, K.S. (2017). Let's rework our approach with 'angry young people'. *Social Work with Groups*. doi:10.1080/01609513.2016.1219837.

McFerran, S. K. and Wölfl, A. (2015). Music, violence and music therapy with young people in schools: A position paper. *Voices: World Forum for Music Therapy*, **15**(2).

Neumann, F. (2008). *Musik als Schutzimpfung. Thesen des Kriminologen C. Pfeiffer über den Zusammenhang zwischen Medienkonsum, Schulleistungen und Musikausübung bei Kindern und Jugendlichen*. [Music as a Vaccination. Theses of the Criminologist C. Pfeiffer on the Connection between Media Consumption, School Performance and Music Education in Children and Adolescents]. Available at: www.hs-burgkirchen.de/Musik_als_Schutzimpfung.pdf (accessed 24 March 2018).

Nöcker-Ribaupierre, M. and Wölfl, A. (2010). Music to counter violence: A preventative approach for working with adolescents in schools. *Nordic Journal of Music Therapy*, **19**, 151–161. doi:10.1080/08098131.2010.489997.

Rickson, D. and McFerran, K. S. (2014). *Creating Music Cultures in the Schools: A Perspective from Community Music Therapy*. Gilsum, NH: Barcelona Publishers.

Scrine, E. (2016). Enhancing social connectedness or stabilising oppression: Is participation in music free from gendered subjectivity? A position paper. *Voices: World Forum for Music Therapy*, **16**(2).

Smetana, M. (2017) Recurring similarity: The meaning of musical objects in music therapy for adolescents with structural disorders. *Nordic Journal of Music Therapy*, **26**(2), 105–123. doi:10.1080/08098131.2015.1117123.

Stige, B., Ansdell, G., Elefant, C., and Pavlicevic, M. (2010). *Where music helps: Community music therapy in action and reflection*. Surrey, UK: Ashgate.

Stige, B. and Aarø, L. E. (2012). *Invitation to Community Music Therapy*. New York: Ashgate.

Strange, J. (2012). Psychodynamically informed music therapy groups with teenagers with severe special needs in a college setting: Working jointly with teaching assistants. In J. Tomlinson, P. Derrington, & A. Oldfield (Eds), *Music Therapy in Schools: Working with Children of All Ages in Mainstream and Special Education* (pp. 179–193). London: Jessica Kingsley.

Viega, M. (2013). "Loving me and my butterfly wings:" a study of hip-hop songs written by adolescents in music therapy. Unpublished doctoral dissertation. Temple University. Available at: http://pqdtopen.proquest.com/pubnum/3552365.html (accessed 24 March 2018).

Wahl, K. (2009). *Aggression und Gewalt*. [Aggression and Violence]. Heidelberg: Spektrum.

World Health Organization (2002). World report on violence and health: Summary. Available at: www.who.int/violence_injury_prevention/violence/world_report/en/summary_en.pdf (accessed 24 March 2018).

Wölfl, A. (2014). *Gewaltprävention mit Musik: Empirische Wirkungsanalyse eines musiktherapeutischen Projektmodells.* [Violence Prevention through Music: Empirical Impact Analysis of a Music Therapy Project Model]. Wiesbaden: Reichert-Verlag.

Wölfl, A. (2016). DrumPower—music for a better community in the classroom. Group music therapy program for violence prevention, social integration and empowerment in schools. Suggestions from community music therapy approaches. *International Journal of Community Music*, **9**(1), 65–75.

Wölfl, A. (2017). Musik und Gewalt: musiktherapeutische Gewaltprävention [Music and violence: Music therapy as prevention of violence]. In T. Timmermann and H.-U. Schmidt (Eds), *Förderung von Kindern und Jugendlichen durch musiktherapeutische Vorgehensweisen—Ausgewählte Schriften zur Musiktherapie der Universität Augsburg* [Fostering Children and Young People through Music Therapy Approaches—Chosen Texts for Music Therapy of the University of Augsburg]. Wiesbaden: Reichert-Verlag.

Part 2

Identity

Chapter 8

Music as a resource for agency and empowerment in identity construction

Suvi Saarikallio

Introduction: music as a resource for identity construction

Identity formation is the critical, defining process of youth. Many of the core elements of self-definition are in a state of negotiation: sexuality, significant relationships, career paths, core values, and world views. It is a time of many choices and yet young people are still searching for the wisdom and authority to make major (or even minor) life decisions. Fortunately, adolescents are equipped to face the challenging changes of their identity formation and music is one of the most readily available tools used by this age group. It has been identified as a multifaceted psychosocial resource for performing identity, gaining a sense of agency, negotiating relationships, and supporting the related emotional processing (Laiho, 2004; Ruud, 1997). The chapters in this section discuss music as a resource for adolescents' identity construction: as a reflection of their personality (Chapter 9), a bridge from youth to adulthood (Chapter 11), and a medium for exploring their gender and sexuality (Chapter 14), and as a resource for their social identity construction (Chapter 10), participation (Chapter 12), and even—and perhaps particularly—when experiencing disability (Chapter 13).

Authors in this section mostly approach music with a resource-oriented perspective: in contrast to viewing music as something that would passively impact a listener. Music engagement is considered as an act of creating, re-constructing, and cultivating the self and the social world, emphasizing the agency of the person engaging in music (DeNora, 1999; Krueger, 2011). Christopher Small (1998) was one of the pioneers of this line of thinking, transforming music into a verb—musicking—thus placing the ownership of action into the person who engages with music. Several other authors have argued for the relevance of understanding music as a technology of self-reconstruction (DeNora, 1999), as affective scaffolding (Krueger, 2011), as a resource for health and identity (Ruud, 1997), and as an affordance, the health impacts of which depend on the young people themselves (McFerran and Saarikallio, 2014). This introductory chapter for the Identity section elaborates on how music functions as a source of personal agency, and why the affordances of music play such an important role during the formation of youth identity.

Identity construction and agency in youth

Identity construction is a challenge for one's sense of agency

Adolescent identity development occurs in a context of several other fundamental changes in the body, in capacities for cognitive and emotional processing, in behaviour regulation skills, in significant relationships, and in societal demands. Ronald Dahl (2004) discusses adolescence as a period that starts from the biological changes of puberty and ends with the social domain of life: the attainment of adult roles and responsibilities. He argues that youth vulnerability is partly due to this transition occurring at a time when the biological changes of puberty heighten the motivational drive systems, creating needs for sensation seeking, ecstasy, and increased sexual arousal. At the same time societal expectations increase, concerning responsible decision-making of demanding life choices, for example starting a career, owning a home, or choosing to become a parent. Adolescents are balancing the often conflicting demands of their bodies, their personal aspirations for the future, the opinions of their friends and family, and the views of the wider society.

Both internal and external factors pose challenges for identity construction. In terms of cognitive-emotional development youth is a time when self-regulatory skills are still only developing (Seiffge-Krenke, 1995), illustrated by the frontal lobes only maturing towards late adolescence (Steinberg, 2005). This sometimes becomes visible in strong emotions 'hijacking' the young person's decision-making (Dahl, 2004). In terms of external demands, while being expected to develop independence and take responsibility of their life, young people are not often given the opportunities to think independently, make personal choices, and take ownership of their actions.

Constructing identity is a complicated task of synchronizing the internal and external demands and resources, and taking ownership of the various emerging aspects in oneself from body image to adult roles. All this is particularly challenging for adolescents' sense of agency, self-control, and self-esteem. If we consider a regular day of an adolescent life, it is not that easy to feel a thorough agency over one's thoughts, feelings, and actions when your body shouts one thing, when your teachers and parents tell you to think, feel, and behave in a certain way, when your friends demand and tempt you into something different, and when you should know who you are and who you want to be in the future.

Agency as a critical competence and resource for the young

Sense of agency is a concept that refers to the subjective experience of being the actor in one's life, of having ownership of one's actions, feeling, and thoughts (Jeannerod, 2003). It is closely linked to the concept of internal locus of control (Rotter, 1966), which refers to a belief that one's own abilities, efforts, or actions—not external factors—determine what happens. It is also closely related to self-efficacy (Bandura, 1977), which refers to a person's belief that he or she can accomplish a particular activity. It can indeed be considered as the critical resource for the development of independence and identity accomplishment.

Agency can be defined in many ways and be considered either as an individual characteristic, or in terms of acts and behaviours that a young person can take. James Côté

(1997), for instance, discussed agency in terms of *personal qualities* that constitute an agentic personality, developing a Multimeasure Agentic Personality Scale (MAPS) that contains features of self-esteem, purpose in life, internal locus of control, ego strength, self-actualization, and ideological commitment.

On the other hand, agency has been linked to the development of behavioural regulation (Ford and Thompson, 1985), and the concept has been understood as *acts* of intentional self-regulation. For instance, Richard Lerner and his colleagues (Lerner et al., 2001) discussed adolescents' self-regulation in terms of three agentic behaviours: selection (choosing opportunities that match with one's sense of self and personal potential), optimization (refining one's resources to reach goals), and compensation (being able to 'change course' if resources fail). These regulatory competencies of selection, optimization, and compensation were further shown to predict self-esteem, competence, and purpose across grades 7–10 (Gestsdottir et al., 2009).

Furthermore, while sense of agency intrinsically refers to the personal ownership and self-directedness of action, it must be acknowledged that young people are certainly not always able to make any choice they like or realize all the goals they are setting for themselves, and this is also due to external influences. Indeed, agency is always exercised within contextual constraints (Côté and Levine, 2002), and it can also be considered as a dialogue of personal capacities and the social structures and cultural factors that both provide support but also place limits on agency. Just as more ecological explanations of resilience are emerging that consider the ways young people navigate and negotiate multiple contexts and realities as they endeavour to cope (Ungar, 2005), contexts significantly shape and influence agency.

The relevance of agency for identity construction

Researchers who study youth and emerging adulthood have made an important sociological observation: the breadth of materials and alternative options available for identity construction concerning careers, relationships, and world views is expanding in Western societies, while the collective support for the identity formation is decreasing (Côté and Levine, 2002). This creates a situation that highlights identity construction as a process during which young individuals have to find their *own* path to adulthood, essentially placing agency, self-determination, and self-directedness in a heightened position (Schwartz et al., 2005; Arnett, 2007). Seth Schwartz and his colleagues argue that the unstructured transition to adulthood, prevalent particularly in current Western societies, may be extremely fruitful for those who are able to capitalize on the breadth of opportunities, but can be extremely difficult and distressing for those who are unable to exercise personal agency at this stage (Schwartz et al., 2013).

It is easy to consider sense of agency as an integral resource for identity construction, which, in essence, is a process of self-definition. The relevance of self-determination is embedded already in the writings of Erik Erikson (1994) and James Marcia (1966) who discuss identity formation as self-directed exploration of, and commitment to, adult identity. More recently however, there has been research that systematically demonstrates the relatedness of sense of agency and identity status. For instance, a composite measure of agency, consisting of self-esteem, purpose in life, ego strength, and internal locus of control, was found to be positively related to identity achievement and negatively related to identity diffusion (Côté and Schwartz, 2002). Similarly, identity status has been shown to correlate with the locus of control: identity achievement correlates positively with an internal locus of control, while moratorium, foreclosure, and diffusion statuses are associated with an external locus of control (Lillevoll et al., 2013).

Declines of agency as a risk factor

The correlates of agency such as internal locus of control and self-efficacy are highly relevant for wellbeing (Roddenberry and Renk, 2010) and link to experiences of self-esteem (Judge et al., 2002). Considering the amount of change and maturation required in one's conception of self during the adolescent years, it is no wonder that youth is a period of heightened insecurity about self-perception and self-esteem. Early studies of adolescent self-esteem suggest it is particularly low during early adolescence (Harter, 1990; Hirsch and DuBois, 1991) and then increases again during middle and late adolescence and early adulthood (Savin-Williams and Demo, 1983; Harter, 1990). While temporary fluctuations and low levels of self-esteem are part of the normal development in youth, they also become a risk factor for outcomes ranging from delinquency to dropping out of school, and depression. Low levels of perceived control, self-efficacy, and competence have been shown to correlate with depressive symptoms in youth (Gomez, 1998; Herman-Stahl and Petersen, 1999; Muris et al., 2001; Seiffge-Krenke, 2000). It appears that individuals differ greatly in the personal and social resources they have available to face the challenges of identity development, and those in vulnerable situations may deserve additional support (Savin-Williams and Demo, 1983; Sadovnikova, 2016).

Music as a resource to achieve agency

Music as an affordance for adolescents' personal agency

Why does music have such a captivating and intense presence in youth? One answer to this puzzling question relates to the sense of agency. Western adolescents are faced with the paradox of a growing need for independence combined with being granted limited skills and external opportunities for taking ownership of their behaviour. Music offers a much more encouraging context. Music is the playground and the kingdom of young people, in which they can shout and be silly, be fragile and search to understand themselves, and identify their own, personal, choices.

The chapters in this section on identity address the potential of music to serve as a source of personal agency in many ways. In Chapter 9 Dave Miranda discusses music, particularly music listening, as a reflection of adolescents' personality. Music preferences and the ways of using music and engaging with music serve to mirror our personalities, our inner selves, allowing us to act and perform our identity. Alexandra Lamont and David Hargreaves in Chapter 10 take this discussion into the field of performing social identities through music listening preferences, and discuss the formation of music preferences as a reflection of identity formation. They describe a process that moves from musical open-earedness towards preference commitment, just as identity moves from moratorium and role confusion towards commitment to adult identities. Lamont and Hargreaves discuss this in relation to the idea of everyone being musical—the musicianship of listening—which refers to everyone being able to use their daily music listening as an act of showing their knowledge and personal competence; in essence, using music listening as an act of personal agency. Tia DeNora then expands on the capacity of music in Chapter 11 to reflect our inner selves and inner identities from an age-linked meta-level perspective on personal experience. She argues that music can capture our age-specific identities and serve as a form of age-band travel to our prior experiential worlds, helping us to return to performing the identity of our 'inner teen', which may sometimes serve as an asylum and shelter from the daily stress, facilitating coping and adaptation.

These three chapters provide a convincing picture of music as an easily accessible daily resource for young people to perform and re-organize their inner selves, to serve as a natural affordance for agency in terms of defining and performing their personal thoughts and feelings about who they are, and who they wish to be. Indeed, music is effortlessly available for everyone, serving as an accessible forum for the young people to act as agents of their experience and behaviour. Prior research has noted that music listening choices function to personalize daily activities (Sloboda and O'Neill, 2001) and one of the main reasons people find music pleasurable in their daily life may be because it provides feelings of self-determination (Saarikallio et al., in press). Music listening allows young people to have control over the sound environment, to take their own space, to feel secure in uncertain situations, and to train their impulse control and emotional self-regulation (Laiho, 2004). In music listening, the young can experience freedom about choosing the mental content of what to think, how to feel, and what to pay attention to, which may be a much-needed break from the related conflicting pressures from their parents, school, and peer group. And if we go beyond listening to musical hobbies, it can offer adolescents opportunities for mastery and, importantly, allow the young people themselves to participate in defining their personal goals and the criteria for their successful goal accomplishment (Laiho, 2004). Recent research in music education has begun to emphasize the relevance of involving the young themselves as agentic actors of their own learning (Karlsen, 2011).

Overall, it can be concluded that adult control of music is typically loose enough for the adolescents to feel agency and to explore independence whether in self-regulation of thoughts, feelings, or goal-oriented behaviour. Dahl (2004) also points out that while the heightened activation of the motivation networks in youth may create emotional turbulence, it also fuels passion in a healthy way, fostering creativity, aspiration, and accomplishment.

When agency fails—can music help?

However, young people are not always capable of being such agentic actors in their own music engagement. Katrina McFerran and I (McFerran and Saarikallio, 2014) observed that adolescents who were receiving support for depression, anxiety, or emotional and behavioural problems appeared relatively unable, in comparison to their healthy peers, to identify, take responsibility for, and change their maladaptive patterns of music use towards more helpful patterns. The descriptions of the vulnerable adolescents painted an alternative narrative about agency in music use. The adolescents did not always act as agents of their own music-related feelings and behaviours, but instead found relying on music to be the agent: they were sometimes trying to feel better but ending up feeling worse, or continuing to listening to the same songs even when such songs were fuelling their negative thoughts and feelings. These findings are similar to theories about music being used for rumination (Garrido and Schubert, 2013; Garrido et al., 2017), which refer to listening to sad music without the ability to find resolution or contemplative clarity and instead sinking deeper into hopeless and helpless negative thought patterns often associated with rumination.

The experience of agency failing is a clear signal of problems in youth development. It is close to the concept of learned helplessness, which is integrally linked with depression (Seligman, 1975). The inability to exercise agency over one's music use is to some extent captured by the Unhealthy subscale of the Healthy-Unhealthy Uses of Music Scale (HUMS) (Saarikallio et al., 2014), which contains elements of rumination, avoidance, and inability to achieve mood improvement through music, and correlates relatively strongly with youth depression. In such situations, the young people themselves may no longer have the resources to use any tools, not even listening to their favourite music, in constructive ways. Such situations call for supportive interventions, such as music therapy, as a medium to restore agency.

The last three chapters of this section address music therapy as an example of a context for working with young people in situations that propose extra challenges to identity development. These situations also pose extra challenges for the adolescents' sense of agency, and very often music therapy aims at restoring the lost sense of agency. In Chapter 12 Viggo Krüger addresses the overall problem of child welfare contexts not necessarily supporting children and adolescents to participate, and presents music therapy as a type of activity that can restore such affordances and make it available for the young people. Krüger argues that when music therapy is used to let the young people speak through music and music performances it serves not only as a structuring resource of their personal identity formation, but also of their involvement with their daily social environment and even their surrounding society, its values, rights, and attitudes. Daphne Rickson, in Chapter 13, addresses case examples of working with adolescents who have conditions that may result in marginalization and jeopardize their sense of agency, such as adolescents who have attention-deficit/hyperactivity disorder (ADHD) and intellectual disability. Rickson describes music as an enjoyable, motivating resource that can highlight the adolescents' capabilities, and foster both their autonomy and connectedness. Finally, in Chapter 14, Elly Scrine discusses music therapy as a forum for exploring gender and sexuality, particularly with adolescents not conforming to the sexual 'norm', but also highlighting the importance of addressing sexual identity development with a dialogical, anti-oppressive attitude through music.

As a whole, the last three chapters of the identity section all emphasize working with adolescents in a therapy context with an overarching aim of youth empowerment. The potential of music in fostering the sense of agency seems to be ever more valuable in situations when agency, self-directedness, internal locus of control, and self-esteem have, for whatever reason, become fragile or compromised. Persons with a long-term illness, for instance, seem to appreciate music listening particularly because it provides them an experience of personal empowerment, a means to survive the disempowering difficulties of daily life (Batt-Rawden et al., 2005). One pioneer emphasizing the relevance of agency in music as a resource for health, whether in the clinical therapy context or in the daily-life context, was Even Ruud (1997). He criticized the medicalization of health promotion in our society particularly because it easily increases the feeling of being disempowered. Ruud connected the sense of agency to health resources as defined by Aaron Antonovsky: feeling that life is comprehensible (predictable), manageable (conceivable), and meaningful. He argued that agency is about responsibility for one's life and actions, including self-management, competency, achievement, feeling of mastery, and self-esteem, and suggested that music serves as a daily resource for a sense of agency by providing experiences of controlling the environment, 'being somebody', and perceiving life as being manageable and meaningful.

Conclusion

Healthy individuals show effortless agency in their daily use of music. For instance, they seem to efficiently use music for affective self-regulation in adaptive ways, even with relatively little conscious awareness of the goals of their behaviour (van Goethem and Sloboda, 2010; Saarikallio, 2011). Music can thus be considered as an effortless and powerful resource for the daily sense of agency. However, as noted in this chapter, this affordance may not be so available in all situations and for all adolescents. Recent programmes in preventive care have particularly aimed to increase young people's personal awareness of their music engagement and its impact on them; in essence, their agency in music use (Gold et al., 2017; Dingle et al., 2006). Preliminary results of these studies indicate that increased awareness of the impact of music seems to foster vulnerable adolescents' ability to engage in more helpful music use strategies (McFerran Hense et al., 2018). It may well be that in situations where agency is lacking there is an increased need for reflective awareness about music use. Small steps in 'musical agency' (e.g. understanding how music impacts me, how I would want it to impact me, and how I can achieve that) may lead to further steps in agency in general.

If we turn back to Richard Lerner and colleagues' (2001) discussion about agency as selection, optimization, and compensation, we can argue that music fluently serves as a resource for each of these aspects. Music is a rich material for choosing opportunities that match our sense of self and personal potential (selection). Through musical learning and musicianship of listening we can with small steps, yet almost endlessly, refine our resources to reach goals (optimization) and, by increasing awareness of how we allow music to impact us, we can also become better in 'changing course' if resources fail (compensation). If we recall Côté and Levine's (2002) critique about acknowledging the role of contextual factors and social structures as barriers or facilitators of agency, we can certainly see how that relates to us as researchers or practitioners working and making dialogues with young people. All this relates to the broader discussion of increased awareness in our society about the importance of fostering individuals' own capacity and responsibility for their health promotion. And yes, youth is certainly a fundamental period for this, a period in which music can be one of the best tools for making identity formation an act of agency and empowerment.

References

Arnett, J. J. (2007). Emerging adulthood: What is it good for? *Child Development Perspectives*, 1(2), 68–73.

Bandura, A. (1997). *Self-efficacy: The Exercise of Control*. New York: W. H. Freeman.

Batt-Rawden, K. B., DeNora, T., and Ruud, E. (2005). Music listening and empowerment in health promotion: A study of the role and significance of music in everyday life of the long-term ill. *Nordic Journal of Music Therapy*, 14(2), 120–136.

Côté, J. E. (1997). An empirical test of the identity capital model. *Journal of Adolescence*, 20, 421–437.

Côté, J. E. and Levine, C. G. (2002). *Identity Formation, Agency, and Culture: A Social Psychological Synthesis*. Mahwah, NJ: Lawrence Erlbaum Associates.

Côté, J. E. and Schwartz, S. J. (2002). Comparing psychological and sociological approaches to identity: Identity status, identity capital, and the individualization process. *Journal of Adolescence*, 25, 571–586.

Dahl, R. E. (2004). Adolescent brain development: A period of vulnerabilities and opportunities. Keynote address. *Annals of the New York Academy of Sciences*, 1021(1), 1–22.

DeNora, T. (1999). Music as a technology of the self. *Poetics*, 27(1), 31–56. doi:10.1016/S0304-422X(99)00017-0.

Dingle, G. A., Hodges, J., and Kunde, A. (2016). *Tuned In* emotion regulation program using music listening: Effectiveness for adolescents in educational settings. *Frontiers in Psychology*, ??, ???–???. Published online 2016 Jun 7.

Erikson, E. H. (1994). *Identity: Youth and Crisis* (no. 7). New York: WW Norton & Company.

Ford, M. E. and Thompson, R. A. (1985). Perceptions of personal agency and infant attachment: Toward a life-span perspective on competence development. *International Journal of Behavioral Development*, 8(4), 377–406.

Garrido, S. and Schubert, E. (2013). Adaptive and maladaptive attraction to negative emotions in music. *Musicae Scientiae*, 17(2), 147–166.

Garrido, S., Eerola, T., and McFerran, K. (2017). Group rumination: Social interactions around music in people with depression. *Frontiers in Psychology*, 8, 490. doi:10.3389/fpsyg.2017.00490.

Gestsdottir, S., Lewin-Bizan, S., von Eye, A., Lerner, J. V., and Lerner, R. M. (2009). The structure and function of selection, optimization, and compensation in middle adolescence: Theoretical and applied implications. *Journal of Applied Developmental Psychology*, 30, 585–600.

Gold, C., Crooke, A. H. D., Saarikallio, S., and McFerran, K. (2017). Group music therapy as a preventive intervention for young people at risk: Cluster-randomized trial. *Journal of Music Therapy*, ??, ???–???.

Harter, S. (1990). Identity and self development. In S. Feldman and G. Elliott (Eds), *At the Threshold: The Developing Adolescent* (pp. 352–387). Cambridge, MA: Harvard University Press.

Hirsch, B. and DuBois, D. (1991). Self-esteem in early adolescence: The identification and prediction of contrasting longitudinal trajectories. *Journal of Youth and Adolescence*, **20**, 53–72.

Jeannerod, M. (2003). The mechanism of self-recognition in human. *Behavioral Brain Research*, **142**, 1–15.

Judge, T. A., Bono, E. A., and Thoresen, C. J. (2002). Are measures of self-esteem, neuroticism, locus of control, and generalized self-efficacy indicators of a common core construct? *Journal of Personality and Social Psychology*, **83**(3), 693–710.

Karlsen, S. (2011). Using musical agency as a lens: Researching music education from the angle of experience. *Research Studies in Music Education*, **33**, 2.

Krueger, J. W. (2011). Doing things with music. *Phenomenology and the Cognitive Sciences*, **10**, 1–22. doi:10.1007/s11097-010-9152-4.

Laiho, S. (2004). The psychological functions of music in adolescence. *Nordic Journal of Music Therapy*, **13**(1), 49–65.

Lerner, R. M., Freund, A. M., De Stefanis, I., and Habermas, T. (2001). Understanding developmental regulation in adolescence: The use of the Selection, Optimization, and Compensation model. *Human Development*, **44**, 29–50.

Lillevoll, K. R., Kroger, J., and Martinussen, M. (2013). Identity status and locus of control: A meta-analysis. *Identity: An International Journal of Theory and Research*, **13**, 253–265.

Marcia, J. E. (1966). Development and validation of ego-identity status. *Journal of Personality and Social Psychology*, **3**(5), 551.

McFerran, K. and Saarikallio, S. (2014). Depending on music to feel better: Being conscious of responsibility when appropriating the power of music, *The Arts in Psychotherapy*, **41**(1), 89–97.

McFerran, K. S., Hense, C., Koike, A., and Rickwood, D. (2018). Intentional music use to reduce psychological distress in adolescents accessing primary mental health care *Clinical Child Psychology and Psychiatry*, **??**, ???–???.

Roddenberry, A. and Renk, K. (2010). Locus of control and self-efficacy: Potential mediators of stress, illness, and utilization of health services in college students. *Child Psychiatry and Human Development*, **41**(4), 353–370.

Rotter, J. B. (1966). Generalized expectancies of internal versus external control of reinforcements. *Psychological Monographs*, **80**(1), 1–28.

Ruud, E. (1997). Music and the quality of life. *Nordic Journal of Music Therapy*, **6**(2), 86–97.

Saarikallio, S. (2011). Music as emotional self-regulation throughout adulthood. *Psychology of Music*, **39**, 307–332.

Saarikallio, S., McFerran, K., and Gold, C. (2015). Development and validation of the Healthy-Unhealthy Music Scale (HUMS). *Child and Adolescent Mental Health*, **??**, 210–217.

Saarikallio, S., Maksimainen, J., and Randall, W. (in press). Relaxed and connected: Insights on the emotional-motivational constituents of musical pleasure. *Psychology of Music*. Accepted for publication on 26.3.2018.

Sadovnikova, T. (2016). Self-esteem and interpersonal relations in adolescence. *Procedia—Social and Behavioural Sciences*, **233**, 440–444.

Savin-Williams, R. and Demo, D. (1983). Situational and transitational determinants of adolescent self-feelings. *Journal of Personality and Social Psychology*, **44**, 824–833.

Schwartz, S. J., Donnellan, M. B., Ravert, R. D., Luyck, K., and Zamboanga, B. L. (2013). Identity development, personality, and well-being in adolescence and emerging adulthood. Theory, research, and recent advances. In Editors? *Handbook of Psychology* (2nd edn, pp. ???–???). Place?: Wiley.

Schwartz, B. (2000). Self-determination: The tyranny of freedom. *American Psychologist*, **55**, 79–88.

Schwartz, S. J., Côté, J. E., and Arnett, J. (2005). Identity and agency in emerging adulthood: Two developmental routes in the individualization process. *Youth & Society*, **37**, 201–229.

Seiffge-Krenke, I (1995). *Stress, Coping, and Relationships in Adolescence*. Mahwah, NJ: Lawrence Erlbaum Associates.

Seiffge-Krenke, I. (2000). Causal links between stressful events, coping style, and adolescent symptomatology. *Journal of Adolescence*, **23**, 675–691.

Seligman, M. E. P. (1975). *Helplessness: On Depression, Development, and Death*. San Francisco, CA: W. H. Freeman.

Sloboda, J. A. and O'Neill, S. A. (2001). Emotions in everyday listening to music. In P. N. Juslin and J. A. Sloboda (Eds), *Music and Emotion: Theory and Research* (pp. 415–429). New York: Oxford University Press.

Small, C. (1998). *Musicking: The Meanings of Performing and Listening*. Middletown, CT: Wesleyan University Press.

Steinberg, L. (2005). Cognitive and affective development in adolescence. *Trends in Cognitive Sciences*, **9**(2), 69–74.

Ungar, M. (2005). Pathways to resilience among children in child welfare, corrections, mental health and education settings: Navigation and negotiation. *Child and Youth Care Forum*, **34**(6), 423–444.

van Goethem A. and Sloboda, J. (2011) The functions of music for affect regulation. *Musicae Scientiae*, **15**, 208–228.

Chapter 9

Personality traits and music in adolescence

Dave Miranda

Introduction

Personality was a neglected topic in music psychology for quite some time (Kemp, 1999). However, since the early 2000s, personality research has seen an outburst of contributions to music psychology (e.g. Rentfrow and Gosling, 2003). These contributions were facilitated by comprehensive models that clarify how traits are organized within our human nature (e.g. 'Big 5'). The Five Factor Model (or Big 5) signifies that individual differences in personality are a matter of degrees on five trait dispositions within each person: extraversion (e.g. being sociable, being active, feeling positive emotions); agreeableness (e.g. being sympathetic, kind, cooperative); conscientiousness (e.g. being organized, responsible, efficient); neuroticism (e.g. feeling tense, anxious, depressed); and openness (e.g. being sophisticated, artistic, intellectual; John et al., 2008). Notably, personality traits are understood as *relatively stable* patterns of emotions, cognitions, and behaviours that combine stability with just enough change to be reasonably flexible across situations in everyday life (Fleeson, 2001) and across developmental periods throughout the life span (Roberts et al., 2006).

Personality traits and music listening

In music psychology in adolescence, research on personality traits and music listening behaviours can be described according to at least four lines of research: (1) personality traits as correlates of music listening behaviours; (2) personality traits as antecedents of music listening behaviours; (3) music listening behaviours as markers of personality traits; and (4) personality traits as outcomes of music listening behaviours.

Personality traits as correlates of music listening behaviours

Are personality traits associated with the degree of liking for different music styles in adolescence? The cartography of interrelations among personality traits and music preferences in adolescence has been increasingly studied in recent years. For example, Peter Rentfrow and Samuel Gosling (2003) conducted a series of studies on large samples of undergraduate students[1]. More precisely, they examined the interrelations between the Big 5 and four music factors: reflective/complex music (e.g. classical), intense/rebellious music (e.g. heavy metal), upbeat/conventional music (e.g. pop), and energetic/rhythmic music (e.g. rap/hip hop). Extraversion was associated with intense/rebellious music, with upbeat/conventional music, and with energetic/rhythmic music. Agreeableness was linked to upbeat/conventional music and to energetic/rhythmic music. Conscientiousness was associated with upbeat/conventional music. Emotional stability (neuroticism reserved) was associated with reflective/complex music. Openness was associated with reflective/complex music, with intense/rebellious music, and (but negatively) with upbeat/conventional music. Overall, it must be said that the effect size of most correlations was rather small. Nevertheless, the correlations between openness and reflective/complex music showed the largest (i.e. a medium) effect size.

More recently, Arielle Bonneville-Roussy et al. (2013) examined relationships between the Big 5 and cross-sectional age trends (adolescence, young adulthood, and middle adulthood) in five music factors (mellow, unpretentious, sophisticated, intense, and contemporary) among several thousand Internet users. Mellow music (which is related to, for instance, soft rock and R&B/soul) was associated with openness. Unpretentious music (which is associated with, for instance, country music) was linked to extraversion, agreeableness, and conscientiousness. Sophisticated music (which was linked to, for example, classical music) was associated with openness. Intense music (which was associated with, for instance, classic rock and punk) was related to conscientiousness and also openness. Contemporary music (which was linked to, for instance, rap music) was associated with extraversion. Overall, openness (as related to mellow music) and extraversion (as related to contemporary music) seem to have the largest effect sizes. Moreover, openness had more significant relationships with music preferences than did the other four traits.

Are personality traits associated with the reasons for which adolescents engage in music listening? Our knowledge of relationships between personality traits and music motives in adolescence has been scarcer but has been improved in recent years. In a series of studies Tomas Chamorro-Premuzic and collaborators examined the interrelations between the Big 5 and three basic motives for listening to music in late adolescence: emotional use, cognitive use, and background use. First, Tomas Chamorro-Premuzic and Adrian Furnham (2007) conducted a study among students who were on average late adolescents (mean age = 19.9 years) at the time they attended American and British universities. They found that extraversion and conscientiousness were both associated with less emotional use of music. Neuroticism was associated with more emotional use of music. Openness was associated with more cognitive use of music. Overall, openness had the largest (i.e. medium) effect size, but it was closely followed by neuroticism's rather similar

---

[1] Unfortunately, their study did not report the age of participants for those samples with which they examined personality traits and music. Nonetheless, those undergraduate students were enrolled in an introductory course in psychology and thus most of them were probably late adolescents (i.e. 18–21-year-olds).

(also medium) effect size. Subsequently, Tomas Chamorro-Premuzic et al. (2009a) sought to replicate and extend their findings with Spanish (Catalonian) university students who were also on average late adolescents (mean age = 20.1 years). Extraversion was associated with more emotional use and more background use of music. Neuroticism was associated with more emotional use of music. Openness was associated with more cognitive use of music, which was still the largest (i.e. medium) effect size. Tomas Chamorro-Premuzic et al. (2009b) aimed to further replicate their findings among Malaysian undergraduate and graduate students who were on average in the closing stages of late adolescence and starting emerging adulthood (mean age = 21.5 years). Extraversion was associated with more emotional use and more background use of music. Neuroticism was associated with more emotional use of music. Openness was associated with more cognitive use of music. However, in this last study, it was neuroticism that had the largest (i.e. medium) effect size. Hence, in terms of music motives, this corpus of research seems to suggest that not only openness—but also neuroticism—can have the largest effect size.

Other studies have examined more specific personality traits in relation with various music listening behaviours in adolescence. In particular, sensation seeking has caught the attention of researchers studying personality and music in adolescence. For example, in the United States, Jeffrey Arnett (1992) found a relationship between sensation seeking and liking for more defiant and rebellious music (hard rock and heavy metal music) among middle adolescents. Lately, the relationship between trait empathy and music behaviours in adolescence has also received attention. In Japan, for instance, Ai Kawakami and Kenji Katahira (2015) studied four facets of empathy (empathic concern, personal distress, perspective taking, and fantasy), emotional reactions, and liking for sad music among children who were on average early adolescents (11.9 years). Their findings indicated that some—but not all—facets of empathy played a role. More specifically, fantasy was associated with a liking for sad music, while perspective taking was associated with three emotional reactions from listening to sad music (sweet emotion, tragic emotion, and heightened emotion). In sum, this kind of research highlights that more specific traits (i.e. empathy can be a trait subsumed by agreeableness) can reveal more nuanced links with music listening behaviours (i.e. only some facets of empathy were significant correlates).

Personality traits as antecedents of music listening behaviours

Can personality traits predict the music listening behaviours that adolescents will adopt later in their life? Personality traits have also been studied as antecedents (i.e. predictors) of music preferences. Longitudinal studies have the most appropriate design for testing traits as antecedents of music listening behaviours. Unfortunately, as often the case in psychology, there are very few of such longitudinal studies, but they nonetheless report two basic observations.

First, it seems that personality traits can predict music preferences in adolescence, at least in the short term. Dave Miranda and Michel Claes (2008) conducted a 6 month longitudinal study among participants who were on average middle adolescents living in Canada (the province of Québec). The longitudinal design enabled examination of whether the Big 5 could predict five factors of music preferences: metal (e.g. heavy metal); soul (e.g. hip hop); electronic (e.g. techno); pop (e.g. pop); and classical (e.g. classical). Findings indicated that extraversion predicted more liking for soul music. Conscientiousness predicted more liking for pop music but only among girls. Openness predicted more liking for both metal and classical music. That said, openness also predicted less liking for soul music in girls whereas it predicted more liking for electronic music in boys. Interestingly, openness predicted more eclecticism (i.e. diversified liking across many different music genres). Extraversion (linked with soul music in girls) and openness (linked with electronic music in boys) showed the largest effect sizes. Nonetheless, openness had the greatest number of significant relationships with music preferences. Moreover, the study also suggested that the potential influence of personality traits on music preferences might also include some gender differences in adolescence.

Second, it also seems that personality traits may predict music preferences in the long term during adolescence. In a 3 year longitudinal study spanning early to late adolescence among adolescents living in the Netherlands, Marc Delsing et al. (2008) tested if the Big 5 could predict four factors of music preferences: rock (e.g. heavy metal), elite (e.g. classical), urban (e.g. hip hop/rap), and pop/dance (e.g. Top 40/charts). Results from latent growth curve modelling revealed predictive links in terms of both actual levels and growth rates across time. Extraversion predicted higher levels of urban and pop/dance music, but also a decrease in the growth of liking for rock. Agreeableness predicted higher levels of elite and pop/dance music, but also a decrease in the growth of liking for pop/dance. Conscientiousness predicted lower levels of rock music. Emotional stability (neuroticism reversed) predicted lower levels of elite music. Openness predicted higher levels of rock and elite music, as well as a decrease in the growth of liking for urban and pop/dance music. Overall, openness had the largest effect size.

Music listening behaviours as markers of personality traits

Do adolescents' music listening behaviours give away their personality to others? Music preferences were also examined as markers of personality traits, more specifically in the context of young people judging the personality of others. In the United States, Peter Rentfrow and Samuel Gosling (2006) examined if late adolescents (undergraduate students who were on average 18.9 years of age) could accurately assess the personality traits (Big 5) in complete strangers (whom they did not see or know) just by listening to their top 10 favourite songs without any further indication. Overall, people could accurately judge the traits in others from their favourite songs, with the exception of conscientiousness. That said, the effect sizes for relationships between the personality judgements and the actual self-report of personality were small/medium, but medium/large for openness. In other words, people are especially able to estimate others' degree of openness by merely knowing their music preferences. In sum, Rentfrow and Gosling conclude that music preferences may literally serve as cues of someone's personality traits.

Personality traits as outcomes of music listening behaviours

Can music listening behaviours influence the personality development of adolescents? Music listening behaviours have rarely been studied as having an impact on personality traits. Nevertheless, Dave Miranda et al. (2010) revisited data from the Miranda and Claes (2008) study with the new objective of examining if different strategies of coping with stress through music listening could predict changes in neuroticism within the 6 month longitudinal follow up of middle adolescents. Findings indicated that coping by music listening predicted changes in neuroticism. More specifically, for those adolescents with high neuroticism at baseline and who engaged in less avoidance coping, problem-solving coping predicted less neuroticism. For those adolescents with high neuroticism at baseline and who engaged in more avoidance coping, problem-solving coping predicted more neuroticism. Furthermore, for adolescent girls who engaged in more avoidance coping, emotional coping predicted more neuroticism. In sum, the potential influence of coping by music listening on personality traits is liable to depend on prior levels of traits, coping styles, and gender differences.

Furthermore, Maja Djikic (2011) conducted an experiment with Canadian late adolescents (mean age = 18.3 years) enrolled in their first year at university. The aim of this study was to examine if music and/or lyrics could have some kind of transformative impact on the Big 5, at least in a laboratory setting. The experimental design essentially consisted of a pre-test and post-test for the Big 5 across three groups: (1) music only; (2) lyrics only; and (3) music and lyrics. Intriguingly, findings showed that music enhanced (whereas lyrics suppressed) traits' total fluctuation from pre-test to post-test. In other words, the personality traits of those who listened to music (as opposed to lyrics) fluctuated (i.e. changed) more during the experiment. Unfortunately, the unique impact of music and/or lyrics on each trait was unspecified.

Summary of findings

From the recent literature, it is possible to make at least three remarks. First, personality traits are associated with music listening behaviours in adolescence. That being said, the effect size is usually small. Second, of all personality traits, openness (e.g. being sophisticated, artistic, intellectual) often displays the strongest (medium effect size) and broadest (diverse music genres) associations with music listening behaviours (e.g. music eclecticism, cognitive use of music). Perhaps this is why, of all traits, openness is the easiest one to judge in others from simply knowing their tastes in music. Third, we know more about personality traits and music listening in late adolescents (i.e. young university students) than in younger adolescents (i.e. high school students).

Implications for wellbeing

Implications from this literature for wellbeing are tentative at this stage. A research direction could be to test emotion regulation through music listening as a mediator between personality traits and wellbeing. In terms of personality, Openness would be an obvious choice as a predictor because it displays the most potent relationships with music listening behaviours in adolescence. Moreover, extraversion and low neuroticism would also be judicious predictors as they are well known to predict wellbeing (Ozer and Benet-Martínez, 2006). Therefore, in light of the present review, it seems reasonable to suggest that at least openness and neuroticism would be trait predictors.

Emotion regulation through music listening could be a mediator between personality traits and wellbeing given that music listening behaviours are often used as emotion regulation strategies that can either positively or negatively impact wellbeing in adolescence and emerging adulthood (e.g. Miranda and Claes, 2009; Saarikallio and Erkkilä, 2007; Saarikallio et al., 2015; Thomson et al., 2014). For the sake of example, the potential role of emotion regulation through music listening as a mediator can be illustrated using a known two-factor model of emotion regulation: cognitive reappraisal and emotional suppression (Gross and John, 2003). First, it is known that wellbeing can be associated with more reappraisal and less suppression (e.g. Aldao et al., 2010). Second, the Big 5 can be associated with both of these two emotion regulation strategies in adolescence, with the exception of the link between openness and suppression (Gullone and Taffe, 2012). Third, it has recently been found, but in an older sample of (primarily) emerging adults (mean age = 23.93 years), that reappraisal mediated relationships between music engagement and wellbeing, whereas suppression mediated relationships between music engagement and less wellbeing (Chin and Rickard, 2014). In sum, for instance, future studies could examine if openness might increase cognitive reappraisal while listening to music, which, in turn, may promote wellbeing. Conversely, neuroticism might respectively decrease cognitive reappraisal and increase emotional suppression while listening to music, which, in turn, may hinder wellbeing.

Personality traits and music making

Personality research in music psychology, among other things, has included studies of people who play music, as well as performance issues (e.g. performance anxiety) in musicians (Kemp, 1999)[2]. In adolescence, there are at least two emerging lines of research on personality traits and music making: (1) personality traits and music involvement and (2) personality traits and music performance.

Personality traits and music involvement

Personality traits and music involvement often refers to an area of research pertaining to how traits influence how much people engage in music making activities. In Canada, Kathleen Corrigall et al. (2013) aimed to better understand links between the Big 5, cognitive ability, and music involvement. Participants across two studies consisted of undergraduate students who on average were in late adolescence (mean age = 20 years) as well as early adolescents (10–12-year-old children; mean age = 11.5 years). Notably, in early

---

[2] For example, Kemp (1999) had noticed that musicians have traditionally been reported as low in extraversion, but perhaps as a result of years of solitary practice.

adolescents, openness was associated with lifetime exposure to music training, even after controlling for age, family income, parents' education, non-musical activities, and cognitive ability. In late adolescents, openness was associated to lifetime engagement in music playing despite controlling for parents' education and cognitive ability. In sum, openness seems distinctively linked to greater music involvement.

Personality traits and music performance

Personality traits and music performance often refers to a research field related to how traits can impact how well people perform in their music making activities. In Japan, Satoshi Kawase (2016) studied links between the Big 5, empathy, and ensemble (and solo) performance aptitude in university music students who were on average late adolescents (mean age = 20.2 years). Extraversion was associated with positive ensemble self-evaluation and greater ensemble preference. Agreeableness was linked to more positive ensemble self-evaluation and greater ensemble preference. Conscientiousness was associated with greater ensemble preference. Openness was related to more positive ensemble self-evaluation, greater ensemble preference, and more positive solo self-evaluation. Interestingly, agreeableness had the largest (medium/large) effect size, perhaps because of its interpersonal quality. That said, empathy's facets (perspective taking, fantasy, emphatic concern, and personal distress) were not associated with any aptitudes in ensemble (or solo) performance. Many other music behaviours were examined. Playing for fun with others was associated with extraversion and openness. Studying music theory was associated with openness. Having professional conversations about music was tied to extraversion and openness. Frequency per year of solo performance recitals was associated with openness. Practising with other performers, practising alone, taking music lessons, reading books on or browsing the Internet about music, and number of annual ensemble concerts were not associated with the Big 5 nor empathy. Intriguingly, it is playing for fun alone that was related to empathy (i.e. fantasy, emphatic concern, and personal distress). Moreover, listening to music was also linked to empathy (i.e. perspective taking, fantasy, and personal distress), as well as to agreeableness and neuroticism. Hence, this study seems to call for more research comparing the role of empathy across different kinds or settings of musical activities.

Jason Thomas and Ted Nettelbeck (2014) found that trait anxiety was associated to music performance anxiety (MPA) in Australian middle adolescents. In fact, although it was also found that bivariate relationships between MPA and lower extraversion and higher neuroticism were significant, these links became non-significant when trait anxiety was statistically controlled. In a rare longitudinal study, Michael Sadler and Christopher Miller (2010) studied whether personality traits could predict MPA in university music students who were on average late adolescents (mean age = 20 years). The prospective design was based on 15 diaries that were filled out over the course of one academic year. It was found that trait negative emotionality (a temperamental dimension related to the trait of neuroticism) was associated with more MPA. Interestingly, it also seems that having cumulated a substantial amount of music study experience may buffer against that putative aggravating effect of negative emotionality on MPA.

In Germany, Joachim Stoeber and Ulrike Eismann (2007) examined different facets of perfectionism (striving for perfection, negative reactions to imperfection, perceived parental pressure, and perceived teacher pressure) in middle adolescents who attended high schools for musically talented students. Among many observed relationships, overall, it seems possible to summarize that more adaptive forms of perfectionism (i.e. striving for perfection) were linked to positive outcomes (e.g. more time spent practising), whereas more maladaptive forms of perfectionism (notably negative reactions to imperfection) were related to negative outcomes such as distress (i.e. performance anxiety, somatic complaints, and emotional fatigue).

Summary of findings

From the recent literature, it is possible to make at least three comments. First, openness seems to be a robust correlate of music involvement in adolescents. Second, the music performance of adolescents might be affected by neuroticism, maladaptive forms of perfectionism, and trait anxiety. Third, unfortunately, there is a lack of research on personality traits and music making in adolescence.

Implications for wellbeing

Implications from this scant literature for wellbeing are speculative at this stage of research in adolescence. However, it seems plausible that—just like for people in general—the wellbeing of young musicians might be hindered by neuroticism and trait anxiety. Future studies could also test moderation models that involve interaction effects. For example, it could be tested whether a thwarted music performance may aggravate the negative effects that certain traits (e.g. neuroticism, trait anxiety) have on the wellbeing of adolescent musicians. Furthermore, conversely, it could also be examined whether maladaptive levels on those traits (i.e. neuroticism, trait anxiety) may worsen the possible negative impact that music performance difficulties may have on the wellbeing of adolescent musicians.

Conclusion

The current literature supports that personality traits are associated with various music behaviours in adolescence. However, personality research is still scant and fragmented in music psychology, especially in adolescence. In particular, more research is needed to establish how the personality–music interface has clear implications for wellbeing in adolescence. However, an open-minded way to reappraise this situation is that more research on personality traits is a pertinent, intriguing, and original contribution to music psychology.

References

Aldao, A., Nolen-Hoeksema, S., and Schweizer, S. (2010). Emotion-regulation strategies across psychopathology: A meta-analytic review. *Clinical Psychology Review*, 30(2), 217–237.

Arnett, J. (1992). The soundtrack of recklessness: Musical preferences and reckless behavior among adolescents. *Journal of Adolescent Research*, 7(3), 313–331.

Bonneville-Roussy, A., Rentfrow, P. J., Xu, M. K., and Potter, J. (2013). Music through the ages: Trends in musical engagement and preferences from adolescence through middle adulthood. *Journal of Personality and Social Psychology*, **105**(4), 703–717.

Chamorro-Premuzic, T. and Furnham, A. (2007). Personality and music: Can traits explain how people use music in everyday life? *British Journal of Psychology*, **98**(2), 175–185.

Chamorro-Premuzic, T., Gomà-i-Freixanet, M., Furnham, A., and Muro, A. (2009a). Personality, self-estimated intelligence, and uses of music: A Spanish replication and extension using structural equation modeling. *Psychology of Aesthetics, Creativity, and the Arts*, **3**(3), 149–155.

Chamorro-Premuzic, T., Swami, V., Furnham, A., and Maakip, I. (2009b). The big five personality traits and uses of music: A replication in Malaysia using structural equation modeling. *Journal of Individual Differences*, **30**(1), 20–27.

Chin, T. and Rickard, N. S. (2014). Emotion regulation strategy mediates both positive and negative relationships between music uses and well-being. *Psychology of Music*, **42**(5), 692–713.

Corrigall, K. A., Schellenberg, E. G., and Misura, N. M. (2013). Music training, cognition, and personality. *Frontiers in Psychology*, **4**, 222.

Delsing, M. J., ter Bogt, T. F., Engels, R. C., and Meeus, W. H. (2008). Adolescents' music preferences and personality characteristics. *European Journal of Personality*, **22**(2), 109–130.

Djikic, M. (2011). The effect of music and lyrics on personality. *Psychology of Aesthetics, Creativity, and the Arts*, **5**(3), 237–240.

Fleeson, W. (2001). Toward a structure-and process-integrated view of personality: Traits as density distributions of states. *Journal of Personality and Social Psychology*, **80**(6), 1011–1027.

Gross, J. J. and John, O. P. (2003). Individual differences in two emotion regulation processes: Implications for affect, relationships, and well-being. *Journal of Personality and Social Psychology*, **85**(2), 348–362.

Gullone, E. and Taffe, J. (2012). The Emotion Regulation Questionnaire for Children and Adolescents (ERQ–CA): A psychometric evaluation. *Psychological Assessment*, **24**(2), 409–417.

John, O. P., Naumann, L. P., and Soto, C. J. (2008). Paradigm shift to the integrative Big Five trait taxonomy: History, measurement, and conceptual issues. In O. P. John, R. W. Robins, and L. A. Pervin (Eds), *Handbook of Personality: Theory and Research* (3rd edn, pp. 114–158). New York: Guilford Press.

Kawakami, A. and Katahira, K. (2015). Influence of trait empathy on the emotion evoked by sad music and on the preference for it. *Frontiers in Psychology*, **6**, 1541.

Kawase, S. (2016). Associations among music majors' personality traits, empathy, and aptitude for ensemble performance. *Psychology of Music*, **44**(2), 293–302.

Kemp, A. E. 1999. Individual differences in musical behaviour. In J. Hargreaves and A. C. North (Eds), *The Social Psychology of Music* (pp. 25–45). New York: Oxford University Press.

Miranda, D. and Claes, M. (2008). Personality traits, music preferences and depression in adolescence. *International Journal of Adolescence and Youth*, **14**(3), 277–298.

Miranda, D. and Claes, M. (2009). Music listening, coping, peer affiliation and depression in adolescence. *Psychology of Music*, **37**(2), 215–233.

Miranda, D., Gaudreau, P., and Morizot, J. (2010). Blue notes: Coping by music listening predicts neuroticism changes in adolescence. *Psychology of Aesthetics, Creativity, and the Arts*, **4**(4), 247–253.

Ozer, D. J. and Benet-Martinez, V. (2006). Personality and the prediction of consequential outcomes. *Annual Review of Psychology*, **57**, 401–421.

Rentfrow, P. J. and Gosling, S. D. (2003). The do re mi's of everyday life: The structure and personality correlates of music preferences. *Journal of Personality and Social Psychology*, **84**(6), 1236–1256.

Rentfrow, P. J. and Gosling, S. D. (2006). Message in a ballad: The role of music preferences in interpersonal perception. *Psychological Science*, **17**(3), 236–242.

Roberts, B. W., Walton, K. E., and Viechtbauer, W. (2006). Patterns of mean-level change in personality traits across the life course: A meta-analysis of longitudinal studies. *Psychological Bulletin*, **132**(1), 1–25.

Saarikallio, S. and Erkkilä, J. (2007). The role of music in adolescents' mood regulation. *Psychology of Music*, **35**(1), 88–109.

Saarikallio, S., Gold, C., and McFerran, K. (2015). Development and validation of the healthy-unhealthy music scale. *Child and Adolescent Mental Health*, **20**(4), 210–217.

Sadler, M. E. and Miller, C. J. (2010). Performance anxiety: A longitudinal study of the roles of personality and experience in musicians. *Social Psychological and Personality Science*, **1**(3), 280–287.

Stoeber, J. and Eismann, U. (2007). Perfectionism in young musicians: Relations with motivation, effort, achievement, and distress. *Personality and Individual Differences*, **43**(8), 2182–2192.

Thomson, C. J., Reece, J. E., and Di Benedetto, M. (2014). The relationship between music-related mood regulation and psychopathology in young people. *Musicae Scientiae*, **18**(2), 150–165.

Thomas, J. P. and Nettelbeck, T. (2014). Performance anxiety in adolescent musicians. *Psychology of Music*, **42**(4), 624–634.

Chapter 10

Musical preference and social identity in adolescence

Alexandra Lamont and David Hargreaves

Introduction

Is everyone musical? What do we mean when we call someone a musician? Based on over 50 years of research, the field of music psychology is coming to a consensus on these two important questions. Firstly, humans have an innate capacity to respond to music from birth. Mothers around the world sing spontaneously to their infants in a way which induces calm, familiarity, and bonding (Tafuri, 2008; Trevarthen and Malloch, 2017). Given the right opportunity, time, and instruction, all children can benefit and make progress with technical and expressive aspects of performing and making music and the consequent cognitive gains this brings (e.g. Hanna-Pladdy and MacKay, 2011). Importantly, the definition of a musician has now broadened to encompass the perception and understanding of music through listening and imagining as well as the more traditional understanding involving composition, performance, or improvisation (Hargreaves, 2012). Informal exposure begins at home and continues through school, peer groups, neighbourhood associations, religious groups, and community organizations across the lifespan (Green, 2008; Marsh and Young, 2016). Rickard and Chin (2017) label this the 'musicianship of listening', and we focus here on how this operates in the critical adolescent period in terms of musical preferences and allegiances.

Theories of identity in adolescence

Adolescence is a turbulent period of development, and one key theoretical concept is that of identity formation. Erikson (1968) first identified adolescence as a critical period in identity where role confusion is experienced; adolescents go through the processes of identification with the characteristics of others, individuation of their own identity across contexts, and integration of these new characteristics into a stable personal identity. Strong social allegiances are formed, in terms of friendships, fledgling romantic relationships, and political ideologies, setting the stage for subsequent later development in terms of intimacy, generativity, and integrity. Marcia's work (1980), applied usefully to adolescents' and young adults' musical performer identity by Davidson and Burland (2006) and Evans and McPherson (2017), proposed that identity developed through the twin processes of exploration and commitment. Exploration refers to the extent to which we try to discover and find out more about different activities and attitudes while searching for a new sense of self. Commitment, on the other hand, refers to the extent to which we take on these beliefs and values.

Social identity theory (or SIT; see e.g. Tajfel and Turner, 1986) helps explain how identification takes place. Social identity theory proposes that people categorize themselves as members of certain groups, which become 'ingroups' for them, automatically excluding other people who belong to corresponding 'outgroups'. Ingroup members are favoured and outgroup members discriminated against, thus shaping behaviours and attitudes. From a different perspective, the sociocultural approach to understanding adolescence emphasizes different aspects of social behaviour, informed by Vygotsky, cultural-historical activity theory, and cultural psychology, which all share a focus on context as fundamentally shaping people's ways of thinking and concepts through a process of cultural apprenticeship (see Hargreaves and Lamont, 2017). One key feature of this approach is the means by which social engagement is expressed, namely through talk. Vygotsky (1978) emphasized language as one of the most fundamental and central cultural tools that people use in forming social relationships, and more recently psychologists, educators, and linguists have investigated the discourses and patterns of dialogue that shape society.

Identity and musical preferences

As noted, our key focus in this chapter is musical listener identity, and one of the most obvious applications of identity is in understanding the music that adolescents listen to and the functions that this fulfils for them (Lamont, 2017). Considering the adolescent period in relation to the rest of the lifespan, we can establish some key differences that illustrate the importance of identity in relation to music listening behaviours.

First, it is now well established that music forms an important part of life, routine, ritual, and celebration from birth. Children are exposed to more music than adults (Juslin et al., 2008; Lamont, 2008), and adolescents seem to listen to more music (around 25 hours a week) than people of any other age, whether younger or older (Bonneville-Roussy et al., 2013). Secondly, passion for music is also reportedly higher in adolescence (Bonneville-Roussy et al., 2013). Music preferences are a way for adolescents to explore various identities, and once they have committed, Frith's (1981) suggestion that music serves as a 'badge of identity' at this point in development clearly encapsulates the notion that these—related to clothing styles, leisure interests, and other values and attitudes—can then be communicated to other people. Thirdly, the music itself is critical. Different kinds of music are liked at different ages. Young children tend to prefer to listen to children's music, music from films and television programmes, and pop music (Lamont, 2008). Pop music in its many incarnations (including hip hop, rap, DJ-based music, dance/house, R&B, indie, and chart pop) is the most preferred style for young adults, while older adults gravitate more to the pop of their adolescent period as well as musicals and opera (North and Hargreaves, 1995). We return to the issue of the kind of music later in the chapter, but first consider the stability of music preferences over time.

Whatever music is liked, individual preferences do not change much over short time periods. In a 3 year longitudinal study with adolescents aged 12 and 16, Delsing et al. (2008) found that music preference dimensions remained stable. The older group was more consistent across the time period, but both groups showed a consistency in their preferences for the four musical style factors (rock, elite, urban, and pop/dance). Similarly, Mulder et al. (2010) found highly consistent preferences for different styles in adolescents and young adults over 21 months.

Preference for specific pieces of music may also be stable over the lifespan, reflecting the notion of a critical period for establishing deeply held music preferences which occurs some time in adolescence or early adulthood. Krumhansl and Zupnick (2013) found some evidence of this in their studies of 'reminiscence bumps' in liking for music. Their 20-year-old participants recognized and liked songs that were at the top of the charts both when they themselves were in adolescence and early adulthood, and when both their parents and grandparents were at the same ages, in comparison to music popular in the intervening years. Krumhansl and Zupnick make a strong argument that the reminiscence bumps for these pieces are caused by transmission through generations, while acknowledging that the 'grandparent' bump might be more to do with the quality of the music at that particular period in time. Similarly, North and Hargreaves (1995) found that some popular artists, notably Elvis Presley and The Beatles, are consistently rated as eminent by all age groups over the last 30 years or so, supporting the idea of eminence in preferences for pop music. While Krumhansl and Zupnick do not link this explicitly to identity, it seems likely that these strong memories make a significant contribution in terms of musical identity during adolescence (see Rathbone et al., 2008).

When considering these longer-term patterns of engagement with music, we need to distinguish between preference for broad styles of music—often termed 'taste'—and preferences for individual pieces. Specific pieces of music have connections to the wider sociocultural context through association with popular culture, and we all have individual memories associated with different pieces of music, which both affect memorability and thus preference. For instance, 'Eye of the Tiger' was used on the soundtrack for *Rocky III*, and has become synonymous with the trope of training against the odds and physical endurance. Thus it has become an extremely popular song for athletes and sportspeople (Hallett and Lamont, 2015), whatever their age when the track was first released. Following the 'Darling they're playing our tune' theory first coined by Davies (1978), specific pieces will also have highly personal connections, such as one's first dance at a wedding or one's first important breakup, which are likely to cloud any clear results. In support of this, Mulder et al. (2010) found considerable variation in liking for individual pieces of music within styles over that time period from their adolescent listeners, highlighting the complexity of this area.

One attempt to go beyond the distinction between preference for individual pieces and that for artists, styles, and genres is the approach to studying music preferences championed by Rentfrow and Gosling (2003). Through a number of large-scale studies they have re-fined their enquiry to five musical categories. In the so-called MUSIC model, these five styles (derived through rigorous experimental work) are defined as Mellow (e.g. soft rock and adult contemporary music; seen as romantic, relaxing, and slow); Unpretentious (e.g. uncomplicated and relaxing; country and western or folk music); Sophisticated (e.g. clas-sical, opera, and jazz; seen as aspiring, intelligent, and complex); Intense (e.g. punk and heavy metal; characterized by distorted, loud, and aggressive sounds), and Contemporary (e.g. pop, rap, and dance). Broad changes to preference for these kinds of music are found with age. Bonneville-Roussy et al. (2013) studied over 254 000 participants aged between 12 and 65, finding changes in the kinds of music preferred at given ages. Preference for the unpretentious and sophisticated dimensions increased linearly with age, preference for the mellow dimension showed a peak in early adulthood and a slight decline in later adulthood, and preference for the intense and contemporary factors gradually declined across the age range.

Bonneville-Roussy et al. ascribe these changing preferences to life stage and age-related processes. Rock and heavy metal was preferred more in adolescence than at other ages, perhaps again reflecting adolescents' search for identity and independence. Continuing the theme of identity development and following Erikson's stages, preference for mellow music in early adulthood, for instance, might reflect the intimacy of building lasting so-cial and family relationships. We move on next to the notion of open-earedness to help explain how identity formation in music preferences might work at a more generalizable level in adolescence.

Preference, tolerance, and exploration

Hargreaves (1982) coined the term 'open-earedness' to explain the overall pattern of re-sults in a study of children's and adolescents' willingness to listen to and their liking for a wide variety of different styles of music at different ages, based on an original study of 126 children aged 7–15. The original formulation of the term open-earedness was used to explain the finding that younger children were more readily able to listen to and maybe also enjoy unconventional or unusual (e.g. 'avant garde', aleatory, or electronic) musical forms, as they may 'show less evidence of acculturation to normative standards of "good taste" than older children' (Hargreaves, 1982, p. 51). LeBlanc (1982, 1991) later adopted the concept more formally, extending its definition to include 'listener tolerance', and op-erationalizing it in terms of music preferences. He also formulated a model of age-related changes in open-earedness, based on his literature review, which included four general-izations across the lifespan:

younger children are more open-eared ... open-earedness declines as the child enters adolescence ... there is a partial rebound of open-earedness as the listener matures from adolescence to young adulthood ... open-earedness declines as the listener matures to old age.

(LeBlanc 1991, pp. 36–38)

Since then, much research has been carried out based on this concept and its development across the lifespan: the literature published in English was recently reviewed by Hargreaves et al. (2016) and Hargreaves and Lamont (2017). With one or two exceptions, LeBlanc's generalizations receive general support. The 'dip' in open-earedness in later childhood seems to occur at around the age of 10 or 11 years. This typically shows itself in very strongly expressed preferences for a narrow range of pop styles, and strong general dislike for all other styles, and may well be related to changes in self-identity. The 'rebound' of open-earedness in early adulthood is often a phase in which adults are seeking to acquire music, whether recordings or downloads (Greasley et al., 2013). After this, there seems to be a general decline in liking for popular music styles across the rest of the lifespan, and a corresponding general increase for 'classical' styles.

More recent research has attempted to explore the validity of the earlier stages of development, looking at open-earedness in childhood. Gembris and Schellberg (2003), for example, explored the music preferences of 591 children between ages of 5 and 13, assessing their likes or dislikes for a set of eight short excerpts from four different styles (classical music, pop music, 20th century art (avant garde) music, and ethnic music). They found highly significant age-related declines in liking for all of these styles across the age range. Pop music was preferred most, and younger children were more positive about classical, avant garde, and ethnic music, but with increasing age all the ratings became strongly negative. Some studies suggest that classical music might be the main driver of these results. For instance, Kopiez and Lehmann (2008) found that the decline in open-earedness with increasing age in their results disappeared when classical music was excluded from their analyses, which led them to suggest that other factors may also have influenced their results. Other studies suggest that tolerance and liking for a range of styles may decrease across childhood: Busch et al. (2016) explored primary school children's music preferences, collecting data from both children and parents over 4 years, finding declines in open-earedness for both conventional and unconventional styles across this age range.

These generalizations about age differences in open-earedness with respect to 'popular' and 'classical' or 'serious' styles may be valid because they work at a high level of generality: they refer to broad genres rather than to specific styles within those genres, and thus sidestep the problems of cohort or historical effects. Children spontaneously use these kinds of labels to describe music, although we found young adults resisted categorization of their own music preferences (Greasley et al., 2013). Nonetheless, as we have seen, preference for specific pieces also seems to follow a similar pattern of waxing and waning between breadth and depth (Greasley and Lamont, 2013). Adolescence might be a critical period at which lasting preferences for both styles and specific artists and pieces are formed: in Marcia's terms, this would represent a process of identity commitment.

Holbrook and Schindler's (1989) seminal study of preferences for specific songs over time demonstrated a general preference for artists/musicians who were popular during the listeners' late adolescence/early adulthood. They introduced a useful concept of song-specific ages (the year of release of the song minus the listener's year of birth) to explore preferences against historical context from a range of participants of different ages. Based on a relatively small number of participants aged 16–86, their study involved playing 30 second extracts from 28 different music examples from the charts, taken from 2 year intervals between 1932 and 1986, asking participants to rate their liking for these songs, and exploring the most popular song-specific ages. From their results, they argued that the age of 24 was the peak of the critical period for defining music preferences. A more recent replication of this work by Hemming (2013), with a larger sample of 473 listeners and music extracts drawn from 1960 to 2008 in the same manner but with some different treatment of data, has suggested this peak might occur earlier, at about 17 years. Hemming is somewhat ambivalent about whether the peak might exist at all, given the need to treat the data in different ways to achieve this set of results, and while Holbrook and Schindler (2013) disagree with his conclusions, his findings do seem to provide more weight for the importance of the adolescent period in forming important and long-lasting musical preferences.

The studies into open-earedness vary widely with respect to their theoretical rationales, their participant groups and age ranges, the actual genres and styles under investigation, and the assessment techniques employed. Louven (2016) suggested open-earedness should be better understood as openness, curiosity, and tolerance rather than preference, while Hargreaves and Bonneville-Roussy (2018) refute this with new evidence from adults showing an increase in number of styles liked in early adulthood. These differences in definition and approach notwithstanding, LeBlanc's original generalizations do seem to broadly hold true. Considering adolescence as a period of extreme 'closed-earedness' fits clearly with the theories of identity development, which suggest that narrowing of taste and developing strong links to peers is somehow necessary to achieve this stage of identity development. Although not uncontroversial, the research evidence mostly supports the importance of music liked and listened to around the age of 16–17 as likely to be highly influential in shaping future preference and listening behaviours, and may even have consequences in terms of negotiating difficulties in general development (Schwartz and Fouts, 2003).

A return to theory

As noted, there are two core theories that can help explain musical behaviours, allegiances, and preferences in adolescence. The first links clearly to mainstream social psychology and the social identity approach, while the second relates to the influence of specific sociocultural contexts of development.

Tarrant and colleagues' research explores how music preferences play a role in in- and outgroup discriminations. For instance, Tarrant et al. (2001) found that adolescents believed pupils from the same school—the ingroup—would show greater preferences for what they called prestigious musical styles (such as pop music, valued by this age group) and lesser preference for non-prestigious music than pupils from a different school—the outgroup. Music was found to be more influential than other activities such as media interests and sport, suggesting that the decline in open-earedness illustrated by their music preferences plays a role in helping adolescents form judgements about one another. Liking for musical styles thus forms a key defining feature of social identity, which can predict many other aspects of teenagers' values and attitudes. These social identity judgements can also be used to recognize clear and distinct stereotypes about fans of different types of music (Rentfrow et al., 2009).

The second, sociocultural approach to understanding adolescence has been applied to adolescent musical identity in research on how teenagers talk about pop music. For instance, MacKinlay and McVittie (2017) explore how young people talk about different styles and genres of pop music as a way of demonstrating their identifications with particular genres. Taking a broader approach, Miranda et al. (2015) argue for the need for a cultural-developmental psychology of music in adolescence which includes a consideration of elements 'in the world' (cultural products and objects) as well as those 'in the mind' such as social identity, and a global as well as local perspective on what culture is. Looking at adolescent musical preferences, while we can assume that they have some underlying psychological dimensions, the question of how these might apply within different cultures and with those with disturbed or hybrid identities remains unaddressed in contemporary research.

A paper by Cogo-Moreira and Lamont (2018) uncovered evidence for both these influences in mapping and theorizing exposure to music earlier in childhood. From factor analysis of a range of questions asked to over 1000 Brazilian school children, two factors emerged in 5–13-year-olds' responses. The first factor brought together activities such as personal music listening, the home music environment (including live singing from parents and children themselves), and influences from the media, television, and the Internet. The second factor reflected the more commonly focused on social types of musical activity such as playing a musical instrument, having music lessons, and attending live events (notably not all of these are performing activities). These data support the importance of personal and private music experiences in early adolescence, and confirm findings from many earlier studies that music listening provides powerful mood-regulation capabilities for adolescents (Saarikallio and Erkkilä, 2007).

In summary, considering identity provides some useful theoretical frameworks for understanding music preference in adolescence which tie together different social and sociocultural explanations of development. First, social identity theory relates more closely to the social musical activities, such as going to concerts, which are likely to be important in adolescents' lives and play a central role in forming their badges of identity. Secondly, sociocultural approaches relate more to the more personal musical development where children and adolescents are taking messages from home, peers, and the media and integrating them into their own developing sense of musical identity. More research is urgently needed on this second approach to help uncover the complexities of music use among adolescents and to discover why our musical tastes and identities could be so critically shaped by this period in life.

References

Bonneville-Roussy, A., Rentfrow, P. J., Xu, M. K., and Potter, J. (2013). Music through the ages: Trends in musical engagement and preferences from adolescence through middle adulthood. *Journal of Personality and Social Psychology*, **105**(4), 703–717.

Busch, V., Bunte, N., and Schurig, M. (2016). Open-earedness, musical concepts, and gender identity. In O. Krämer and I. Malmberg (Eds), *European Perspectives on Music Education VI: Open Ears—Open Minds, Listening and Understanding Music* (pp. 151–165). Innsbruck: Helbling.

Cogo-Moreira, H. and Lamont, A. (2018). Multidimensional measurement of exposure to music in childhood: Beyond the musician/non-musician dichotomy. *Psychology of Music*, **46**, 459–472. doi:10.1177/0305735617710322.

Davidson, J. W. and Burland, K. (2006). Musician identity formation. In G. E. McPherson (Ed.), *The Child as Musician: A handbook of Musical Development* (pp. 475–490). Oxford: Oxford University Press.

Davies, J. B. (1978). *The Psychology of Music*. London: Hutchinson.

Delsing, M. J. M. H., ter Bogt, T. F. M., Engels, R. C. M. E., and Meeus, W. H. J. (2008). Adolescents' music preferences and personality characteristics. *European Journal of Personality*, **22**, 109–130.

Erikson, E. H. (1968). *Identity, Youth, and Crisis*. New York: W. W. Norton & Company.

Evans, P. and McPherson, G. E. (2017). Processes of musical identity consolidation during adolescence. In R. A. R. MacDonald, D. J. Hargreaves, and D. E. Miell (Eds), *Handbook of Musical Identities* (pp. 213–231). Oxford: Oxford University Press.

Frith, S. (1981). *Sound Effects: Youth, Leisure, and the Politics of Rock'n'Roll*. New York: Pantheon.

Gembris, H. and Schellberg, G. (2003). Musical preferences of elementary school children. *Abstracts of the 5th ESCOM conference* (p. 324). University of Hanover.

Greasley, A. E. and Lamont, A. (2013). Keeping it fresh: How listeners regulate their own exposure to familiar music. In E. King and H. Prior (Eds), *Music and Familiarity: Listening, Musicology and Performance* (pp. 13–31). Basingstoke: Ashgate.

Greasley, A. E., Lamont, A., and Sloboda, J. A. (2013). Exploring musical preferences: An in-depth study of adults' liking for music in their personal collections. *Qualitative Research in Psychology*, **10**(4), 402–427.

Green, L. (2008). *Music, Informal Learning and the School: A New Classroom Pedagogy*. Aldershot: Ashgate.

Hallett, R. and Lamont, A. (2015). How do gym members engage with music during exercise? *Qualitative Research in Sport, Exercise and Health*, **7**, 411–427.

Hanna-Pladdy, B. and MacKay, A. (2011). The relation between instrumental musical activity and cognitive aging. *Neuropsychology*, **25**(3), 378–386.

Hargreaves, D. J. (1982). The development of aesthetic reactions to music. *Psychology of Music, Special Issue*, 51–54.

Hargreaves, D. J. (2012). Musical imagination: Perception and production, beauty and creativity. *Psychology of Music*, **40**(5), 539–557.

Hargreaves, D. J., North, A. C., and Tarrant, M. (2016). How and why do musical preferences change during childhood and adolescence? In G. McPherson (Ed.), *The Child as Musician: A Handbook of Musical Development* (pp. 303–322). Oxford: Oxford University Press.

Hargreaves, D. J. and Lamont, A. (2017). *The Psychology of Musical Development*. Cambridge: Cambridge University Press.

Hargreaves, D. J. and Bonneville-Roussy, A. (2018). What is 'open-earedness', and how can it be measured? *Musicae Scientiae*, **22**, 161–174. doi:10.1177/1028764917697783.

Hemming, J. (2013). Is there a peak in popular music preference at a certain song-specific age? A replication of Holbrook & Schindler's 1989 study. *Musicae Scientiae*, **17**(3), 293–304.

Holbrook, M. B. and Schindler, R. M. (1989). Some exploratory findings on the development of musical tastes. *Journal of Consumer Research*, **16**(6), 119–124.

Holbrook, M. B. and Schindler, R. M. (2013). Commentary on "Is there a peak in popular music preference at a certain song-specific age? A replication of Holbrook & Schindler's 1989 study" *Musicae Scientiae*, **17**(3), 305–308.

Juslin, P. N., Liljeström, S., Västfjäll, D., Barradas, G., and Silva, A. (2008). An experience sampling study of emotional reactions to music: listener, music, and situation. *Emotion*, **8**(5), 668–683.

Kopiez, R. and Lehmann, M. (2008). The "open-earedness" hypothesis and the development of age-related reactions to music in elementary school children. *British Journal of Music Education*, **25**(2), 121–138.

Krumhansl, C. L. and Zupnick, J. A. (2013). Cascading reminiscence bumps in popular music. *Psychological Science*, **24**, 2057–2068.

Lamont, A. (2008). Young children's musical worlds: Musical engagement in three-year-olds. *Journal of Early Childhood Research*, **6**(3), 247–261.

Lamont, A. (2017). Musical identity, interest, and involvement. In R. A. R. MacDonald, D. J. Hargreaves, and D. E. Miell (Eds), *Handbook of Musical Identities* (pp. 176–196). Oxford: Oxford University Press.

LeBlanc, A. (1982). An interactive theory of music preference. *Journal of Music Therapy*, **19**, 28–45.

LeBlanc, A. (1991). Effect of maturation/aging on music listening preference: A review of the literature. Paper presented at the Ninth National Symposium on Research in Music Behavior, Cannon Beach, OR, 7–9 March.

Louven, C. (2016). Hargreaves' "open-earedness": A critical discussion and new approach on the concept of musical tolerance and curiosity. *Musicae Scientiae*, **20**(2), 235–247.

MacKinlay, A. and McVittie, C. (2017). 'Will the real Slim Shady please stand up?' Identity in popular music. In R. A. R. MacDonald, D. J. Hargreaves, and D. E. Miell (Eds), *Handbook of Musical Identities* (pp. 137–151). Oxford: Oxford University Press.

Marcia, J. E. (1980). Identity in adolescence. In J. Adelson (Ed.), *Handbook of Adolescent Psychology* (pp. 159–187). New York: Wiley.

Marsh, K. and Young, S. (2016). Musical play. In G. E McPherson (Ed.), *The Child as Musician: A handbook of Musical Development* (2nd edn, pp. 462–484). Oxford: Oxford University Press.

Miranda, D., Blaise-Rochette, C., Vaugon, K., Osman, M., and Arias-Velanzuela, M. (2015). Towards a cultural–developmental psychology of music in adolescence. *Psychology of Music*, **43**(2), 197–218.

Mulder, J., ter Bogt, T. F. M., Raaijmakers, Q. A. W., Nic Gabhainn, S., and Sikkema, P. (2010). From death metal to R&B? Consistency of music preferences among Dutch adolescents and young adults. *Psychology of Music*, **38**, 67–83.

North, A. C. and Hargreaves, D. J. (1995). Eminence in pop music. *Popular Music and Society*, **19**(4), 41–66.

Rathbone, C. J., Moulin, C. J. A., and Conway, M. A. (2008). Self-centered memories: The reminiscence bump and the self. *Memory & Cognition*, **36**(8), 1403–1414.

Rentfrow, P. J. and Gosling, S. D. (2003). The do re mi's of everyday life: The structure and personality correlates of music preferences. *Journal of Personality and Social Psychology*, **84**(6), 1236–1256.

Rentfrow, P. J., McDonald, J. A., and Oldmeadow, J. A. (2009). You are what you listen to: Young people's stereotypes about music fans. *Group Processes and Intergroup Relations*, **12**(3), 329–344.

Rickard, N. S. and Chin, T. (2017). Defining the musical identity of 'non-musicians'. In R. A. R. MacDonald, D. J. Hargreaves, and D. E. Miell. (Eds), *Handbook of Musical Identities* (pp. 288–303). Oxford: Oxford University Press.

Saarikallio, S. and Erkkilä, J. (2007). The role of music in adolescents' mood regulation. *Psychology of Music*, 35, 88–109.

Schwartz, K.D. and Fouts, G. T. (2003). Music preferences, personality style, and developmental issues of adolescents. *Journal of Youth and Adolescence*, **32**(3), 205–213.

Tafuri, J. (2008). *Infant Musicality: New research for Educators and Parents.* Farnham: Ashgate.

Tajfel, H. and Turner, J. C. (1986). An integrative theory of intergroup conflict. In S. Worchel and W. G. Austin. (Eds), *Social Psychology of Intergroup Relations* (pp. 2–24). Chicago: Nelson-Hall.

Tarrant, M., North, A. C., and Hargreaves, D. J. (2001). Social categorization, self-esteem, and the estimated musical preferences of male adolescents. *Journal of Social Psychology*, **141**(5), 565–581.

Trevarthen, C. and Malloch, S. (2017). The musical self: Affections for life in a community of sound. In R. A. R. MacDonald, D. J. Hargreaves, and D. E. Miell (Eds), *Handbook of Musical Identities* (pp. 155–175). Oxford: Oxford University Press.

Vygotsky, L. S. (1978). *Mind in Society: The Development of Higher Psychological Processes.* London: Harvard University Press.

Chapter 11

'Forever piping songs forever new': The musical teenager and musical inner teenager across the life course

Tia De Nora

Introduction

The idea of the life course and its stages is deeply embedded in cultures around the world (Aries, 1973). As a narrative structure, the life course delineates categories and stages. These categories have been and continue to be subject to extensive elaboration in the arts and popular culture, perhaps nowhere more famously than in William Shakespeare's reference to the seven ages played out over the course of a full life (Shakespeare, 1623):

> All the world's a stage,
> And all the men and women merely players,
> They have their exits and entrances,
> And one man in his time plays many parts,
> His acts being seven ages.

Thinking about the life course as a construction over long and short-term history illuminates age bands and the things we associate with them as, to some extent, plastic, as taking shape in relation to a social distribution of resources for the configuration of age-specific identities, as constructions that are spatially and temporally situated. The meaning of ageing, in this view, is more complex than any linear typology implies; it is possible, in other words, to 'time travel' from one age band to another according to circumstances and to experience 'young days' or 'old days' from moment to moment of lived experience. As identity, in other words, age is figured from a matrix of resources and practices and it is in relation to these things that age becomes—for all practical purposes—a reality, in time and for a time. The contents of that matrix, therefore, and access to those contents, is of considerable significance since it is in relation to those things that people (individuals, groups) are able to access opportunities for action and experience and, in relation to age, to produce age-specific 'scenes' in daily life and real time.

If the realities of age are contextual and if they emerge, develop, retract, and mutate in relation to contingencies, then age can be explored for how, at different times and in different situations, people may experience and perform themselves as different kinds of age-identified beings. If so, we may speak of enfolded moments of age; for example, times when a child must, or is forced, to function as an adult (such as child slavery and other forms of oppression but also when children function within the family as carers for sick parents or siblings and also when children place themselves in the subject positions of older people as part of play, e.g. playing house, playing dressing up) just as a parent might behave, or be reduced to behaving, like a child. Questions of interest related to these anachronistic adoptions of age-linked roles should perhaps therefore include under what circumstances, and in relation to what kinds of materials, including music, do we come to inhabit age-linked social categories that are at odds with the conventions typically associated with our chronological ages. This question opens up further questions about the nature of age-linked, culturally mediated experience in real time. In particular, it opens up questions about kairotic, rather than chronological time: how are age-linked identities both performed and experienced as 'inner' matters, phenomenologically, and in what ways can this experience be understood to be underwritten musically?

Exploring these questions in relation to the age band known as adolescence opens up, arguably, an especially rich seam for research. As the adage puts it, 'you are as young as you feel' and youth, while it can be over-rated ('it is wasted on the young', etc.), is typically associated with vibrancy, physical health and fitness, freedom (albeit 'freedom from' (responsibilities) rather than 'freedom to'), beauty, and love. Conversely, it is also associated, typically, with turmoil, anxiety, heightened emotions, and raging hormones. To what extent, then, and under what conditions, and with what qualitative and temporal parameters, may the amalgam of emotions and stances that we associate with adolescence recur in later life? And how might exploring these questions shed light on the more general question of how age is a sociotechnical, cultural construction? And specifically, the topic of this chapter, how is music implicated in this process of identity performance?

Age within age: the 'inner adult' and the 'inner teen'

In keeping with the focus on age-linked identity as plastic constructions, it is important to consider adolescence as itself an internally heterogenous category or life stage. We know that the time of being a teenager is a time of becoming emotionally autonomous, independent, developing networks of friends and close associates, and generally a phase of transition (Laiho, 2004). This transition activity means that at times adolescents affiliate with the 'grown up' world while at other times they may orient to earlier, childhood times. These varieties of age orientation in turn imply that the adolescent engagement with music will itself proceed in ways that perform at times anachronistic moments, and enfold features, behavioural stances, or attitudes, and emotional orientations, from any other age band. This enfolding involves both forward- and backward-looking stances wherein young teens may shift age roles in ways that allow them to adopt nostalgic stances and to long for 'olden times' in much the same way that people 30 or more years senior to them might:

Elisa: The Strokes, 'You Only Live Once', it's really nostalgic for me, it's quite, like, summery, I find the summery ones, like, kind of the most memorable and nostalgic ... just generally memories, but, like music related with summer I find very nostalgic. ...

(Bergh et al., 2014, p. 323)

Here, age-linked identity is performed but, within the performance of one's own age band, it is, as this quote from Elisa illustrates, also possible to see individuals performing themselves in anachronistic fashion.

In this respect, however, adolescents are by no means unique. Every age band is heterogeneously configured and situated socially over time. For example, sociomusic studies have described how older care home residents may be subject to musical stereotyping by visiting musicians who assume that their audiences or clients want to hear 'the good old' songs and in ways that may be unappealing or unpleasant for those audiences (Hara, 2011; Bergh, 2011. p. 275). So too, in music, musicians' personae and performance practices may fuse being 'old' (in vocal timbre for example or in terms of repertoire) with being chronologically 'young' (Leppert and Lipsitz, 2000).

Age-linked identity is performed but, within the performance of one's own age band, anachronistic performances are also common. So just as teens may perform themselves as 'older' than they are, so too, 'older' people may perform themselves, through music, as younger than they are. They may attach themselves to music as part of the means for feeling rejuvenated. Indeed, music may gain enhanced importance for adults seeking to connect to their 'inner teen' because it offers an important resource for time travel, for configuring and reconfiguring age-linked forms of experience. Exploring this question allows us to explore in turn transgression or 'breaching' of age and the regulation (and gendered) regulation of age: it allows us to consider social rebellion (or imagined or 'controlled' rebellion) and to explore some of the ways that 'reversion' to adolescence in later life is both personal and political.

The 'old teen' in other words may be a figure that allows us to consider how established people engage in acts of play, how they engage, if fleetingly and if in musically mediated— and therefore bounded—ways with otherwise lost dreams or utopian fantasies. As such, and contra to the conventional wisdom that derides such moments (labelling them as lapses or indiscretions or acts of bad judgement or bad taste), I shall examine these kind of musically mediated moments in terms of how they showcase musically assisted strategies for reclaiming age-segregated (and gender-segregated) opportunities for action. Linked to this, I suggest that these moments offer different forms of refuge and 'asylum', and in ways that connect with what we already know more generally about music's role in relation to the promotion of mental wellbeing (DeNora, 2013; Ansdell and DeNora, 2016).

By 'asylum' I mean a physical or symbolic 'space' that may offer some kind of solace or pleasure, either because it temporarily 'removes' the individual from noxious stimuli (it is a form of 'removal'; DeNora, 2013, p. 56) or because it allows the individual (or cluster of individuals operating as groups) to renegotiate some feature of the social space(s) they regularly (and maybe must regularly) inhabit. Of interest here is the question of to what extent might music, more so than other forms of art or cultural pursuit, afford asylum-seeking strategies and enhance our understanding of how music is, in the broadest sense, a political resource. Just as in situations of music therapy and community music therapy music can become politics by other means, just as it can offer a 'safe' medium for the consideration of social-psychological issues, so too in daily life music offers a means by which to negotiate and sometimes challenge seemingly 'given' presumptions about what is appropriate, expected, required, and even 'natural'.

The 'inner teen': anachronistic identities in and through music in later life

Teenagers frequently employ music to solder new social connections, to break with dependent family ties, and to heighten emotion. But so do adults. And perhaps especially so do 'vulnerable' adults; for example, adults experiencing crisis, bereavement, trauma, or ill health. In our research with adult service users of a mental health facility in London, Gary Ansdell and I described (Ansdell and DeNora, 2016) how the various ways in which people at a community day centre made use of and engaged with music was integral to the forging of pathways 'to' and pathways that were understood—by the individuals themselves but also by professionals—to be 'developmental'. Music offered a way of gaining emotional support and self-validation and it offered a way of regulating mood (McFerran et al., 2014), individual, and group. And just as with young people, these uses or appropriations of music were not unilaterally a 'good thing'. At times the vehement cleaving to music was a practice that performed illness rather than recovery, as when one client recurrently cleaved to the music of his beloved mother and thus could be seen to be—in Ian Hacking's sense (1995, p. 351)—caught in a process of identity 'looping':

….a causal understanding, if known by those who are understood, can change their character, can change the kind of person that they are. This can lead to a change in the causal understanding itself.

(Hacking, 1995, p. 351)

Hacking describes how looping is facilitated by the creation of ecological niches, that is places where conditions are conducive for things to flourish. In the case of the mental health client and his strong attachment to the music of his mother, the repeated engagement with that, and only that, kind of music held the individual in an identity from the past (one in which he was an adolescent). Affiliation with that music also held him back from engaging, musically and therefore protosocially, in Simon Procter's (2011) sense, with other members of the mental health centre and wider community who, though respectful, did not share this man's musical sensibilities (and without some shared sensibility—protosocial capital—the more overt forms of socialization—verbal media, cooperation, coordination—are more difficult). Music, in other words, 'performed' functions that solidified an age-linked identity for this mental health service user by preventing him from developing contacts and experiential horizons capable of lifting out of a living (and obsessing perhaps) in the past (for more detail see Ansdell and DeNora, 2016, pp. 63–65, 235). Thinking about this issue highlights more generally how there is a need to think about how people shift, and are helped to shift, from narrow and vehement musical attachments to being more musically, and therefore socially, open.

Beyond the teenage years people turn to music at times when they find themselves in situations of role conflict and at times when they are seeking to 'reconnect' or 'rediscover' earlier/new rejuvenated selves or when they desire change and novelty, perhaps relief from responsibilities and ties, often a degree of distance from spouses and/or family. For example, Diana, in her fifties, remembers how music was integral to the heightened form of awareness and couple culture associated with a love affair, one that made her feel young again:

'Whiter Shade of Pale', oh yes. I had an affair with . . . and we used to go out in the evenings . . . to . . . and they had music there and 'Whiter Shade of Pale' was our tune and I just loved it . . . and of course it was on the radio all the time . . . we just sort of . . . held hands or—looked at each other intently, something like that . . . .

And, Lesley (in her late thirties at the time of her interview), describes how, near the end of her relationship with her ex-husband, she would sometimes, when she was angry, play a song by Soft Cell called 'Say Hello, Wave Goodbye'. She played the track loudly so that it would be audible from any room in the house. As she puts it, 'It was a hint really', though, as she reflected upon this statement she added that she was not sure her husband understood as 'he didn't say anything'.

Here we see the middle-aged Lesley using music to convey a message, perhaps about her evolving aesthetic and stylistic stance: but to whom? To her husband, so she says, but perhaps more importantly, to herself and in this sense Lesley can also be seen as engaging in refurnishing activity, that is in attempt to alter the acoustic furniture of her daily surroundings in ways that would be conducive to altered forms of imagination, and action and change. Importantly, this was a message that she had not yet formulated in words; she was formulating a sense of how she was 'different' from her partner, thinking through musical practice about leaving that partner and in this sense the music helped her to do that. Her eventual line of action was, it could be said, music-led.

By this point, and as I have suggested in earlier work, I mean that Lesley may also have been undermining the aesthetic basis of their relationship, preparing the aesthetic ground for her departure. As such, there were different steps in this process, the first of which was to move away from the music that had hitherto been located in the centre of their relationship (albeit weakly). The second step was:

---

to turn, instead, to the sort of music her husband had always frowned upon, 'raucous or heavy metal or something', as she puts it, or else something conducive to introspection (and alienation), such as Leonard

Cohen or Susanne Vega, to the sort of music that did not signify, from her partner's point of view, 'happy families'. In a sense, Lesley presaged her leap from a social relationship—her marriage—by trying it out 'virtually' in the aesthetic sphere. Changes in musical practice provided, in other words, a practice genre for the 'real' or social and economic move that was to follow—leaving home.

(DeNora, 2000, p. 128).

In short, Lesley was engaging with music, one might say, 'like a teenager' and these two examples of Lesley and Diana highlight some of the ways that the 'grown up' uses of music afford teenage musical practices and with them, for better or worse, teenage 'moments' in later life. In other words, the categories of the life course do not proceed inexorably in stages but rather can be seen next to and within each other, such that at any one time, and in relation to music, it is possible to be both old and young.

Performing 'inner' ages: asylum and opportunities for action

In the midst of daily life, in the midst of perhaps mild depression or anxiety, burdened with responsibilities, worries, chores, and other people's needs, and as part of accepted everyday practices of health promotion, people seek asylum, understood as refuge, respite, or refreshment. Musically assisted forms of asylum have been studied with approbation by many scholars and in relation to personal musical practices as well as collaborative musicking (Batt-Rawden et al., 2005; Skånland, 2011; DeNora, 2013). The kind of musically assisted time travelling that I have been discussing can be viewed as just such an asylum-seeking attempt. On the one hand, as we saw with Diana, it is oriented to a way of gaining distance from the paramount reality of daily life and a way of attaining an alternate reality, if only temporarily, if even for only as long as the music lasts, clandestine, for the evening. On the other hand, as we saw with Lesley the music provides the leverage for effecting change, for actually shifting the circumstances of daily life, for a kind of 'adult' rebellion employing, 'like a teenager', music for rebellion. In both cases, however, music's powers are double edged: they are simultaneously constructive and destructive.

Most of the time, perhaps, musical time travel serves more incremental and adaptive functions linked to music's role in the care of self (DeNora, 2000). In particular, music may form part of the complex assemblages that both maintain wellbeing and promote recovery from mental illness. For example, in their study of the mid-life experiences of women who self-identified as 'recovered' from depression, Simone Fullagar and Wendy O'Brien (2014) describe how, for women who chose to disengage with medicalized models of depression and treatment, it was important to find ways of creating 'imaginative space', and in ways that could shift the self's relationship to self. One respondent, Mary, described using music for this purpose. It was, the authors suggest, ultimately less helpful than perhaps it might have been. This was not because music can't work—to the contrary, the research shows that it can work indeed as an everyday technology of health—but because Mary could not explain how or why music helped her, and 'had not been encouraged to explore what a musical relation to self might generate in terms of different emotions, relations with others'. Learning what to do with music, informal and peer-linked and/or formal or music therapeutic is, in short, vital if music is enabled and empowered as a 'health technology'.

Conclusion: musically enhanced ageing?

We are always ageing, even when we are young. And yet we are never fully any particular age. Rather, age, to the extent that it is the inner experience of outer performance, should be understood as a plastic category. We flow in and out of different age-linked subject positions (and with them different physical and mental capacities that can be quantitatively assessed; Langer, 2009). Examining music's role in this process offers a way of exploring age-based emotions and relations with others and may offer insight into age-linked conflicts, such as those between adolescents and their parents or teachers, in so far as music can be seen to heighten or diminish the differences between these groups. Musical engagement can be catalytic for major life change and for smaller processes of adaptation and coping. Musical engagement can shift us, making us younger or older for a while. How this process, and specific micro-events of musical rejuvenation happen, and specifically how they are judged and by whom, is a topic for critical sociology. To the extent that it is always possible, within music to be 'young', music affords connection and reconnection with all of our aged selves, all our days. Like Keats' youth painted on the Grecian urn ('child of silence and slow time ... forever piping songs forever new') the younger person within each of us, in other words, never dies; they are always there and capable of being revived, re-experienced, and managed in music—if we know how.

References

Ansdell, G. and **DeNora, T.** (2016). *Musical Pathways in Recovery: Community Music Therapy and Mental Wellbeing.* London: Routledge.

Aries, P. (1973). *Centuries of Childhood.* New York: Penguin.

Batt-Rawden, K. B., DeNora, T., and **Ruud, E.** (2005). Music listening and empowerment in health promotion: A study of the role and significance of music in everyday life of the long-term ill. *Nordic Journal of Music Therapy,* **14**(2), 120–136.

Bergh, A. (2011). Emotions in motion: Transforming conflict and music. In I. Deliege and J. Davidson (Eds), *Music and the Mind: Essays in Honour of John Sloboda* (pp. 363–378). Oxford: Oxford University Press.

Bergh, A, DeNora, T., and **Bergh, M.** (2014). 'Forever and ever': Mobile music in the lives of young teens. In S. Gopinath and J. Stanyek (Eds), *Oxford Handbook of Mobile Music Studies,* vol. 1 (pp. 317–334). Oxford: Oxford University Press.

DeNora, T. (2000). *Music in Everyday Life.* Cambridge: Cambridge University Press.

DeNora, T. (2013). *Music Asylums: Wellbeing Through Music in Everyday Life.* Farnham: Ashgate.

Fullagar, S. and **O'Brien, W.** (2014). Social recovery and the move beyond deficit models of depression: A feminist analysis of mid-life women's self-care practices. *Social Science & Medicine,* **117**, 116–124.

Hacking, I. (1995). The looping effect of human kinds. In D. Sperber (Ed.), *Causal Cognition: An Interdisciplinary Approach*. Oxford University Press: Oxford.

Laiho, S. (2004). The psychological functions of music in adolescence. *Nordic Journal of Music Therapy*, **13**(1), 47–63.

Langer, E J (2009). *Counterclockwise: Mindful Health and the Power of Possibility*. New York: Ballantine Books.

Leppert, R. and Lipsitz, G. (2000). 'Everybody's lonesome for somebody': Age, the body, and experience in the music of Hank Williams. In R. Middleton (Ed.), *Reading Pop* (pp. 307–328). Oxford: Oxford University Press.

McFerran, K. S., Garrido, S., O'Grady, L., Grocke, D., and Sawyer, S. M. (2014). Examining the relationship between self-reported mood management and music preferences of Australian teenagers. *Nordic Journal of Music Therapy*, **24**(3), 187–203.

Procter, S. (2011). Reparative musicing: Thinking on the usefulness of social capital theory within music therapy. *Nordic Journal of Music Therapy*, **20**(3), 242–262.

Shakespeare, W. (1623). As You Like It. *The Complete Works of William Shakespeare*. Available at: http://shakespeare.mit.edu/asyoulikeit/full.html (accessed 2 May 2017).

Skånland, M. S. (2011). Use of MP3 players as a coping resource. *Music and Arts in Action*, **3**(2), 15–33.

Chapter 12

Music as a structuring resource in identity formation processes by adolescents engaging in music therapy—a case study from a Norwegian child welfare setting

Viggo Krüger

Introduction

In this chapter I will focus toward how music therapy may function as an approach for working with young people's identities in various contexts. The following question is asked: How can music function as a structuring resource in identity formation processes by adolescents using music therapy in a child welfare context? To answer this complex question, I will combine perspectives from modern identity theory and sociocultural theory and reflect their implications for music therapy practice in the context of child welfare. The reflections will result in a proposal for a three-stage approach, in which music therapy can be seen to support the identity development of a young person at levels that range from individual experience to societal participation.

I will describe a case narrative taken from the population of adolescents living under care in the Norwegian child welfare context. The story of Javid, an 18-year-old adolescent, and his peers, joining a music workshop group illustrates how music therapy can be a resource for individual and collective identity-formation processes. The individual and collective identity-formation process of Javid will be used as a basis for a reflective discussion about recent child welfare research, sociocultural theory, and music therapy literature. An increasing number of children and adolescents receive help from Norwegian Child Welfare Services (www.ssb.no/). As seen from a Norwegian perspective, one challenge is that the child welfare systems lack practices that can improve the quality of participation in child welfare work (Christiansen et al., 2015). Some scholars have demonstrated that the system is not sufficiently designed to facilitate dialogue and communication among young people and their supporting adults (Kayed et al., 2015). Others have even implied that the rules, procedures, and programmes provided by the child welfare system may actually hinder participation processes (Tjelflaat and Ulset, 2007). The situation of adolescents under welfare care is not aligned with the rights and values set out by the

United Nations Convention on the Rights of the Child (UNCRC; United Nations, 2009). According to the UNCRC, children and adolescents have several rights, including rights concerning participation, provision, and protection, which include the right to be protected against any threats in the society, the right to take part in everyday activities such as leisure and culture, and the right to be heard concerning important decisions.

I will also turn to sociocultural theory, especially to the concept of structuring resources. Cultural psychology, as seen from a philosophical point of view, builds on a tradition that can be traced back to Hegel (1807/1977) and Marx (1845/1970). Hegel and Marx argued for the developmental perspective that human knowledge is related to historical and sociocultural change. Taking this into consideration, sociocultural theory argues that values, sentiments, attitudes, ideas, beliefs, and choices should be used to explain and predict human behaviour (Stige and Aarø, 2012).

Using a sociocultural perspective on music therapy allows us to focus on the changing attitudes, lifestyles, and values as important factors in the research process. A sociocultural perspective implies that various forms of identity construction are linked to each individual's possibilities and power to employ and transform sociocultural structure (Giddens, 1991). Human structuring resources such as knowledge, language, art, and music can be used for reproduction of structures needed for development of identity, creativity, and change. On the other hand, the production of human resources may also influence identity formation in a negative way as, for example, in institutions with asymmetrical power relations amongst staff members and the young persons who receive the child welfare service.

Identity formation has been subject of investigation in music therapy literature over recent years. Research report that music facilitates social relationships and thus for the development of collective identity. Gold et al. (2012) have shown how adolescents use music to develop an emotional framework and human relations. The way that adolescents inform us about the role of music can also be seen in relation to what has been known as resource-oriented music therapy (Rolvsjord, 2010), where music can be used to transform autobiographical experiences into dialogues and performances. Other studies, by Laiho (2004) and Saarikallio and Erkkilä (2007), show how music is used by young people to give shape to personal and social identity processes. The use of music provides continuity of autobiographical stories that include stories about places, people, and events (Ruud, 1997). Music may also facilitate help and support from adults and peer relations (Krüger and Stige, 2015). Moreover, music therapy gives opportunities to establish meeting places where young people experience that their skills and knowledge may be used in new communities of practice, such as school or work (McFerran, 2010).

The music workshop

As a background for the case example, I will describe the music workshop. In the workshop children and adolescents from the aforementioned population receive instruction on instruments, write songs, play together in rock bands, or perform in concerts. Music therapy activities are offered on an individual and a collective basis. Often individual music activities are offered as preparation for participation in a group. It is also possible to invite family members, social workers, or teachers from school as participators or as audiences. Activities consist of many different tasks, with possibilities for the development of many associate social roles and social identities. It is possible to take different positions and roles in a range from being an active to a more passive participant. The passive participant has a prominent role such as audience member, sound technician, or stage worker whereas the active participant can be an actor, guitarist, singer, or rapper, for example. Another active role in the music workshop is to be the leader of processes and to stimulate the progress of a current workflow. The active roles are increasingly involved in influencing what happens and what choices are made. Another role, the chairperson, shall, for example, ensure that everyone's voice is expressed and contributes to the structuring of different topics that are brought forward. The role of a leader requires the ability to safeguard the interests of others and takes great responsibility. The chairperson and head of the process in the music workshop may be the adults, but it may also be necessary to allow the young people to be leaders. When young people take the role of leaders, it is important to offer guidance and close supervision.

Through these music workshops, young people can take part in activities with peers and adults such as social workers, family, or friends. Participation may create opportunities for individual skill development, self-understanding, and social participation. The way the music workshop is organized makes it possible for the participants to find the balance between the individual and communal, and between structure and improvisation. The way that music therapy proceeds may be described as developing through various phases: preparing, working, performing, and evaluating. The phases do not necessarily develop successively, but often overlap and can occur at irregular intervals. The phases are not governed by rules and procedures. Instead, inspired by a UNCRC perspective on participation it is very important that the participants themselves are involved in determining the progress and content of the different phases (Krüger, 2012).

Planning phase

This phase is about identifying individual needs and seeking practical solutions. The music therapist will take part in relevant meetings, and find out about the young people to map relevant aspects such as social network, power relations, and skills needed for the process. Those involved in the phase may be the participants themselves, representatives of the children and adolescents, instructors, and students. It is also appropriate to invite people from school and social work institutions.

Preparation phase

The preparation phase is about getting to know the adolescents. The phase includes activities such as activities for getting acquainted, presentation rounds, a 'low-threshold' (i.e. highly accessible) music café, or tours. At this stage we get to know the young people's interests and goals. The participants are able to get to know how the music workshop works and in which ways they can influence the activities by offering their own ideas. Participants are encouraged to come with their own suggestions for activities. Throughout this phase, relationships and trust among participants can develop. Potential conflicts among members and personal interests are included in further planning, as well as making individual adaptations and adjustments.

Working phase

During this phase, efforts are actively made to meet the needs identified in the previous phase. The phase includes activities such as music rehearsal, songwriting, recording, and performance. Participators collaborate with music therapists to find artistic expressions through which they can convey their meanings. Central to this stage is the need to facilitate the individual so that they can cope with the activities in a group. An example of this would be to play a 4/4 beat on the drums or to learn one-finger guitar chords. Another example might be to write lyrics or record music using music technology.

Realization phase

This penultimate phase is about turning our attention towards the environment, the local community, and the society at large. The phase concerns facilitating performance of songs, texts, or recordings. The phase depends on an active audience that may provide feedback on what is written, rehearsed, or recorded. Music, text, and drama are used to convey stories which are listened to by an audience consisting of friends, family, professionals who are working in the school or child care, peers, relatives, and other important people.

Evaluation phase

Central to the evaluation phase is feedback from the audience and the participants themselves as a basis to adjust and adapt new ideas and practice. It is crucial that the young people's voices are heard in terms of changing practice. Evaluation is conducted through focus groups and/or as individual interviews.

Case narrative

Javid[1] is 18 years old and has a multicultural background. He has lived in Norway for about 3 years and spent most of this time in various institutions. As a 15-year-old boy he fled to Norway from his home country as a refugee. He travelled alone and experienced many dangerous situations and unpleasant experiences during his journey. Some of these experiences have given him symptoms of trauma and he continues to receive treatment for this. He has repeatedly reported having unstable sleep at night as well as having

---

[1] To maintain anonymity this case is constructed from several cases.

problems in concentrating at tasks in school. He is well taken care of by the staff where he lives, but he has problems when it comes to participation in recreational activities and thus to make friends.

When Javid first came to Norway he was quickly offered the opportunity to play musical instruments at the various institutions where he lived. He was introduced to rock bands such as Metallica and Sepultura by adult social workers at one institution, which he came to like. After some time, he was introduced to Norwegian black metal music. By talking about music with adult male social workers and, because of his fascination with metal music, Javid became interested in learning to play the drums. He was allowed to play drums in school after hours.

When I first met Javid it was quite difficult to understand him verbally. Working through the first phase of music therapy, as already outlined, I tried to map Javid's musical identity, his social network and identified needs. I went to meetings with Javid's caregivers to plan and organize the music therapy sessions. At the start of music therapy, Javid talked really quickly and it was necessary to ask him to repeat his words slowly. Even though it was difficult to understand Javid through his words, it was easy to understand his body language. Javid had gestures that clearly communicated his feelings and state of mind; he often communicated that he was frustrated and sorry about his life situation. He talked about his difficult childhood experiences and travel to Norway. He had not seen his parents in a very long time and, although he presumed that they were not alive anymore, he could not be sure. He knew that he had some distant relatives living in Europe, but did not have very much contact with them.

Music was a natural part of the sessions with Javid. They would include listening to music, for example songs by the American punk band The Ramones, and Javid and I would try to compose, record, and perform music together. This was not always a planned intervention, but was part of an on-going activity. Either Javid's own music would be the centre of the process, or I would suggest music for him. The end result was often something other than that planned at the start. Work with the music could be described as a collaborative process. After playing music, Javid and I would usually talk for five minutes and then continue playing again.

During the working phase of music therapy Javid brought lyrics with him. Through a collaborative process of trying and failing, I found a way to sing his lyrics. Based on this process, we made recordings and performances. Javid used his songwriting to express his feelings and thoughts. He would write at home and bring lyrics to music therapy sessions. We could use the time to look at grammar and fix any language mistakes. Working with lyrics could last for months before Javid was satisfied. Javid seemed to use songwriting as a form of diary account, but he also had ambitions of being a songwriter and performer. Both of the goals were taken care of: Javid told me that it was easier for him to express himself through a song than through a conversation. Writing songs helped him to articulate thoughts that otherwise would be difficult to communicate directly through conversation. The following song was written in music therapy by the end of this phase:

Moving
Keep going on from station to station
Tried to flag a ride and go from nation to nation
Standing at the borderline feeling so uncertain
Trying to find out what is hiding behind the next curtain

Left my mum and dad in a small town
They told me to go on even though I was a little kid
Travelled on with a boat that was all too crowdy
Didn't make any friends there even though I tried to say hi and send my love

Javid also wrote songs together with his peers and together they would spend time exploring technology related to recording and performing. In the realization phase of music therapy, Javid and his peers organized a concert where they invited an audience consisting of social workers and friends. The concert became a venue where they could perform lyrics written during the earlier phases of music therapy. At the concert, they were able to convey messages of being stigmatized and marginalized as child welfare users.

The invited audience, including social workers and teachers from school, responded to the young performers and told them that it was very useful to get these messages from the stage. The audience for Javid's and his peers' story, the most important people and closest to them, could take part in their storytelling and be able to acknowledge the performance. It became a way for the adolescents to show an alternative to their well-established identity as 'child welfare users'. Through their music they could stand out as young people worth listening to, people with a voice and a story to tell. In the aftermath of music therapy, Javid was invited to join a conversation where he, together with the music therapist, could evaluate the process of music therapy. Javid described various aspects of the process that he felt had been useful and, in some cases, had not been useful. The feedback Javid provided were used to facilitate practice for both him and other adolescents.

Songwriting as a way of articulating an identity

The story about Javid teaches us how individual and social resources can be used strategically in child welfare work. As the story informs us, music can become an important resource for the forming, expressing, and communicating different personal views. Through Javid's song, 'Moving', and the message that the song gave to adults in the child welfare system, it can be said that Javid used music to articulate a set of resources that helped him organize and make meanings in his everyday life situations. His music making could be understood as a way of creating space for personal reflection in developing a social environment. The use of music also provided Javid with a continuity of autobiographical stories including narratives about places, people, and events. Moreover, music gave Javid opportunities to challenge established positions of power, namely the positions of adults in the child welfare system. By giving Javid a voice to be heard through his music, acceptable protest actions, such as creating an alternative child welfare identity, could be attained.

If we look to sociocultural theory, Lave (1988) uses the concept of structuring resources to describe how individuals create an identity over continuity and make meaning in the transitions between different everyday life situations and contexts. Lave's understanding of structuring resources is complex and she presents different explanations of the term in relation to various contexts. Play is an example of a set of social practices where resources structured at different levels come into play simultaneously. A specific example that she gives is chess (Lave, 1988). To play chess offers opportunities to learn the rules of the game and the names of objects, while there is simultaneously a social interaction between players who can experience humour, frustration, or joy together. By taking part in the activity of playing chess, the participants also take part in the activities of constructing an identity by thinking and feeling. The game is not just about moving pieces according to certain rules, but also about observing body language and facial movements, listening to the other's breath, and so on. Each situation offers resources that the individual can use to solve advanced problems.

Lave's point is that one type of activity can trigger a different type of activity and that they influence each other reciprocally. The activity of playing a game gives form to the activity of doing social activity. Seen in relation to the case narrative of Javid, songwriting could be an example of an activity producing structuring resources on different levels. Songwriting includes the use of physical objects and dialogues, both internal and external. Through the activity of songwriting, the songwriter is equipped with a set of structuring resources that gives structure to dialogues within a relationship and a cultural community. The story of Javid shows that structuring resources produced as a result of a songwriting process could help him construct an identity influenced by social participation.

Music therapy as a collective experience

Javid's experiences can be understood in light of modern identity theory. Sociocultural theory will tell us that identity is always socially and relationally produced. Identity is shaped in dialogue with other people where one can both confirm and test new understandings of who you are. Responses from peers and adults from public performances can be seen as very important in terms of identity as a social and relational product. Identity and adolescents' experience of other people's view of them is ever changing, and the music workshop is an arena where such changes can be experienced, expressed, and performed (Krüger, 2012). This line of thinking is also in line with Giddens' (1991) theory on identity. According to Giddens, a person's identity formation includes a sense of being the same over time and in different situations. Giddens emphasizes the term self-reflexivity. Self-reflexivity implies that we constantly think about and speculate on whom we will be, and that we have the opportunity to rewrite our own history and envision another. The reflexive self implies various sets of opportunities. As a result of Javid's participation in the music workshop, Javid's identity as a refugee could be nuanced and changed. He did not always have to be a 'foster child' or a 'child in care'. Music therapy gave him tools and an arena to rewrite histories about himself with the support of others.

In order to construct an identity, adolescents need others, especially peers. If we look to research on child welfare, the ability to make relationships with peers is an important factor for psychological development in adolescents (Collins and Laursen, 2004). Hence it is worrying that adolescents with experiences from Norwegian child welfare institutions report less positive experiences with friends than other adolescents (Kayed et al., 2015). One reason for the lack of friendship is that adolescents with a child welfare background have to move more frequently than others: adolescents with child welfare experiences move three times more often than their peers (Backe-Hansen et al., 2014). Such practice makes it difficult for lasting friendships to be formed.

On the positive side, research studies show that participation in leisure activities helps adolescents participate in school and to join in with peers (Pecora et al., 2006). Other research also provides evidence that participation in organized leisure activities may prevent crime, drug use, and marginalization (Caldwell and Witt, 2011; Persson et al., 2007). Others point to the fact that organized leisure activities facilitate social problem-solving and increase creativity (Säfvenbom, 1998). Organized leisure activities may also lead to increased self-regulation, motivation, and satisfaction of individual needs (Caldwell and Witt, 2011). In the implementation and evaluation of such approaches, it is important that there is continuity in the activities (Fong et al., 2006). As we saw in the case example of Javid, the music workshop functioned as a community where reciprocal trust and belonging could be found. It is then possible to argue that participation in the music workshop offered the necessary continuity and structure for friendships to form and to be sustained.

Implications for music therapy practice

The use of music therapy in a child welfare setting has many possibilities and may imply different strategies. Drawn from the story of Javid, we can outline three strategies (Fig. 12.1).

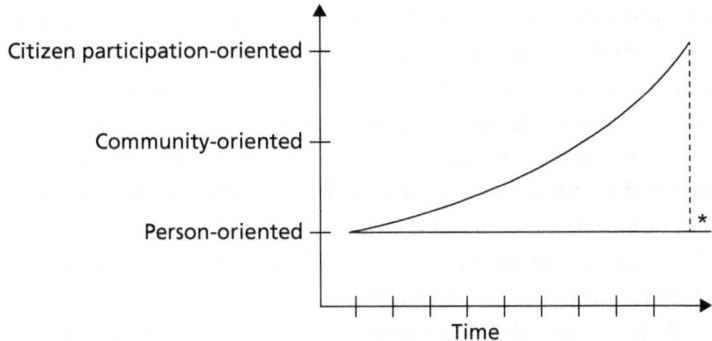

Fig. 12.1 The three strategies for the use of music therapy in a child welfare setting. The asterisk denotes the co-play of strategies in Javid's music therapy development.

First of all, there is the need for a person-oriented strategy. This strategy includes person-oriented activities such as conversation, songwriting, and the use of music technology. This strategy is aligned with Julie Sutton's (2002) description of music therapy as an approach to provide opportunities for the strengthening of communication and relationships. Sutton's approach is related to a perspective on trauma treatment. In many ways, music therapy seems very consistent with recent trauma understanding, suggesting that the ability to regulate difficult emotions is not developed primarily through language and understanding, but through bodily movement and face-to-face communication in relationships (Nordanger and Braarud, 2014).

Secondly, from the case example of Javid we learned that there is the need for a community-oriented strategy wherein activities such as playing in a band or performing at a concert come into focus. The community-oriented approach is important because it implies the facilitation of peer-group relations and contact with family members or adults from child welfare institutions.

Thirdly, music therapy can function as a form of citizen participation. This strategy involves the promotion of community-related aspects such as values, rights, and attitudes (Krüger and Stige, 2014). Music therapy oriented towards this strategy makes it possible to establish meeting places where, for example, music can be used as a resource to challenge established positions of power (Krüger, 2012). Letting young people speak through music and music performances provides a structure and affords acceptable protest actions, such as communicating an alternative identity. Different views on participation may be seen as mutually constitutive and music may be regarded as giving structure to a complex set of participatory practices, including aspects related to community, health, wellbeing, and values related to democracy (Krüger and Stige, 2015). Furthermore, I suggest that the three strategies should be combined to meet the needs of participants. This means that children and young people should be given the opportunity to receive individual guidance through the attainment of protection and support, and that they should have the opportunity to spend time with peers where friendship, participation, and social support can be found. Put another way, it is important that adolescents experience a balance between support, protection, and boundaries, and are given freedom to create an autonomous identity as young people.

Conclusion

In summary, the strategies in music therapy that I have outlined provide opportunities to work in the tension between the individual and the community, between dependence and independence, between the need for protective measures and mesures that facilitate participation, all of these tensions that can be seen in relation to the many paradoxes and dilemmas inherent to the UNCRC (United Nations, 2009). The strategies outlined provide multiple perspectives, where work with the individual can be seen in relation to the community and social environment. As we have seen from the case of Javid, music is a structuring resource which links personal strategies to community and citizen participation.

While strategies may vary over a period of time, the goal set for music therapy can be the same, namely to enhance the individual's ability to succeed in relation to society's opportunities and limitations. Whatever strategy is chosen for the implementation of music therapy in any given context, the need for individual adaptation should always be the guiding factor in the development of music therapy practice.

Acknowledgement

The chapter is written as part of an ongoing research project called 'Towards independent living in a community, a qualitative research study of music therapy practice in the phase of aftercare in child welfare'. I would like to thank Aleris Omsorg Norge for financial support, and I would also like to thank my collegues at GAMUT, Grieg Academy at the University of Bergen for much appreciated help and support in writing this chapter.

References

Backe-Hansen, E., Madsen, C., Kristofersen, L. B., and Hvinden, B. (Eds) (2014). Barnevern I Norge 1990–2010 En longitudinell studie Norsk institutt for forskning om oppvekst, velferd og aldring [Child Welfare in Norway 1990-2010 A longitudinal study, Norwegian Institute for childhood, welfare and aging]. NOVA Rapport 9/2014.

Caldwell, L. L. and Witt, P. A. (2011). Leisure, recreation, and play from a developmental context. *New Directions for Youth Development*, **130**, 13–27.

Christiansen, Ø., Bakketeig, E., Skilbred, D., Madsen, C., Skaale Havnen, K. J., Aarland, K., and Backe Hansen, E. (2015). Forskningskunnskap om barnevernets hjelpetiltak. [Research-based knowledge about child welfare services]. Uni Research Helse,Regionalt kunnskapssenter for barn og unge (RKBU Vest). [Uni Research Health, Regional Center for Childhood and Adolescence].

Collins, W. A. and Laursen, B. (2004). Changing relationships, changing youth: Interpersonal contexts ofadolescent development. *Journal of Early Adolescence*, **24**(1), 55–62.

Fong, R., Schwab, J., and Armour, M. (2006). Continuity of activities and child wellbeing for foster care youth. *Children and Youth Services Review*, **28**, 1359–1374.

Giddens, A. (1991). *Modernity and Self-Identity, Self and Society in the Late Modern Age.* Cambridge: Polity Press.

Gold, C., Saari Kallio, S. H., and McFerran, K. (2012). Music therapy. In R. J. R. Levesque (Ed.), *Encyclopedia of Adolescence* (pp. 1826–1834). New York: Springer.

Hegel, G. W. F. (1807/1977). *Phenomenology of Spirit*, translated by A. V. Miller (1977). Oxford: Oxford University Press.

Kayed, N. S., Jozefiak, T., Rimehaug, T., Tjelflaat, T., Brubakk, A. M., and Wichstrøm, L. (2015). Resultater fra forskningsprosjektet Psykisk helse hos barn og unge i barnevernsinstitusjoner, Regionalt kunnskapssenter for barn og unge—psykisk helsevern [Results from research project of mental health for children and adolescents living in child protection institutions, Regional Centre for Children and Adolescents' Mental Health]. NTNU.

Krüger, V. (2012). Musikk—fortelling—fellesskap: En kvalitativ undersøkelse av ungdommersperspektiver på deltagelse i samfunnsmusikkterapeutisk praksis I barnevernsarbeid [Music—narrative—community: A qualitative study of adolescents' perspectives of a community music therapy project in context of child welfare work]. Doctoral thesis, Grieg Academy, University of Bergen.

Krüger, V. and Stige, B. (2014). Between rights and realities—Music as a structuring resource in the context of child welfare aftercare. A qualitative study. *Nordic Journal of Music Therapy*, 2(24), 99–122. doi:10.1080/08098131.2014.890242.

Krüger, V. and Stige, B. (2015). Music as a structuring resource: A perspective from community music therapy. In H. Klempe (Ed.), *Cultural Psychology of Music Experiences* (pp. 235–250). Charlotte, NC: IAP: Information Age Publications.

Laiho, S. (2004). The psychological functions of music in adolescence. *Nordic Journal of Music Therapy*, 13(1), 47–59.

Lave, J. (1988). *Cognition in Practice*. Cambridge: Cambridge University Press.

Marx, K. (1845/1970). Theses on Feuerbach. In J. Elster and E. Lorenz (Eds), *Verker i Utvalg [Collected Works]*, vol. 2 (pp. 13–15). Oslo: Pax Forlag AS.

McFerran, K. (2010). *Adolescents, Music and Music Therapy: Methods and Techniques for Clinicians, Educators and Students*. London: Jessica Kingsley Publishers.

Nordanger, D. Ø. Braarud, H. C. (2014). Kompleks traumatisering hos barn: En utviklingspsykologisk forståelse [Complex childhood trauma, a developmental perspective]. *Tidsskrift for Norsk psykologforening*, 48(10), 968–972.

Pecora, P., Williams, J., Kessler, R. C., Hiripi, E., O'Brien, K., Emerson, J., Herrick, M. A., and Torres, D. (2006). Assessing the educational achievements of adults who were formerly placed in family foster care. *Child & Family Social Work*, 11, 220–231.

Persson, A., Kerr, M., and Stattin, H. (2007). Staying in or moving away from structured activities: Explanations involving parents and peers. *Developmental Psychology*, 43(1), 197–207.

Rolvsjord, R. (2010). *Resource-Oriented Music Therapy in Mental Health Care*. Gilsum, NH: Barcelona Publishers.

Ruud, E. (1997). *Music and Identity*. Oslo: University Press.

Saarikallio, S. and Erkkila, J. (2007). The role of music in adolescents' mood regulation. *Psychology of Music*, 35(1), 88–109.

Säfvenbom, R. (1998). *Four Thousand Hours a Year, Leisure Time and Its Developmental Potential for Adolescents That Youth Protection Institutions*. Oslo. Norwegian School of Sport Sciences.

Stige, B. and Aarø, L. E. (2012). *Invitation to Community Music Therapy*. New York: Routledge.

Sutton, J. (Ed.). (2002). *Music Therapy and Trauma, International Perspectives*. London: Jessica Kingsley Publishers.

Tjelflaat, T. and Ulset, G. (2007). Barn og unges medvirkning i institusjon, Rapport nr. 11 i skriftserien til Barnevernets utviklingssenter i Midt-Norge.

United Nations. (2009). *Rights of the Child*. Resolution adopted by the General Assembly, A/RES/64/146, December. United Nations.

Chapter 13

Working in music with adolescents who experience disability

Daphne Rickson

Introduction

Adolescents have varying individual physical, mental, or psychological resources to draw on as they negotiate the social process of discovering what it means to be an adult. Those who experience disability can be particularly challenged to develop the skills that will enable them to become increasingly independent and responsible for their own actions. A process of music therapy that takes account of their individual physical, cognitive, social, and emotional strengths and challenges in the context of their social and cultural networks can support them to develop the resources they need to grow and maintain a positive sense of wellbeing.

The following vignettes from music therapy practice demonstrate how young people with disabilities have drawn on the affordances of music to reduce stress and anxiety and to regulate affect; to develop individuation, self and group awareness, and social competence; and to feel safe enough to engage and connect with others. This in turn led them towards cultural integration. They have used their strengths and musical intelligence to achieve and experience success, and to create positive and robust memories that have enhanced their self-esteem.

Adolescents living with attention-deficit/hyperactivity disorder (ADHD) working in a special school setting—a case vignette

As humans we have a basic need to be able to participate and to feel as if we belong within our communities. We become unwell, not only because of differences or changes in our bodies, but when we are badly treated, ignored, or misunderstood. Adolescents experiencing disability are faced with multiple challenges as they move towards adulthood (Groce, 2004; Pineda, 2014) and are particularly vulnerable in this regard. They have to negotiate their identities through disability labels and specialized educational, medical, and psychological services (Pineda, 2014) and regular confrontations with stigma, inequality, and discrimination (United Nations Children's Fund, 2013; World Health Organization and The World Bank, 2011). Powerlessness and lack of authority can force them into cycles of dependency, unable to know themselves, their needs, capabilities, and options, and this leads to their exclusion in many and varied ways (Charlton, 2000). It can be difficult for them to understand the situations they find themselves in, and they need assistance to develop the strength and skills they need to cope.

The following paragraphs describe the experiences of a group of six adolescents who were diagnosed as having ADHD and were working at a special school for learners who experienced significant social and emotional difficulties. All struggled to manage their academic work, to respond appropriately to rule-governed behaviour, and to develop social relationships. They each frequently demonstrated aggression in socially inappropriate ways. They attended 16 weekly sessions which were held in a music room at the school. This vignette summarizes their music therapy process.

An anxious beginning

On first meeting the boys were quiet, anxious about the new situation they found themselves in. Gradually they began to communicate more overtly but remained focused on their own needs and desires and appeared unaware of the feelings of other group members. They made inappropriate remarks about each other, without any apparent malicious intent, and were consistently putting down their own ideas. They talked simultaneously and raised their voices to be heard above the others. Yet when music was introduced, they were immediately engaged.

The need for structure

Early music activities were highly structured, specifically inviting the boys to attend more overtly to each other. For example, they would be asked to play a particular instrument for one verse of a song before passing it along. The pulse or rhythm of the accompanying music supported their internal organization and they were more 'settled'. As they developed the skills to maintain a steady beat they were more able to play simultaneously and support each other to solo, using a framework such as the 12-bar blues. This challenged them to work hard to ensure they were playing quietly enough for their peer's contribution to be heard—and they were not always successful. There were times when they would complain about each other's playing, someone would feel they were being 'picked on', and it would become necessary to deal directly with their frustrations. Importantly though, the boys experienced music as containing. During one chaotic moment when they were changing and trying out instruments while preparing to improvise, the music therapist began to play a simple blues riff on the piano. This caught their attention and brought them back to their seats, where they were quiet and ready to attend more carefully to each other.

Developing independence

Gradually the group were able to work with less overt direction or musical containment from the music therapist. In their fifth session they decided to improvise on the theme of a train. This involved them thinking of the sounds encountered on a train ride, and reproducing those sounds on their musical instruments to develop an original group composition. The suggestion of a concrete theme supported their engagement. Someone suggested they begin slowly, increase speed, and return to a slow pace—to mimic the sounds of a train leaving and returning to a station. The boys were enthusiastic and paid considerable attention to each other's musical contributions. They had previously shown a tendency to copy one of the more able boys, particularly when he soloed during body percussion activities. During the train improvisation, however, it was clear that the boys were developing more individuality by establishing their own 'role' in the group, and were beginning to evaluate the strengths of all the group members.

Developing meaningful relationships

During subsequent sessions the group continued to enjoy improvising, became increasingly attentive to each other, and created fleeting but meaningful periods of silence, particularly at the end of their improvisations. The more reluctant participants gradually increased their musical and verbal contributions as they began to trust the group to support their risk-taking, and in turn to sense the groups' appreciation and support for their efforts. They began to pat each other on the back in gestures of encouragement and congratulations, and their comments to each other became increasingly meaningful. Instead of saying 'he was good' for example, they began to say things like 'he was listening well'.

Developing a shared identity

Their increasing abilities with self-expression and cooperation were evident in their song writing too. Initially their lyrics were unimaginative, grounded in the here and now, and consisted of concrete stories about what they had done and where they had been.

In an early session for example, using a 12-bar blues framework to contain their song, they wrote:

> We went riding; we went riding last night (riding last night)
> We went riding; we went riding last night (riding last night)
> We saw rabbits and possums and cats and it was cool.
> We went riding; we went riding last night (riding last night)
> We went riding; we went riding last night (riding last night)
> We went up a hill and skidded in the school van.

Over time as they began to share and laugh about specific incidents that had occurred at school, they began to take more risks in their communication with each other. Their singing became stronger. They composed increasingly sophisticated lyrics, and were able to communicate meaningful messages and to express their frustration through their songs. Their composition, 'Laundry Blues', was one example. They were all asked to take a turn working in the school laundry, in what they described as a 'hot', 'smelly', and 'boring' environment. During the seemingly cathartic process of writing and singing about this experience the boys shouted and swore, but also laughed. In the further example below, the boys are expressing their confusion regarding their 'incarceration' in a special residential school.

People think that our school is nothing
People think that our school is nothing
People think that but I know it's not true

People say that we're wasting our precious time
People say that we're wasting our precious time
But do they know? Do they know what we're talking about?

Do they know what we are talking about?
Do they know what we are talking about?
When we say they are our friends? I don't think so!

We need to be kind to others and treat them with respect
We need to be kind to others and treat them with respect
These are the things that help us in life, and that's the school rules!

We're jumping and thumping at music bro and that's ok
We're jumping and thumping at music bro and that's ok
Music is cool and it's a safe and happy place!

We know that we are lucky to be at our school
We know that we are lucky to be at our school
They pay for our outings, and also for our food

Reflections on the vignette

The success of group work with this population depends on deliberate and careful planning of specific tasks that bring relationship issues to the fore and give the adolescents opportunities to alter their feelings towards others and themselves (Malekoff, 2006). Group music making provides excellent opportunities for this development as it provides inherent boundaries and directions, as well as opportunities for creative expression. This non-directive and non-confrontational approach respects the adolescents' autonomy and offers many opportunities for self-expression and development of positive identity (Frisch, 1990). It seemed important for initial sessions to be highly structured and to involve direct teaching of appropriate group social skills until the boys developed their abilities to cooperate independently.

When making music the group became unified. While they were playing they remained involved and their music making was cohesive. However, during transition times, between music making tasks, they were less able to focus. They engaged relatively easily in the sessions because they viewed music positively, it was an important part of their subculture, and they considered it non-threatening compared with other 'interventions' they were exposed to. The process of group music making increased the boys' awareness of the existence and feelings of others, and helped them to develop relationships based on respect and trust. As they began to recognize the benefits of collaborative musicking they needed less external reinforcement. Learning to get along with others and developing friendships in a small group setting would enable them, to a certain extent, to transfer their new skills to a natural social environment.

Adolescents living with intellectual disability as music leaders—a case vignette

Adolescence generally brings opportunities coupled with uncertainties, challenges, and risks which can lead to emotional turbulence, a reduced sense of control, and feelings of insecurity, all of which can be intensified for young people experiencing disability (Blacher, 2004; King et al., 2006). They usually have limited autonomy and are often unable to independently engage with the typical tasks of adolescence which involve spending less time with family and more with friends, learning to independently regulate emotions, developing coping skills, and becoming increasingly responsible for one's own actions. They are often held back by parents and other professionals who have low expectations of what they can achieve (Shifrer, 2013) and overprotect, control opportunities, and inhibit their independent decision-making capabilities and coping strategies (Dos Santos et al., 2016; Pineda, 2014). If they are not sufficiently supported during this time, they can develop feelings of apathy, doubt, dependency, and depression (Pineda, 2014), and isolation, lowered self-esteem, and lack of hope for the future (King et al., 2006). They may need particular help to reduce their levels of anxiety, to express their emotions in constructive ways, to regulate their affect, and to develop conflict-resolution skills.

The following paragraphs are drawn from ACTIVE Music, a collaborative music research project involving three music therapists and 12 young people with intellectual disability, which took place in a university setting. All participants were both musicians and co-researchers. The music sessions took place in a well-equipped music room, and the young people were asked to make suggestions about the music they would like to listen to and the instruments they would like to play. The primary focus of the research was to find out from the young people themselves the ways music making might support them as they transitioned from school to work. We aimed to develop a culture of interdependence which recognized that mutual support is beneficial for everyone. One of the main manifestations of our interdependence is our carefully co-constructed research findings (Rickson et al., 2014). The themes presented here, even though they represent only some of the findings, have therefore been reproduced verbatim[1]. Hearing the young people's voices is more powerful than reading a summary of their work. Their findings clearly indicate what they value, and the impact of musicking on their developing identities, relationships, and independence.

---

[1] I acknowledge and thank the team: Axel Evans, Natasha Ratitihuia Claydon, Patrice Dennis, David Cree, Kate Dovey, Tess Kiernan Francis, Janiece Pollock, Shafiq Sos, Erin Upjohn-Beatson, Kwame Williams, Jacob Dombroski, Sarah McMahon, Tessa Haanen, Edward Watkins, and Daphne Rickson.

Music groups can be fun

We enjoyed doing a wide variety of musical activities. We like music, we believe it is good for us to go to music, and we feel as if we have achieved a lot of things. Music group was mostly a fun and happy place.

Music groups are good places to develop social skills (fun but hard work)

The music group was both fun and hard work. We had different ideas about what we liked at music, and it was often hard choosing what music to do. We learnt a lot about how to work together. We found out quickly that very noisy places were not helpful for some people because it hurt their ears, or because they couldn't hear each other. We learnt to adjust the volume and tempo of our music to fit in with what others in the group were playing. The size of the music group meant that people could not always do what they would choose to do. We had to be patient and tolerant while waiting for our turn. We got better at listening to each other, helping each other in practical ways, and working out what we would do as a group.

Music groups can be good places to develop independence

At first we liked familiar things. New things can be scary for us. Being in a new place and trying new things was difficult for most of us. The university was a confusing and daunting place to be in and some of us found it hard to talk with staff and other students, especially at first. When we started our music research we liked having our support people with us. Later we were keen to be at music without them because we wanted to be independent. Over the 20 weeks we became more relaxed. We explored the university a bit more when we had been going there for a while, and some of us talked to other students and staff when we had jobs to do like photocopying the data in the staff room. We like being with friends, but meeting new people can be good too. We began to enjoy being in the university environment. It might take a bit longer for us to be completely comfortable, but we like lots of things about it now.

It is hard when we want to be independent but still need help. The music group was a place where we were encouraged to ask for help, and we could practice asking for help when we needed it. We asked Daphne, Patrice, and Erin to help us to play our favourite instruments by showing us ways we could join in. Trying new things was hard, but when someone suggested a new music activity, most people wanted to 'give it a go'. We thought it was good to learn how to do something different. We made mistakes but it was good to learn by practising. We wanted to learn new things, and we worked hard to get them right. Over time we became more independent. We decided by ourselves that we wanted to put on a concert for family and friends. We sent invitations, booked the room, borrowed some instruments, and organized supper by ourselves. Tash took a very important role to be the 'master of ceremonies' on the night.

Music groups are good places to practice teamwork

In music groups we learnt to notice what other people were doing. We learnt to accept that people contribute in different ways and that everyone's contribution is important and helpful. Sometimes someone did a solo, and others listened and watched. Listening and watching is important. Some people found it hard to join in but they kept trying to. We learnt which part to play, practiced our parts, played together, and took turns.

Some of us were able to do things that we had never done in the group before, like doing a solo song, or playing an instrument on our own without help. One person liked doing the filming. We all had individual parts to play, but we felt as if we were a team when we were playing music together. We made mistakes but it was good to learn by practising. We liked it when other people were good at music. Someone wrote in their journal 'Being respectful and nice is good'.

Music groups can be safe places to express emotions

A fierce spring storm is being recreated ... The music rolls in waves, building steadily to a gusty roar, before dying away. The musicians watch each other for cues, responding to the sounds of drums and chimes and adding their own textures. When they finish the room is silent. Then it is smiles all round.

(Harding, 2013)

These words were written by a reporter who heard our music early on. It shows how we were able to improvise on musical instruments to express ourselves. We made the music up as we went along. We worked together, listening and watching each other, we told a story, and it made us feel good.

Our music and research group was a place where we felt safe. We trusted each other. This was important. We could express things that were difficult for us. Sometimes we did this in the music, sometimes we did it with words, and sometimes we did it in other ways. Even though music was mostly a happy place, sometimes we were sad, confused, and even angry. We agreed that doing music, or listening to music, can be helpful when we are feeling upset. People wrote in their journals, 'the music helped, the beat makes people happy' and 'it is good that there were less sad people after music'.

But Tess noticed that she also needed the support of the people at music as well. Having good relationships with other members of the group is important.

I love music because it calms me down when I'm upset. But I can't go to music lessons by myself—I would need you to come with me because I get a bit nervous. If I get upset I go outside for fresh air, or I go near the door of music and I come and sit down. I just sit down and listen. Being at music and listening to it on the tape as well or you know listen to CD ... just listening to nice music and hugging people and all that stuff ... calms me down.

(Tess, interview)

Music reminded Kwame of his family, who live far away, and this made him sad. Listening to music made him feel so sad he felt he couldn't come back to our group after Christmas. He wanted to try, but in the end he stopped coming. Some of us found it hard being at music when our friends were away too. But music can be comforting because it is familiar. So we were mostly relaxed at music.

Music helps us to know people, and connects us

We talked about music that was important to us. We noticed that music is very personal, and that it reflects people's personalities. When we listened and talked about the music that we love, we learnt more about each other. We found that it was very helpful to do music for a friend who died. It helped us to remember her; it helped us to cry; and then it helped us to feel better.

… when our favourite friend passed away on the 4th of October, it was so sad; everyone was really sad. And so I gave everyone a hug, especially (the people) that went to school with her. We were doing songs that she loved.

(Tash, journal entry)

Reflections on the vignette

It is evident that the young people were increasingly empowered as they began to take responsibility for how they participated; negotiated what they wanted to do and for how long, what changes they would make, and what products they would create (Rickson and McFerran, 2014). Three group members presented the findings of the research at an international music research conference, after their abstract was accepted following blind peer review. They reported:

We found out that music groups can be fun. They can also be hard work. They help us develop skills like listening and waiting. They are places where we can be independent. But music groups are also good places to practice working as a team. They can be safe places for people to express emotions. Music helps us to know people. It brings us together. Playing musical instruments can also help physical development. A good life for us would include having the chance to play music with others or to have music lessons. But it is not always easy for us to go to ordinary lessons or music groups. It might be important for young people with intellectual disability to have support from people who understand them at first. We want to be independent but we need help to develop our dreams in practical ways.

(Rickson et al., 2014)

Discussion

Wellbeing is strongly associated with having the necessary resources to meet the demands of daily life and the ability to act and to achieve ones goals. Communities have a duty to remove the hurdles that impede or diminish the participation of adolescents who are experiencing disability. Parents and professionals have the power to expand and nurture their development, and to increase their capacity, freedom, and sense of self-worth (Dos Santos et al., 2016; Pineda, 2014). With adequate supports, they can begin to understand their differences as strengths and not as weaknesses, see themselves as capable, and know that they can play a positive role in society.

Ways need to be found to increase their resilience, competence, feelings of connectedness, and sense of identity. Like all young people they need to be able to reflect positively on what they have been able to do, or might be able to do, in particular contexts over time, and in relation to other people. The stories they imagine and tell about themselves help them make decisions about who they will be as adults. When they are provided with a full range of options, empowered to make their own decisions about what they can and will do, and are enabled to carry through their planning and decision making, they can achieve the sense of agency that is crucial in adolescent wellbeing (Dos Santos et al., 2016; Pineda, 2014). Then, as they are more able to manage themselves, they are more readily integrated within their communities.

Music is a resource that can highlight such capabilities, by providing opportunities for the positive and successful participation of adolescents who are experiencing disability. It can be used to 'regulate, master and influence emotions (as an individual resource) and to inform the construction of identity and socialization (as a social resource)' (Beckmann, 2013, p. 113). It plays an important role in identity formation because it provides access to strong and emotional experiences that define, develop, and change the self (North and Hargreaves, 1999). Our health and wellbeing can be positively influenced when we engage in interpersonal processes such as music making which foster acceptance of personal and cultural diversity, and the development of mutual respect. However, as Gary Ansdell (2014) notes, it is not music per se that helps; rather, it is the things that people do with music and the contexts in which they do them that are important.

Various types of music experiences, such as singing, listening, playing musical instruments, composing music, and talking about music, can be structured to help adolescents who experience disability to develop skills or to relate to others. Music therapists working with adolescents tend to focus on their functional independence and emotional wellbeing, i.e. the ways in which they manage in their homes, schools, and wider communities (Meadows, 2011). Music can provide the motivation, structure, and inherent repetition needed to help them to process and retain information. It can provide them with the resources to interact with and to become more aware of disabled or non-disabled peers, and enable them to offer genuine and meaningful responses and to have a strong experience of connecting with others. Even those living with severe and profound disabilities can negotiate and express issues and emotions in inclusive music groups (Elefant, 2010; Thompson and McFerran, 2015) because music therapy creates engaging conditions that motivate their interaction within relationship (Thompson and McFerran, 2015).

Music is a fun, motivating, engaging, and non-threatening medium for adolescents who experience disabilities to work with. It provides inherent boundaries and directions, and many opportunities for self-expression and the development of positive identity. Music groups provide contexts in which the young people themselves can be more autonomous, take responsibility for their own participation, choose the activities they will participate in, and decide when and how they will participate. However, as the young people in the second vignette noticed, they needed a safe supportive environment in which to rehearse the skills that would foster their developing self-expression, self-awareness, and independence. The success of both groups relied on the careful facilitation of music opportunities that would enable the adolescents experiencing disability to recognize and acknowledge the existence and feelings of others, and provide opportunities for them to rehearse social skills, to give and receive respect, to learn to trust others, and to develop the meaningful relationships that are so essential to their health and wellbeing.

References

Ansdell, G. (2014). *How Music Helps in Music Therapy and Everyday Life*. Farnham: Ashgate.

Beckmann, H. B. (2013). Music, adolescents and health: Narratives about how young people use music as a health resource in daily life. In L. Ole Bonde, E. Ruud, M. Strand Skanland, and G. Trondalen (Eds), *Musical Life Stores: Narratives on Health Musicking* (vol. 6: Centre for Music and Health Publication Series) (pp. 95–116). Oslo: Norwegian Academy of Music.

Blacher, J. (2004). Transition to adulthood for students with severe intellectual disabilities: Shifting toward person-family interdependent planning. *Research & Practice for Persons with Severe Disabilities*, **29**(1), 53–57.

Charlton, J. I. (2000). *Nothing About Us Without Us: Disability Oppression and Empowerment*. Berkeley, CA: University of California Press.

Dos Santos, T. V., Moreira, M. C. N., and Gomes, R. C. (2016). When participation of children and youth with disabilities is not merely activity: A study of the literature. *Ciência & Saúde Coletiva*, **21**(10), 3111–3120.

Elefant, C. (2010). Reflection: Musical inclusion, intergroup relations, and community development. In B. Stige, C. Elefant, M. Pavlicevic, and G. Ansdell (Eds), *Where Music Helps: Community Music Therapy in Action and Reflection* (pp. 75–92)., Farnham: Ashgate Publishing.

Frisch, A. (1990). Symbol and structure: Music therapy for the adolescent psychiatric inpatient. *Music Therapy*, **9**(1), 16–33.

Groce, N. E. (2004). Adolescents and youth with disability: Issues and challenges. *Asia Pacific Disability Rehabilitation Journal*, **15**(2), 13–23.

Harding, P. (2013). In tune with changing times. *Community Moves*. Available from https://ihc.org.nz/our-publications.

King, G. A., Baldwin, P. J., Currie, M., and Evans, J. (2006). The effectiveness of transition strategies for youth with disabilities. *Children's Health Care*, **35**(2), 155–178.

Malekoff, A. (2006). *Group Work with Adolescents: Principles and Practice. Second Edition. Social Work Practice with Children and Families*. New York: Guilford Publications.

Meadows, A. (Ed.). (2011). *Developments in Music Therapy Practice: Case Study Perspectives*. Gilsum, NH: Barcelona Publishers.

North, A. C. and Hargreaves, D. J. (1999). Music and adolescent identity. *Music Education Research*, **1**(1), 75–92.

Pineda, V. (2014). Building capability and functioning: Reframing the rights agenda for adolescents through the lens of disability rights. In J. Bhabha (Ed.), *Human Rights and Adolescents* (pp. 77–101). Philadelphia, PA: University of Pennsylvania Press.

Rickson, D. J., & and McferranMcFerran, K. (2014). *Creating music cultures in the schools: A perspective from community music therapy.* University Park, IL: Barcelona Publishers.

Rickson, D. J., Evans, A., Claydon, N. R., Dennis, P., Dovey, K., Francis, T. K. et al. (2014). *Active Music.* Wellington, NZ: Massey University.

Shifrer, D. (2013). Stigma of a label: Educational expectations for high school students labelled with learning disabilities. *Journal of Health and Social Behaviour,* **54**(4), 462–480.

Thompson, G. A. and McFerran, K. S. (2015). Music therapy with young people who have profound intellectual and developmental disability: Four case studies exploring communication and engagement within musical interactions. *Journal of Intellectual & Developmental Disability,* **40**(1), 1–11.

United Nations Children's Fund. (2013). *Children with Disabilities. The State of the World's Children 2013.* Available at: www.unicef.org/sowc2013/report.html. (accessed 4 December 2018).

World Health Organization and The World Bank. (2011). *World Report on Disability.* Available at: www.who.int/disabilities/world_report/2011/report.pdf. (accessed 4 December 2018).

Chapter 14

Reframing intervention and inclusion: The importance of exploring gender and sexuality in music therapy with all young people

Elly Scrine

Introduction

> We are on the verge of a queer and trans revolution.
>
> *21-year-old Australian trans non-binary author and youth*
> *advocate Nevo (Zisin, 2017)*

Working with adolescents in music-based contexts requires us to think about and explore gender and sexuality for a number of reasons. Discourse is always shifting, and currently these discussions are undergoing significant transformation across health, education, academic, media, and arts contexts. It is in the best interests of those who conduct therapeutic, educational, or community-based work to understand and engage in this discourse. Across these contexts, the violence and systematic exclusion experienced by young people based on their gender and sexual identity is well documented. Lesbian, gay, bisexual, transgender, queer, intersex, asexual (LGBTQIA+) young people are significantly more likely to experience poor mental health than the general population (Robinson et al., 2014). An Australian study found that 21% of trans and gender-diverse adolescents had been physically assaulted on the basis of their gender identity, and that over 90% of those who had been abused had thought about suicide (Smith et al., 2014). A taskforce in the United States showed 61% of transgender respondents had been the victim of physical assault and 64% of sexual assault, and noted that violence disproportionately effects trans women of colour (Grant et al., 2010). Indeed, forces of violence compound and intersect in specific and unique forms, depending on how we are positioned socioculturally (Crenshaw, 1989). Engaging with these alarming statistics often results in seeing LGBTQIA+ young people through a lens of vulnerability and risk. This chapter explores how and why I believe we can adjust this lens.

A deeper look at youth-focused scholarship reveals that young people are in many ways leading gender-based activism: challenging gendered power imbalances and behaviours linked to endemic gender-based violence through creative and digitially-mediated methods (Retallack et al., 2016). Queer youth act as activist educators for their peers (Hackford-Peer, 2010), they challenge heteronormativity and express diverse identity positions in their schools (McGlashan and Fitzpatrick, 2017), and they create dialogues of resistance that better recognize the ways gender, sexuality, race, and class intersect (Grady et al., 2012). The literature also reveals how creative and arts-based modalities can offer young people meaningful and engaging ways to participate in these explorations. British Professor Emma Renold, a leading researcher in gender, sexuality, and violence with young people, describes the powerful potential of creative and arts-based methods to 'safely and creatively communicate and potentially transform oppressive sexual cultures and practices' (Renold, 2017, p. 1). From a theoretical perspective, the literature underscores the need for sociological responses, taking into account the complex relations of power underpinning rigid gender and sexuality norms (Rasmussen et al., 2017).

Locating and defining gender

Gender and sexuality are two complex and distinct markers of identity through which we position ourselves in the world, and the world positions us. Gender and sexuality are defined and understood in myriad ways throughout the world; our understandings of both are increasingly expanding. Broadly, sexuality is understood as a person's orientation and preference(s) for sensuality and sexual activity (Smith et al., 2014). The World Health Organization (2017) defines gender as 'the socially constructed characteristics of women and men—such as the norms, roles and relationships that exist between them'. Queer theorists such as Judith Butler (1990) and María Lugones (2007) have extensively explored gender as a socially and culturally regulated framework. The construction of gender into a rigid classification system of either male or female is referred to as the gender binary. Feminism and queer theory has worked to highlight the deeply embedded imbalances of power between these categories, how the binary discourages and devalues transgression of gender roles, and erases all possible identities that fall outside this binary. The exploration of how gender and sexuality are regulated also requires reflection upon the ways the gender binary has been normalized and naturalized through processes of white dominance and Western imperialism. Theorists such as Lugones illuminate the coloniality of gender, pointing out how gender 'fuses with race in the operations of colonial power' (2007, p. 186). Gender systems that define gender outside of the cisgender[1] male/female binary are neither new nor Western emergings. Non-European examples include identities such as sistergirls and brotherboys in Aboriginal culture in Australia, *fa'afafine* in Samoan culture, two-spirit in Indigenous North American cultures, *hijras* in South Asian cultures, and many, many more.

---

[1] *Cisgender*: a term used to describe gender identity corresponding to sex assigned at birth.

Troubling notions of risk with an 'after-queer' lens

Researchers with queer and gender-diverse youth have recently deepened critique on ways queer, trans, and gender-diverse adolescents are categorically and institutionally positioned as victims. In addressing the existence of queer youth, texts regularly accompany their descriptions with notions of angst, exclusion, and confusion, constructing young people as harmed, innocent, and powerless (Hackford-Peer, 2010). Mary Lou Rasmussen et al. (2017) explore in detail the tendency for such discourse to enable practitioners to see LGBTQIA+ *only* through a lens of injury and powerlessness. Similarly, Audrey Bryan (2017) describes how groups who are marginalized due to their gender or sexuality can be positioned as universally vulnerable by *virtue* of their gender or sexuality. Such discursive positioning can be understood against a backdrop of gendered, raced, and classed cultural anxieties that pathologize, seek to protect, and/or create singular, universalizing narratives about particular adolescent groups. In order to challenge narratives of risk, and avoid practices of othering or abnormalizing queer youth, we can shift the focus to the conditions and effects of normativity which *every young person is subjected to*. This is known as an 'after-queer' approach (Talburt and Rasmussen, 2010). An after-queer approach implies that issues related to gender and sexuality are relevant for *all* who work with young people to consider—not only those working explicitly in this area. Through deconstructing the notion that to be young and queer implies a universal narrative or set of needs, we are better positioned to work with all young people to challenge oppressive constructions of gender and sexuality.

Locating gender and sexuality in adolescent music therapy

While music therapists have an evidence base, training, and skillset equipping us to support adolescents across a wide range of contexts, there is only an emerging body of literature that considers how gender and sexuality norms impact our clients and how we work with them (Rolvsjord and Halstead, 2013; Halstead and Rolvsjord, 2017; Bain et al., 2016). Much of this literature focuses on music therapists' preparedness to work with LGBTQIA+ clients, and recommendations for best practice (Whitehead-Pleaux et al., 2012, 2013; Wilson and Geist, 2017).

Music therapy as an anti-oppressive practice (Baines, 2013) emphasizes the inextricable links between power structures such as patriarchy, colonialism, heteronormativity, white supremacy, and the personal struggles we experience. Importantly, anti-oppressive practice attends to structures of oppression, rather than stigmatizing or pathologizing the people affected by them. Informed by anti-oppressive approaches in music therapy, as well as the key tenets of queer theory, Candice Bain et al. (2016) introduced a queer music therapy model that aims to work beyond simply *including* queer and gender-diverse young people in the therapeutic space. Rather, it requires us to analyse and destabilize fixed and normative notions of gender and sexuality that position queer and gender non-conforming communities as abnormal. Catherine Boggan et al. (2017) have since investigated music therapists' perspectives and reactions to the queer music therapy model, revealing the range of strengths it offers, as well as inherent gaps and silences in regards to integrating intersectionality theory, and addressing structural privilege within the profession. The authors contend these gaps are reflective of the broader music therapy profession and training programs themselves (Boggan et al., 2017). This chapter departs from these critical beginnings, and several key notions from the wider literature. First, that music is a highly influential part of adolescent identity construction, and has the potential to be both harmful, by reinforcing dominant norms, and powerful, as an anti-oppressive force. Second, that through intentionally recognizing and addressing systems of oppression that exist within and outside of the therapeutic space, music therapy can in itself be considered an 'intervention'. The following illustrative case vignettes draw on queer/after-queer and anti-oppressive approaches to music therapy practice. These approaches share a recognition of the overt as well as the hidden violences faced by particular communities of young people, while intentionally avoiding a response that positions those who are marginalized as the problem, and the ones who require 'fixing'.

Confronting our own beliefs

My car approaches the rural school, where I am running one of the very first songwriting workshops of my research project, exploring gender with a group of young people. I am apprehensive about how they will engage with me and the subject matter I am bringing to the workshop. When I enter the classroom, I notice a group of girls on my right, who remain seated. I read them as standoffish and judgmental, as they watch me from the back of the room. They seem to barely register my presence, instead huddling back to their phones, engrossed in their own conversation which is tempered with shrieks and giggles. I feel a little self-conscious, wondering how they perceive me. I assume what they're looking at is unimportant, that perhaps they are gossiping about somebody, and I prepare to interrupt them to introduce myself.

If we are to utilize music therapy as a space to explore gender and sexuality with adolescents, we must begin to critically attend to our own conscious and unconscious beliefs and worldviews. The gendered discourses at play in my description of the girls in the group are, from a feminist perspective, painful to observe. They speak to entrenched narratives of teenage girls as trivial and hypercritical, as well as my own complex, gendered insecurities. The dominant discourses referred to here create unconscious biases in all of us, rooted in stereotypes and prejudices that we may not even actively support or identify with. Our negative biases and beliefs may even be about people from our own identity groups, stemming from internalized forms of oppression, such as (in this case) internalized misogyny. Our biases do not disappear when we step into a professional space with adolescents, even when we are already deeply committed to approaches and paradigms that actively challenge structures of oppression like heterosexism and patriarchy. Confronting our own unconscious bias requires us to ask ourselves questions around power, privilege and beliefs such as:

- How have I benefited from bias in my life? Am I part of a group who is afforded structural power? Do I see myself represented positively in institutions and the media?

- How do my perceptions and descriptions of clients align with gendered, raced, and classed stereotypes, and what am I doing to interrupt these?

- Who are the young people I *like* working with the most? Do I have particular favourites in groups?

- Which clients make me feel uncomfortable, protective, or wary, and why?

- To whom do I give second chances and the benefit of the doubt? Who do I judge as confirming an expectation?

Assessment is political

I am researching at a school in a very low socioeconomic area. It is my first session with a group of 13–14-year-old boys from mixed cultural backgrounds, who have been identified by the social worker and teaching staff as 'violent', and having issues with anger. My plan for the music therapy group is to create a collaborative space to explore masculinity and emotions, through songwriting, instrumental play, and discussion. We are seated in a circle and start with a drumming exercise I call 'Belief Beats'. Whoever is the leader makes a belief statement, and plays a beat on their drum. Whoever else identifies or agrees with the belief echoes the beat on their drums. I start with a few:

'I think men and women should be equal in society.'
I play: THUMP THUMP THUMP-THUMP THUMP
All the boys echo back: THUMP THUMP THUMP-THUMP THUMP
'I think men and women ARE ALREADY equal in society.'
I play: THUMP - - - THUMP - - -
About three quarters of the boys echo back: THUMP - - - THUMP - - -
'If a boy cries, it means he's probably a bit weak'—and the game continues.

In between the activities that follow, I attend to the boys' engagement with each other, and with me. We are in a small room and there is a lot of noise. I notice myself feeling frazzled; I am nervous about how to control the chaos. The boys yell over the top of each other with gendered and homophobic slurs. Numerous times throughout the session they jump off their chairs to face up to each other, seemingly ready for a fistfight. They kick the chair over. And then, punching the other jokingly on the shoulder, they laugh, and pick the chair back up. One of the boys winks at me and grins, 'Are we scaring ya, Miss?'

Part of the way I conduct assessment is reflective of traditional music therapy practice: observing the ways individuals engage musically, and how they respond, relate to, and communicate with each other, in order to shape my therapeutic goals and facilitation style. However, a crucial part of assessment in this work extends *beyond* observing clients' physical, cognitive, and behavioural needs, or their socioemotional engagement with each other, and into the sociopolitical dynamics of the space, which are so often hidden, invisible, or silenced. This means gauging the young people's own attitudes about gender and sexuality, noticing the language they use, the dynamics that you observe at play in the space, and, crucially, how you understand and respond to these. Assessment requires attending to the covert power dynamics at play in any given context; to the young people's subjective positioning within the setting, and outside of it. At the end of the excerpt, one of the boys asked whether I was scared. As the only person coded 'woman'—a white, queer, university-educated woman— alone in a room with eight young men, I did observe myself experiencing fear and apprehension. The origins of of my fear were important to recognize and reflect upon. I contend that assessment also requires mapping *our own* subjective positioning in the space. In this example, assessment required me to critically examine how my constructions of these young people aligned with dominant classed and raced narratives of particular communities of teenage boys as unruly, threatening, or aggressive, and reflect upon the structural power I held over these boys within the school institution, and beyond. Assessment meant unpacking the very notion of 'violence', especially considering 'angry' and 'violent' were labels the boys had been assigned by the institution. Meanwhile, the systemic violence they experienced and power structures they were expected to thrive under went unseen. Assessment in this case meant problematizing the ways their anger was gendered and pathologized, and required thinking deeply about how music therapy could offer intervention into these systemic processes.

Working towards safe(r) spaces

'Ok folks, let's get the drums out!' Each week at the community youth centre, we start with a drumming game to introduce ourselves. This week there are a few new members, so I explain that at the start of music group, we share our names and our pronouns, then play a drum beat for everybody else to echo back. 'This way, everyone has an opportunity to tell the group how they'd like to be referred to on the day, for example as 'he', 'she', 'they', or something else'. After introductions, we commence work on our group song, which is about the young people's vision for the future. One of the young people, Angel, who is a non-binary[2] trans femme[3], and usually very quiet during our group, begins to raise something they have been thinking about this week. 'I've been thinking how, in the future, travel won't be so hard, and—'. Jack, one of the new members interrupts Angel, 'Oh yeah, cause we'll have driverless cars and stuff'. Angel sits back in their chair and mutters, 'No… that's not what I meant. Anyway, don't worry', before falling back into silence.

When working with adolescents to explore issues related to gender and sexuality, the safety of the space is something I prioritize. This subject matter can be sensitive, triggering, and create disagreement among participants; it may relate to their own identities, or touch on complex, painful experiences they have internalized. It is also crucial to recognize that marginalized groups such as queer and gender-diverse young people may experience few spaces that are safe. This vignette illustrates some specific practices I incorporate, such as addressing pronouns, and replacing gendered terms (such as 'guys', 'ladies', or 'boys'), with gender-neutral terms like 'folks', 'mates', 'people', or 'everyone'. Creating a

---

[2] *Non-binary*: a term used to describe gender identity outside of the gender binary.

[3] *Trans femme*: term used to describe an umbrella of queer feminine identities.

group agreement about behaviour and expectations can be helpful for addressing overt issues such as racism, sexism, or interrupting, but also for lesser-understood issues like victim blaming[4], transmisogyny[5], ableism[6], tone policing[7], cissexism[8], and so on. The issues raised in this vignette may have been better navigated had I raised our group agreement at the beginning of the session. After that session, Angel clarified to me that their point was about navigating venues, events, and airports—spaces where they are required to present identification, as a person who visibly transgresses gender norms. Angel's experiences of transphobia and transmisogyny, issues the group were passionate about challenging, were inadvertently erased by the interruption. Sensing a need to attend to the group dynamics, during the next session we had a discussion about visibility and erasure. I invited the young people to share their own experiences, and how we as a group could better support and hold space for these members, and the wider community.

Responding to disclosures

Part of creating a safer space means recognizing the potential for young people to have experienced or be currently experiencing trauma and/or abuse, and the physical, social, cultural, psychological, behavioural, spiritual, and sexual impacts this may have on a young person. While it is beyond the scope of this chapter to delve into the incidence and impacts of abuse and trauma, I note two things here. First, that we must expand the dominant trauma paradigm *beyond* individualized notions of trauma only as a single, catastrophic event, in order to recognize the trauma of historical violence, collective memory, and enduring colonial injustices (Clark, 2016). Second, that as adolescent practitioners we may hear disclosures of harm, especially when we raise topics related to gender and sexuality in our work. The Listen, Reassure, Respect model is a simple guide for responding to young people's disclosure of abuse/interpersonal harm, drawn from the Australian Institute of Family Studies best practice guidelines (Partners in Prevention, 2017):

Listen: If you sense a young person is disclosing abuse, move to a quiet environment free of distractions. Listen patiently and calmly, allowing the young person to feel heard. Avoid leading questions or quizzing the young person about the details.

Reassure: Reassure the young person that it is OK for them to have told you about their experience. Address their current safety. Reassure the young person that they are not at fault, and that any distress you may feel is not their fault.

---

[4] *Victim blaming*: when a victim is held responsible for harm they have been subjected to.

[5] *Transmisogyny*: cultural and systemic devaluing of transgender women.

[6] *Ableism*: discriminatory cultures and practices in favour of 'able-bodied' people.

[7] *Tone policing*: detracting from the validity of a person's statement by attacking the tone in which it was presented, rather than the message itself.

[8] *Cissexism*: discriminatory cultures and practices in favour of cisgender people.

Respect: Respect the young person's choice to tell you the details they have chosen to, but respect their agency by being clear about mandatory reporting procedures and not pressuring them into giving you information. Acknowledge their bravery and strength.

Supporting young people's gender activism through music

The 'Hear Girls' collective is a group of grade eight students from diverse backgrounds who use music to explore issues related to gender and sexuality. Many of the girls have experienced violence at home, and have spoken about their experiences of violence either in group sessions, or privately with me. We start each session by sharing something one of us has found online. This week, Mikki is excited to share a video of a teenage girl performing a poem about girlhood, sexuality, and safety. We discuss the poem, how we relate to the poet's experiences, and one of the girls, Tayla, mentions a pop song that she feels relates to the poet's message.

I ask the girls if they would like to create a playlist, and using my iPad I add a couple of songs that have already been suggested and others that come to my mind, and then I pass it round for the girls to add their ideas. We leave the iPad in the middle and decide to keep adding to the playlist, week to week. They want to share the playlist with their friends online, they want it to be public, and Tayla jokes that perhaps it will go viral. I make a mental note to discuss this playlist with the school staff. I want to enquire as to whether the songs on the playlist could be played over the school loudspeaker system as the bell between classes, which usually features music selected by the office staff.

We move onto our main project—songwriting. The girls want to write an R&B song about gender expectations. I move straight to the board with a pen ready, inviting them to respond to my questions. 'What kind of expectations are we talking about?', 'What do you want to change?' I connect the iPad to the speakers and we listen to their playlist while we brainstorm. The whiteboard fills up quickly, and covers a huge range of issues, from toxic masculinity and family violence, to internalized misogyny, to gender as fluid, and sexuality as a spectrum. Below is an excerpt from their song, 'A Perfect World':

VERSE
In a perfect world, for boys violence isn't a way
If they could show their emotions and not push people away
In a perfect world, girls look past the outside
Accepting each other for what's within
Together share the pride
CHORUS
Be more open with yourselves
And with each other
Open your eyes
And see what you discover
And see what you discover

This excerpt demonstrates the ways existing music therapy frameworks and techniques, such as playlist creation and songwriting, can be applied to this work, inviting young people into music as a form of gender-based activism. Community Music Therapy (Stige and Aarø, 2012) emphasizes social action, participation, and collaboration, and programs are focused on impacting the surrounding culture. Through playlist creation, my aim was initially to stimulate the young people's interest by working within their existing preferences; it then extended into considering how we could share their creation with the school and broader community. Simultaneously, Resource-Oriented Music Therapy (Rolvsjord, 2010) critically informed the way I engaged with and related to the young people in the group, emphasizing mutuality and, again, collaboration. Positioning myself as a collaborator and facilitator, rather than an authority, my goal was to ask questions that created opportunities for the young people to express their experiences and ideas, and that challenged the status quo. Particularly within institutional settings built on regulation and control, I have found that creating space in groups where young people are not just *allowed*, but *invited* to comment on and challenge the power structures that position them, can be central to their authentic participation. At the same time, this work also requires constant attention to the complex, often hidden dynamics which make some young people feel safer and more comfortable to express their views than others.

Conclusion

This chapter is an invitation for those who work with adolescents using music to think reflectively about how our professional approach, and the methods we already use in practice, can be applied to explore gender and sexuality with young people. Music therapists are well placed to intervene in discourses that marginalize communities of young people, alienate them, or position them only as vulnerable victims in need of protection. Contemporary research and literature reveals how practitioners across a range of adolescent contexts can approach their work in ways that emphasize collaboration with young people, uncover and address dominant norms and oppressive structures, and take social action. However, such practice requires ongoing critical and reflexive thinking, and it is deeper and more complex than simply working to include those who have historically been excluded. Supporting young people's wellbeing and healthy development requires us to be conscious of fixed constructions of gender and sexuality, and how these norms intersect with race, culture, class, physical ability, and more. We must strive to better recognize how structures of oppression are upheld and maintained within and beyond the therapeutic space. In doing so, we can locate music therapy itself as an intervention into the conditions and effects of normativity to which each of us are subjected, but which manifest and impact us in different and nuanced ways.

References

Bain, C., Grzanka, P., and Crowe, B. (2016). Toward a queer music therapy: The implications of queer theory for radically inclusive music therapy. *The Arts in Psychotherapy*, 50, 22–33.

Baines, S. (2013). Music therapy as an anti-oppressive practice. *The Arts in Psychotherapy*, 40(1), 1–5.

Boggan, C. E., Grzanka, P. R., and Bain, C. L. (2017). Perspectives on queer music therapy: A qualitative analysis of music therapists' reactions to radically inclusive practice. *Journal of Music Therapy*, 54(4), 375–404.

Bryan, A. (2017). Queer youth and mental health: What do educators need to know? *Irish Educational Studies*, 36(1), 73–89.

Butler, J. (1990). *Gender Trouble: Feminism and the Subversion of Identity*. New York: Routledge.

Clark, N. (2016). Shock and awe: Trauma as the new colonial frontier. *Humanities*, 5(1), 1–16.

Crenshaw, K. (1989). Demarginalizing the intersection of race and sex: A Black feminist critique of antidiscrimination doctrine, feminist theory and antiracist politics. *The University of Chicago Form*, 140, 139–167.

Grady, J., Marquez, R., and McLaren, P. (2012). A critique of neoliberalism with fierceness: Queer youth of color creating dialogues of resistance. *Journal of Homosexuality*, 59(7), 982–1004.

Grant, J. M., Mottet, L. A., Tanis, J., Herman, J. L., Harrison, J., and Keisling, M. (2010). National transgender discrimination survey report on health and health care. Washington, DC: National Center for Transgender Equality and the National Gay and Lesbian Task Force.

Hackford-Peer, K. (2010). In the name of safety: Discursive positionings of queer youth. *Studies in Philosophy and Education*, 29(6), 541–556.

Halstead, J. and Rolvsjord, R. (2017). The gendering of musical instruments: What is it? Why does it matter to music therapy? *Nordic Journal of Music Therapy*, 26(1), 3–24.

Lugones, M. (2007). Heterosexualism and the colonial/modern gender system. *Hypatia*, 22(1), 186–209.

McGlashan, H. and Fitzpatrick, K. (2017). LGBTQ youth activism and school: Challenging sexuality and gender norms. *Health Education*, 117(5), 485–497.

Partners in Prevention. (2017). Responding to disclosures. Available at: www.partnersinprevention.org.au/resources/responding-to-disclosures/. (accessed 6 December 2018).

Rasmussen, M. L., Sanjakdar, F., Allen, L., Quinlivan, K. and Bromdal, A. (2017). Homophobia, transphobia, young people and the question of responsibility. *Discourse: Studies in the Cultural Politics of Education*, 38(1), 30–42.

Renold, E. (2018). "Feel what I feel": Making da(r)ta with teen girls for creative activisms on how sexual violence matters. *Journal of Gender Studies*, 27(1), 37-55.

Retallack, H., Ringrose, J., and Lawrence, E. (2016). 'Fuck your body image': Teen girls' Twitter and Instagram feminism in and around school. In J. Coffey, S. Budgeon, & H. Cahill (Eds.), *Learning Bodies: The body in youth and childhood studies* (pp. 85–103). Singapore: Springer.

Robinson, K. H., Bansel, P., Denson, N., Ovenden, G., and Davies, C. (2014). Growing up queer: Issues facing young Australians who are gender variant and sexuality diverse. Young and Well Research Centre. Available at: www.glhv.org.au/sites/default/files/Growing_Up_Queer2014.pdf (accessed 13 December 2018).

Rolvsjord, R. (2010). *Resource-oriented Music Therapy in Mental Health Care*. Gilsum, NH: Barcelona.

Rolvsjord, R. and Halstead, J. (2013). A woman's voice: The politics of gender identity in music therapy and everyday life. *The Arts in Psychotherapy*, 40(4), 420–427.

Smith, E., Jones, T., Ward, R., Dixon, J., Mitchell, A., and Hillier, L. (2014). *From Blues to Rainbows: Mental Health and Wellbeing of Gender Diverse and Transgender Young People in Australia*. Melbourne: The Australian Research Centre in Sex, Health, and Society.

Stige, B. and Aarø, L. (2012). *Invitation to Community Music Therapy*. New York: Routledge.

Talburt, S. and Rasmussen, M. L. (2010). "After-queer" tendencies in queer research. *International Journal of Qualitative Studies in Education*, 23(1), 1–14.

Whitehead-Pleaux, A., Donnenwerth, A., Robinson, B., Hardy, S., Oswanski, L., Forinash, M., Hearns, M., Anderson, N., and York, E. (2012). Lesbian, bisexual, transgender, and questioning: Best practices in music therapy. *Music Therapy Perspectives*, 30(2), 158–166.

Whitehead-Pleaux, A., Donnenwerth, A., Robinson, B., Hardy, S., Oswanski, L., Forinash, M., Hearns, M., Anderson, N., and Tan, X. (2013). Music therapists' attitudes and actions regarding the LGBTQ community: A preliminary report. *The Arts in Psychotherapy*, 40(4), 409–414.

Wilson, A. and **Geist, K.** (2017). AMTA undergraduate student research award: Music therapy students' preparedness and training to work with LGBT clients. *Music Therapy Perspectives*, **35**(2), 226–227.

World Health Organization. (2017). Gender. Available at: http://apps.who.int/mediacentre/factsheets/fs403/en/index.html. (accessed 13 December 2018).

Zisin, N. (2017). *Finding Nevo: How I Confused Everyone*. Newtown, NSW: Walker Books Australia.

Part 3

Connectedness

Chapter 15

'What's the WiFi code in here?': Connecting with adolescents in music therapy

Philippa Derrington

Introduction

The adolescent's need for a strong sense of belonging, especially from peers, is crucial in the development of self. Connectedness with others is necessary for emotional wellbeing and mental health (Saeri et al., 2017) and, as Andrew Malekoff writes, 'teens who feel connected are less likely to engage in high-risk or internalizing behaviours such as self-harming, violence, early sexual activity, disordered eating, or suicidal behaviour, for example' (2014, p. 142).

This third section of the Handbook allows us to consider how young people use music to connect. Possibilities for connectedness are ever-changing and the following chapters by music psychologists and music therapists focus on young peoples' experiences of connectedness in both face-to-face and online interactions.

With more resources and platforms through which to share and interact than ever before, young people can now choose to experience many different kinds of connectedness, yet adolescence still happens in its own time (and on its own terms) involving physical, emotional, and social growth (Geldard and Geldard, 2004). For a young person who is going through this huge developmental transitional period, many opportunities for online connectedness can be attractive but may also magnify a feeling of isolation that can come with adolescence. The Internet also speeds up communication. It creates a landscape that is fast-paced, immediate, and available on demand. There is a sense that nothing stays the same for long and the speed at which interactions happen and connections are made, and then change, is limitless.

The creative arts offer relational experiences and opportunities for communication and connectedness using multimodal media (Rose, 2017; Ruud, 1998). As the Internet has developed, ways of being involved in and accessing music have changed as well. As Keith Johnstone, a drama teacher writing in 1979, cautioned:

Creating a story, or painting a picture, or making up a poem lay an adolescent wide open to criticism. He therefore has to fake everything so that he appears 'sensitive' or 'witty' or 'tough' or 'intelligent' according to the image that he's trying to establish in the eyes of other people.

(Johnstone, 1979, p. 78).

This creative-expressive dilemma for young people is still alive in the twenty-first century; the framework of the Internet enables the freedom to play, yet the expanded playing field creates a myriad of new complexities.

The diverse voices in this section of the Handbook present a broad view of some of the ways that music offers opportunity for connectedness between young people and others and why that is important. Susan O'Neill (Chapter 16) observes the affordances of spaces in young people's music engagement while Lisa Nikulinsky and Andy Bennett (Chapter 17) outline music scenes for young people, and Helen Oosthuizen (Chapter 18) describes their engagement in group music therapy. Connectedness via online platforms are further explored by Roseann Pluretti and Piotr Bokowsksi (Chapter 19) through the interplay of music and social media in relation to adolescent developmental tasks. Michael Viega (Chapter 20) considers the role of digital music, technology, and media in music therapy. Carmen Cheong-Clinch (Chapter 21) describes an e-platform used in a hospital setting to enable young people to share their preferred music.

In this chapter I present an educational context for music therapy with adolescents who have social, emotional, and mental health needs. Even though the Internet can appear all-consuming, relating offline still has something to offer young people. A research study in this settting showed that young people were, above all, committed to music therapy sessions (Derrington, 2012a) despite the fact that there was not a strong WiFi connection in the room where we worked. I further explore how young people can be empowered to balance their needs for connectedness internally, with others, and to the virtual world. The title of the chapter is inspired by frequent comments about the WiFi connection, or lack of, from the young people I worked with as both researcher and music therapist.

Music therapy in a secondary school

Young people face transition on many levels when they move from primary to secondary school, usually around the age of 11 years in the United Kingdom where I live and work. As well as settling into new schools and establishing new peer groups, they have to adapt to a new school system and get used to different classrooms with a different teacher for each lesson, relying much less on a familiar connection to one particular member of staff (Symonds et al., 2017). These transitions at a vulnerable age can highlight particular needs for some young people.

Having worked as a music therapist at primary and secondary schools for many years, I am aware that integrating therapy within any educational setting can be a complex negotiation between apparently contrasting stances. Back in the 1990s, psychoanalyst

Anton Obholzer (1994) examined how defensive splitting between staff and outside professionals often took precedence over integration and team work. Educationalists Kathryn Ecclestone and Dennis Hayes (2009) have since questioned the therapeutic turn in education and the extent to which teachers are expected to prioritize 'curriculum of the self' and therapeutic approaches to learning, but this could be considered the other extreme.

When working to develop any therapy provision it is important to fully understand the ecology of the school and to find ways to meaningfully share what is happening inside the room outside the room. Generating lines of communication that are open and reciprocal makes a positive impact on the work. For music therapy to be functional in a school, work has to be joined up with teaching staff and fit in with the educational system (Twyford, 2008).

Making therapy available within school is vital (Derrington, 2012a; Alexander, 2012). Having a music therapy space on site can avoid disruption to young people, as well as reduce costs and possible stigma of needing to leave school for an appointment. At such a time of uncertainty, having music therapy as part of the fabric of the school can further engender the young person's sense of security and trust. Equally, being on site means that the therapist can find the most mutually beneficial way to work within an educational assessment system. At one secondary school, I designed accredited learning units for a national award scheme that also helped validate the young person's social and emotional learning through music therapy (Derrington, 2012b).

Although apparently at odds with psychodynamic therapeutic working, the school system and organized structure can actually make an ideal setting for such work: the rules and timetables offer a clear framework and boundaries within which the whole school functions. A school environment offers young people consistency and belonging while they concurrently navigate their changing world.

There has been an increase in understanding of how music therapy can help young people with emotional and social difficulties since the 2000s (Karkou and Sanderson, 2006), with greater emphasis given to schools to intervene early and identify ways to help young people who experience mental health difficulties, as it is recognized that they will have greater difficulty in learning (Department for Education, 2016). Music therapists can respond to this by creating musical school communities and developing music programmes that offer young people opportunities for connectedness, wellbeing, and development (Rickson and McFerran, 2014), as well as providing individual or group music therapy.

The music therapy space

I set up work and conducted research in an old garage within the grounds of the school: a separate brick building that had previously been used as a bike workshop. The space was functional and self-contained; an ideal place for music therapy sessions which was easily accessible yet far enough away from other classrooms. The layout of the garage was important and it housed almost two of every instrument including drum kits. Comfortable chairs were set out next to each other with a range of acoustic and electric instruments within easy reach. A workbench was covered in percussion instruments, a PA system, various microphones, and a video camera on a tripod which the young people were free to use. Even though the garage was tidied up for each new session, it was deliberately left disorderly with the instruments easily available to offer a point of access for young people who might be reticent to play as well as an opportunity to make the space their own.

Together with its uniqueness as a physical space and the resources described, young people—supported in a therapeutic relationship—had room to move physically and metaphorically between childlike and more adult ways of being (Karkou and Joseph, 2017). Analogous to Donald Winnicott's 'holding environment' (Winnicott, 1984) the garage offered a 'potential space' (Winnicott, 1971) and opportunity to play. The space, held within a psychodynamic frame, could also be said to provide 'asylum' which Tia DeNora suggests - recalling its original sense - as 'shelter, safe space, place for living and flourishing, room in which to create, play and rest' (2015, p. 33). As part of the research study (Derrington, 2012a) James, aged 16, spoke about his experience:

Music therapy to me is a sanctuary. It's where I can go at the end of the week to let everything show. . . . It's my time where I play music as I want to.

In order to work with complex emotional responses and sometimes unpredictable behaviour, the space needs to feel safe for both the therapist and the student. Therapists frequently consider how to provide 'a secure base' (Bowlby, 1988) for their clients; however, the therapist also needs to feel secure in order to work effectively. This extends beyond the space and resources available to include the communication systems established with staff.

The music therapy approach

Musical dialogues can happen in many ways. If improvising felt risky and exposing for some of the young people, experimenting with pre-composed musical frameworks could facilitate a sense of security when creatively exploring thoughts and feelings. Young people often chose to listen to music that they liked, sometimes singing along; they wrote their own songs, talked, or initiated playful interactive games without involving music directly (McFerran, 2010; Derrington, 2005). In these dialogues, the balance of initiating, responding, and recognizing when not to play required therapeutic sensitivity. Just as young people can oscillate between needing encouragement while at the same time disregarding adult input, a spontaneous and empathetic response to their musical ideas was often key to their engagement and ability to share their expression in a playful and meaningful way. My approach comes from humanistic roots (Rogers, 1951) and is underpinned by psychodynamic thinking, but has also developed in response to learning from young people. 'Getting alongside' young people, working at their pace and supporting them, with a focus on empowering and listening, can enable young people to gain confidence in working with their own ideas.

The video camera in music therapy

Recording music therapy sessions has become an accepted part of professional practice for a variety of reasons. Carl Rogers introduced recording as a way of reflecting more closely on dialogues within psychotherapy (Hammond, 2015). Mary Priestley (1994) furthered this in music therapy by often listening back to improvisations with clients to further understand and make sense of the work, a process that Gro Trondalen describes as 'self-listening' (2016, p. 43). New technologies offer everyone opportunities in music therapy that did not exist before. As young people tend to store their preferred music on their phones and are likely to bring these to sessions, they can also easily use them to record what happens in sessions, possibly without the therapist's knowledge.

Even with consent, the therapist's privilege of recording sessions and often holding influence over what happens to those recordings can sometimes be overlooked. Ofer Zur (2017) helpfully questions the myth of the 'therapist's omnipotence and the patient's fragility'. In my experience, encouraging young people to be in control of the video camera helped to speak to, and served to minimize, any potential power imbalance in the relationship; it also encouraged an open dialogue about recording.

Making connections in music therapy through the video camera

Young people, who were accustomed to using video recordings as part of their life, enjoyed the camera in music therapy. I noticed that it provided a channel of communication which appeared to be a more indirect way of interacting, so for some young people it proved an easier way to share their thoughts and feelings with me. For videos to be viewed together and witnessed in a different way to how video selfies might be viewed online, for example, gave rich opportunity for exploring emotional expression together.

Jade, 13, used the camera to experiment with different roles. Like many young people, she enjoyed imitating her favourite singers and recreating their music videos. Sessions were spent recording and re-recording different takes of particular songs. She would choreograph these in detail and sometimes ask me to join her in front of the camera, quickly showing me how to do the dance she was planning before we began to film.

She sang along to the songs with great enthusiasm, even when she didn't know the words. Immediately after recording each song she would pore over the footage on the small camera screen hastily reviewing what she saw, and commenting on it, before directing me quickly to begin filming again. Her response was unpredictable and the recordings were met with dismay or delight, largely depending on how she felt.

Jade's use of the camera and her direction over me were important parts of this experience. It felt as if she used sessions to play freely, as she might have done with friends, but the camera allowed her to witness herself repeatedly from outside and to use the process to experiment with different ways of being. Jade's continuous cycle of filming and reviewing throughout a music therapy session became a way for her to organize her emotional responses.

Why recording is important

Creating a recording can allow for something tangible to be taken away from the session, shared, revisited, uploaded, and observed from a distance, in the same way that adolescents instantly record, share, and respond to experiences on social media. It is interesting that all the music therapists' contributions to this section of the Handbook emphasize the importance of producing a recording, which can serve as a reminder of a shared experience and felt connection that can sometimes be difficult to describe. More often than not I was behind the camera, off-screen yet present, but I was clear in my role as facilitator as were the young people. The process of using the camera and creating an artefact is far more effective as a shared experience than in isolation (Pereira et al., 2017).

Young people's ownership of the camera allowed them to decide how to share their stories and, within the robust therapeutic framework of the garage, enabled young people to express and work through strong feelings safely. Acting out fantasies of being performers and playing to huge audiences was held within my sensitive awareness of the risk that the camera could overfeed fantasy, endorse delusions of grandeur and inflate a young person's already fragile self-concept.

On one occasion when Zac, 16, came in to the garage, he seemed unsettled and muttered something to me about another boy. He took off his jacket and chucked it on the floor. He kept his baseball cap on but turned it to face backwards, hunched his shoulders as if preparing for something. Using his phone, he set up a beat through the PA system, and turned up the volume so that the four speakers filled the garage with sound. He asked me to turn the camera on 'cos this needs to be filmed'. He took the microphone off a stand, 'one two, one two', acknowledged me behind the camera, swung the cable free from the desk, and created his space as he looked around him, listened, nodded to the beat, then began:

> *'What you gonna say to me the next time*
> *I come knocking at your door*
> *You gonna say hi?*
> *Fuck the world this is me against yours*
>
> *What am I? I'm my own crew*
> *I'm a free style who wants*
> *to say to you fuck you,*
> *fuck what you think. It's like me against you*
>
> *What are you gonna do the next time*
> *I come knocking at your door.*
> *You gonna run?*
> *Get out my way […]'*

From the start, it was clear that he was challenging someone else. He went on to freestyle about having a fight with another boy and became fully absorbed in the music. It was noticeable from his movement how the aggression built up and moved through him in a piece that lasted more than 10 minutes. Then, as he continued to listen to the accompanying beat for a while, he nodded over to me, to indicate the end and to turn off the camera. As I moved to sit down next to him, he shrugged with some sense of resolution and relief, then quietly asked me 'What did you think?'

Zac was able to address the unknown 'other' through the camera and leave his feelings of anger and confrontation there. He seemed to use the camera as a messenger, but at the same time it was important to him that I listened and witnessed what he was saying. Although he was aware of how he was using the camera for more than just recording, filming for Zac did not seem to be about a desire to share this video with others. For another young person, Josh, the process of creating an object was also the main focus but served a different purpose overall:

Josh, who was 14 at the time, liked songwriting in music therapy. He had been placed into foster care and as a result had to move school and been separated from his siblings. He used the sessions fully, by singing, acting, or talking. In one session he decided that he wanted to record a song for his father with whom he no longer had contact. He directed me to accompany his improvised lyrics on the piano and positioned the camera to the side to capture what he felt was the best possible angle.

Turning to look directly into the camera, he introduced his song with a clear message to his imagined audience. After recording the song, we burned it to disc and he created the sleeve for it. When I gave him the DVD, he took it and immediately snapped it in two. This seemed shocking at the time, as he had spent so long carefully arranging and directing the take. However, his decision to instantly destroy it led us back to talking about what the process had meant for him.

The manner in which Josh was able to vent his anger around his father's absence was pivotal in the therapeutic process. Perhaps, as Johnstone sets out (1979), Josh did not want to lay himself open to criticism from his father, so he had to destroy the recording. As his dad was not around for him to know his feelings, Josh used the camera and the space to share how angry and hurt he was. The process of recording using the video camera and singing to his father appeared to help him to work through aspects of their relationship and the decision to destroy the disc meant that Josh remained in control; he also became aware of some of the anger he was carrying.

What can the video camera add to the therapeutic process?

The camera is shown to act as a container (Bion, 1970) within the contained space of the garage and the therapeutic relationship. As illustrated, the camera could also be said to offer a creative liminal space (Bunt, 2017; Ruud, 1998) to experiment with emerging identities and feelings as young people move between child and adult modes of being and, as Richard Frankel suggests of individual therapy, 'a stillness, which can aid an adolescent in sorting through the differing claims on her being' (1998, p. 47).

Young people use video recordings in music therapy as a way to take risks while not feeling out of control, which Adam Phillips explains is a necessary stage of development leading to an understanding of a new kind of internal environment. Protection from adults 'is both wished for and defied' (Phillips, 1993, p. 26) and using the video camera in music therapy afforded a way for young people to constantly negotiate these boundaries with me. What can return in adolescence is an 'enactment through risk' (Phillips, 1993, p. 26) of the experience of the early holding environment. Risks, Phillips suggests, are indicators of noncompliance that need to be explored in order to re-experience solitude. For Zac, whose holding environment as an infant was not secure, the re-experiencing of this essential phase of infancy (Winnicott, 1984) enabled him to realize how his own body could be a reliable holding environment.

The video camera held different meaning for each young person and the value of recording was not limited to creating an artefact. It was not only about sharing or connecting in a material way but offered opportunities for creating a space within a space in the music therapy garage which could lead to dynamic changes in the therapeutic work. For the young people I worked with, it sometimes appeared that the virtual world was as important as the real world. Their own decisions about sharing any recordings we had made in sessions often led to conversations about trust and vulnerability, when thinking about sharing videos online. Considering the undefined open social arena of the Internet, we were able to explore their own sense of boundaries and those of others, and discuss the consequences of their footprint on social media.

Conclusion

The pace at which young people engage with the Internet is offset by experiencing interactions with others in real time. Regarding online psychotherapy groups, Haim Weinberg refers to the Internet as 'a virtual space with no boundaries' (2014, p. 108). He furthers that 'from a psychological point of view, it can be seen as a giant, boundless potential space (Winnicott, 1987) for reality and fantasy, playing and imagination, closeness and alienation' (Weinberg, 2014, p. 108). The Internet affords young people ideal ways to constantly communicate with their peers and be connected with others, but the therapeutic boundaries within the potential space of the garage offered young people the security to explore new ways of connecting.

In this chapter I have explored how young people used the video camera in music therapy and its integral role in making connections. As a resource in music therapy sessions, the young people used the video camera to embrace the adolescent paradox (Shipley and Odell-Miller, 2012) of seeking freedom while needing direction; experimenting with identity while being held. The camera could help young people to develop awareness of self and other, and lead to positively adaptive interconnectedness and emotional wellbeing.

The integration of music therapy in a secondary school and responsiveness to the structures of the school day, including the creative environment of the garage and the video camera, allowed therapeutic working, communication, and relationships to develop over time. Relational experiences through music in music therapy can enable change (Trondalen, 2016) and the many ways that music therapists respond to meet adolescents in the moment through music can help empower young people to develop autonomy and self-knowledge both internally and in relationship to others. The space to play, experiment, and express themselves in a face-to-face music therapy session that is connected to the vibrant omnipresent virtual world can offer adolescents an extended means of relating and connectedness.

References

Alexander, L. (2012). The adolescent, therapist and school environment. In A. Horne and M. Lanyado (Eds), *Winnicott's Children* (pp. 171-185). Hove: Routledge.

Bion, W. R. (1970). Container and contained. In *Attention and Interpretation* (pp. 72–82). London: Tavistock.

Bowlby, J. (1988). *A Secure Base*. Abingdon: Routledge.

Bunt, L. (2017). Music therapy conversations, episode 2. Podcast. Available from https://www.bamt.org/british-association-for-music-therapy-resources/podcasts.html (accessed 6 December 2018).

Department for Education (2016). Mental health and behaviour in schools. Departmental advice for school staff. Available from www.gov.uk/government/publications/mental-health-and-behaviour-in-schools--2 (accessed 6 December 2018).

Derrington, P. (2005). Teenagers and songwriting. Supporting students in a mainstream secondary school. In F. Baker and T. Wigram (Eds). *Songwriting. Methods, Techniques and Clinical Applications for Music Therapy Clinicians, Educators and Students* (pp. 68-81). London: Jessica Kingsley Publishers

Derrington, P. (2012a). Music therapy for youth at risk: An exploration of clinical practice through research. Unpublished PhD thesis, Anglia Ruskin University. Available from http://arro.anglia.ac.uk/295485/ (accessed 6 December 2018).

Derrington, P. (2012b). "Yeah I'll do music!" Working with secondary-aged young people who have complex emotional and behavioural difficulties. In J. Tomlinson, P. Derrington, and A. Oldfield (Eds), *Music Therapy in Schools: Working with Children of All Ages in Mainsteam and Special Education* (pp. 195–211). London: Jessica Kingsley Publishers.

DeNora, T. (2015). *Music Asylums. Wellbeing through Music in Everyday Life*. Farnham: Ashgate Publishing Ltd.

Eccleston, K. and Hayes, D. (2009). *The Dangerous Rise of Therapeutic Education*. Abingdon: Routledge.

Frankel, R. (1998). *The Adolescent Psyche*. Hove: Routledge.

Geldard, K. and Geldard, D. (2004). *Counselling Adolescents*. London: SAGE Publications.

Hammond, C. (2015). Mind changers: Carl Rogers and the person-centred approach. BBC. Available from www.bbc.co.uk/programmes/b063ztb0 (accessed 6 December 2018).

Johnstone, K. (1979). *Impro: Improvisation and the Theatre*. London: Eyre Methuen.

Karkou, V. and Sanderson, P. (2006). *Arts Therapies. A Research Based Map of the Field*. Edinburgh: Elsevier Science.

Karkou, V. and Joseph, J. (2017). The moving and movement identities of adolescents: Lessons from dance movement psychotherapy in mainstream schools. In R. Macdonald, D. Hargreaves, and D. Miell (Eds), *Handbook of Musical Identities* (pp. 232 – 245). Oxford: Oxford University Press.

Malekoff, A. (2014). *Group Work wth Adolescents*. New York: The Guilford Press.

McFerran, K. (2010). *Adolescents, Music and Music Therapy*. London: Jessica Kingsley.

Obholzer, A. (1994). Fragmentation and integration in a school for physically handicapped children. In *The Unconscious at Work* (pp. 84–93). Hove: Routledge.

Pereira, L. M., Muench, A., and Lawton, B. (2017). The impact of making a video cancer narrative in an adolescent male: A case study. *The Arts in Psychotherapy*, **55**, 195–201.

Phillips, A. (1993) *On Kissing, Tickling and Being Bored*. London: Faber and Faber.

Priestley, M. (1994) *Essays on Analytical Music Therapy*. Phoenixville,: Barcelona Publishers.

Rickson, D. and McFerran, F. (2014). *Creating Music Cultures in the Schools. A Perspective from Community Music Therapy*. University Park, Illinois: Barcelona Publishers.

Rogers, C. (1951) *Client-centered Therapy*. London: Constable and Company.

Rose, S. D. (2017). *The Lived Experience of Improvisation: in Music, Learning and Life*. Bristol: Intellect.

Ruud, E. (1998). *Music Therapy: Improvisation, Communication and Culture*. Gilsum, NH: Barcelona Publishers.

Saeri, A., Cruwys, T., Barlow, F. K., Stronge, S., and Sibley, C. G. (2017). Social connectedness improves public mental health: Investigating bidirectional relationships in the New Zealand attitudes and values survey. *Australian & New Zealand Journal of Psychiatry*, 52(4), 365-374.

Shipley, A. and Odell-Miller, H. (2012). The role of music therapy for anxious adolescent school-refusers: The importance of identity. *British Journal of Music Therapy*, **26**(1), pp. 39-52.

Symonds, J., Hargreaves, J. J., and Long, M. (2017). Music in identity in adolescence across school transitions. In R. Macdonald, D. Hargreaves, and D. Miell (Eds), *Handbook of Musical Identities* (pp. 510 - 526). Oxford: Oxford University Press.

Trondalen, G. (2016). *Relational Music Therapy. An Intersubjective Perspective*. Dallas, TX: Barcelona Publishers.

Twyford, K. (2008). 'Collaborative and transdisciplinary approaches with children'. In K. Twyford and T. Watson (Eds), *Integrated Team Working: Music Therapy as Part of Transdisciplinary and Collaborative Approaches* (pp. 31 -87). London: Jessica Kingsley Publishers.

Weinberg, H. (2014). *The Paradox of Internet Groups. Alone in the Presence of Others*. London: Karnac Books.

Winnicott, D.W. (1971). *Playing and Reality*. London: Tavistock Publications.

Winnicott, D.W. (1984). *Deprivation and Delinquency*. London: Tavistock Publications.

Winnicott, D.W. (1987). *The Maturational Process and the Facilitating Environment*. London: Hogarth

Zur, O. (2017). *Power in Psychotherapy and Counselling*. Zur Institute. Available from www.zurinstitute. com/power_in_therapy.html (accessed 6 December 2018).

Chapter 16

Entangled musical lives: Affordances of spaces in young people's music engagement for connectedness and wellbeing

Susan A. O'Neill

Introduction

Increased fragmentation, mobility, and uncertainty in the world are reflected in the developmental challenges that young people face in what Reed Larson (2011) refers to as 'coming of age in a disorderly world' (p. 330)—a world marked by dissolving boundaries and rapid change (Barnett, 2012). Zygmunt Bauman (2000) describes it as a 'liquid world' that signals a 'fluid modernity' which requires us to rethink old concepts that bind systemic structures and envision new possibilites in their place. In this chapter, I draw on the expression 'entangled musical lives' to explore new possibilities for understanding young people's music engagement by bringing together two dimensions of music making in their entanglement: meaning and materiality. The notion of entanglement has become increasinging popular in theorizing across a range of displines as a way of focusing on processes of becoming and conditions of possibility. Tim Ingold (2010) refers to entanglement as 'a meshwork of interwoven lines of growth and movement' (p. 3). I find this to be a useful starting point for thinking about young people's music engagement (growth and movement) in a world full of 'resistance, improvisation, friction, leakage, and unforeseen consquences' (Anderson, 2016, p. 1). The aim of the chapter is to focus attention on the affordances of spaces where music, modes, and technology converge and are entangled and enacted in ways that provide opportunities for young people to experience connection on a deep and fundamental level that promotes wellbeing.

Setting the scene: materiality and entanglement of young people's musical lives

The complexity and turbulence of today's world, coupled with fast-paced technological innovations, have propelled young people to 'understand themselves anew and to find a new relationship with the world' (Barnett, 2012, p. 9). Today's digital generation are absorbed in social networks and participatory learning cultures. These emphasize connectedness through affinity spaces (Gee, 2004), such as a sense of equity and distributed expertise across networked communities with interest-driven affiliations of people, tools, and resources (Warschauer and Matuchniak, 2010). They also emphasize life-wide learning (Jackson, 2012) that takes place in multiple spaces inhabited simultaneously across physical and virtual worlds (O'Neill, 2017a). These spaces afford contrasting learning experiences; they also entail differences in authorship, power, and boundedness (Barnett, 2010). Young people are increasingly engaged, with an unprecedented amount of autonomy, in technology and media-infused materials and activities that are self-directed, collaborative, transformative, and multimodal (O'Neill, 2014). In addition, learning has become unbundled (Sefton-Green, 2008) from schools or established formal learning contexts and more expansive (Engeström, 2003) as activity systems are transformed 'through reconceptualization of the object and the motive of activity embracing a radically wider horizon of possibilities than in the previous mode of activity' (p. 31).

Along with these changes, we have seen a shift towards theoretical perspectives in human development and education that disrupt the centring and privileging of sociocultural and personal processes and reassert the material (e.g. tools, technologies, bodies, actions, and objects) as entangled in meaning and not separate from it (Fenwick et al., 2011). Recently, this shift has become evident in theorizing about young people's music engagement (O'Neill, 2017a).

Consider, for example, how technological affordances—properties of the environment that offer an action possibility independent of the individual's ability to perceive this possibility—have increased creative and collaborative learning opportunities that have not been available to music learners before. Young people who are interest-driven or have an intense commitment to musical creative pursuits via technology will seek out material and social resources (O'Neill, 2014, 2017b). This is illustrated in the complex music- and technology-related activities described by one male aged 18 years:

I did a piece a while ago that I had grabbed my sister's iPod and mine; I don't have any recording programs or anything so I recorded different tracks through her, both of our iPods and then I lined them up together and did vocals. I don't have a drum set so I had to grab my Rock Band sets, like the video game, and um, I had to play this free-style drum thing in there and make a drum track through that, and played through some strings and piano, and put a little solo in it too.

(O'Neill, 2017a)

This example draws attention to a new style of thought that has taken shape in the digital age. This style of thought emphasizes 'making up' as a social practice that not only influences identity construction; it drives the production of experimental 'hybrids' involving old and new media that are reshaped, recreated, or reinterpreted through technology-enabled tools, resources, and communities (Rose, 2007).

Despite rapid changes in young people's music-making practices, the articulation of this shift conceptually within music research is in its infancy. I agree with Tara Fenwick and colleagues when they argue that the material entanglements of 'energies, processes, motives and outcomes are fully entangled with material practice' and that these entanglements 'are often not acknowledged in the conventional ... preoccupations with understanding human cognition, human activity and intentions, human meaning-making and human relationships' (Fenwick et al., 2011, p. vii). The trio go on to argue that 'attention to the sociomaterial makes visible the mundanity of everyday life'. Add to this the need to reveal the changing patterns of materiality in young people's musical lives, and to study 'the minute dynamics and connections that are continuously enacting the taken-for-granted', (Fenwick et al., 2011, p. vii) and I believe these are compelling reasons to move away from container-like contexts when considering young people's music engagement. I was particularly convinced of the need to take sociomateriality into account in the study of young people's musical lives when I began to see the value of this approach for furthering our understanding of the affordances of spaces in young people's music engagement for promoting a sense of connectedness and wellbeing.

Affordances of spaces

The notion of affordances of spaces that can support or constrain certain behaviours is rooted in James Gibson's (1979/1986) concept of affordances as a reciprocal relationship between the environment and behaviour. People perceive the environment in terms of the actions and activities it suggests or enables. In the case of music, this transactional perspective is linked with the concept of multiplicity since affordances are relative to individuals, and certain features in a given context might afford different musical actions or activities, providing multiple affordances. In music, space can initiate, direct, or organize a musical action or activity (e.g. a music room or a garage band rehearsal space), or it can frame, structure, or give significance (e.g. a popular music song played in a church versus the same song played in a stadium), or it can separate and unite, facilitate, or exclude (e.g. gender-stereotyped associations of musical instruments or songs associated with national identity).

Mobile technologies have done much to 'unmoor' the spaces where music has traditionally been enacted and virtual spaces have opened up online communities that provide new opportunities for young people's music engagement. A framework of the affordances of online communities was proposed by Elizabeth Mynatt et al., (1998, pp. 130–132) as follows:

- persistence, in that these communities are 'durable across time, users and particular uses, providing an ambient and continuous context for activity',
- periodicity is 'established and communicated through a variety of rhythms and patterns' within virtual and physical worlds,
- boundaries, established through 'mutually understood differentiation of units, from single to multiple, from proximate to remote',
- engagement, in which 'the social rhythm and density of engagement necessary for community-building' is enabled through diverse ways of coming together,
- authoring, in which participants are able to 'use and manipulate their space, whether as designers or users' through a broad range of flexible interactions.

In today's digital and media-infused world, these forms of online music engagement are becoming ubiquitous in adolescents' lives. These spaces offer new possibilities for 'supporting the increased forms of mediated sociality of absence-presence beyond the face-to-face' and 'enact[ing] spaces and ecologies of their own—cyberspaces' (Fenwick et al., 2011, p. 137). It is important, however, to also recognize the problematic view of cyberspace, or space more generally, as 'detached from the practices through which it is formed, the materialities through which it is enacted and the constraints it imposes' (p. 139). Fenwick and colleagues adopt instead John Urry's (2007) notion of flux, as 'flux involves tension, struggle and conflict' (p. 25) to emphasize the forms of regulation that characterize cyberspace. In other words, cyberspace only provides metaphorical resources for thinking about space more generally, including the 'new relationship' young people have 'between place, space and the social enabled by these new technologies' (Fenwick et al., 2011, p. 139). Nonetheless, these spaces provide young people with new opportunities for connectedness—'some replace the human material face-to-face interaction, and others facilitate the organization of such interactions' (Fenwick et al., 2011, p. 139). As Scott Bukatman (1996) points out, 'whether cyberspace is a "real" place or not, our experience of electronic space is a "real" experience' (p. 118). As such, these spaces combined with different media technologies offer different affordances and opportunities, often simultaneously. At the same time, opportunities for multimodal sense making or sharing of meaning have become implicated in promoting a deeper sense of musical connectedness that promotes wellbeing (Heydon and O'Neill, 2016).

Within technology-enabled and media-infused lives, musical sound has become a prominent feature in modes of representation, communication, and self-expression (O'Neill, 2014). Increasingly, the literature is documenting how young people experience music multimodally—often describing their musical encounters and creative collaborations as a form of seeing or sensing music through visual images, digital media, mobile devices, and movement (Gauntlett, 2007).

Consider, as an illustration, what Andrew, a 15-year-old guitar student, had to say about why music matters to him:

If you're trying to connect with like young kids you play music that they will identify with if, or if you do something that they identify with, ... you try to incorporate, like, I don't know, something they get so they pick up rhythm, it's in their body, their mind, it's in their soul. And frankly, as a musician I tried to tap that source when I'm composing music. I mean I can see music, I can hear music when I look at it but I don't really feel it and that's what I'm trying to do nowadays is I'm trying to feel the music cuz I feel that if you feel the music and your body is in tune with your mind it brings out a better musical experience, I mean it brings out more musicality through what you do ... and it's really universal this connection and what it means to people.

Increased mobility, social networking, mass media, and globalization have augmented young people's social connections and exposure to diverse musical practices and spaces. These ideas focus on the inherent relationality of young people and music (materiality and meaning) or what I refer to as entangled musical lives.

Entangled musical lives

One way of conceptualizing entangled musical lives stems from the idea that young people's engagement in music activities is thoroughly relational; it is the relational interpretation that we make when we use the tense 'engaging in music' because it refers to an entanglement of the individual agent and the recipient(s) of the musical act, the material objects in use in the musical act, and the conditions under which all these interact. Tim Ingold (2008) refers to this meshwork as SPIDER—Skilled Practice Involves Developmentally Embodied Responsiveness—whereby 'the skilled practitioner is one who can continually attune his or her movements to perturbations in the perceived environment without even interrupting the flow of action' (p. 214). This form of relationality is often taken for granted in thinking about how young people's music engagement affords connectedness on a deep and fundamental level through 'embodied responsiveness'. It reminds us that skill does not come 'readymade'; rather, it 'develops over time as part of a young person's own growth and development in an environment' (p. 115). Further, it is not created through social interaction alone but rather through the various ways that young people engage with non-human, multimodal, and technological objects and the significance of these in their everyday lives (O'Neill, 2017a).

Exploring young people's entangled musical lives began, for me, several years ago with one student's response to a question that probed the value of music in her everyday life. Grace, a 15-year-old violin student, was one of 93 adolescents aged 11–18 years in Vancouver, Canada, who took part in individual interviews about young people's conceptions of music engagement. When asked 'why does music matter to you?', Grace responded:

... it's what we connect through. I think it's a universal language that we all speak in and I don't think without music there's the whole. Like, music always comes back to feelings and I don't know what to say, you know, but umm just feeling, their emotions and everything, they're so connected. So, if it's not there we wouldn't have entertainment, we wouldn't have like true meaning of thoughts, passion, that's a big thing. Just sharing passion and the sympathetic connections between people, I think that's the most important thing that people need to realize.

Like some people take it for granted because it's the simplest thing like piano lessons but umm, I think it's important that every single person needs to feel, like at least have a sympathetic connection with what music gives us and it's like a whole experience that people don't just simply get, which I feel really unfortunate about, but I think it's really important that music should stay with us.

I wondered about the possibilities in Grace's response for understanding how music might be entangled in young people's lives in ways that impact on connectedness and wellbeing. There was a sense of urgency to this project, given growing concerns about adolescent wellbeing in many countries around the world. A recent survey in the UK, for example, showed an increase in the number of young people suffering from mental health and wellbeing issues over the past 5 years (Association of School and College Leaders, 2016). And yet, as Larson (2000) reminds us, young people's disenchantment or low life satisfaction is not necessarily a sign of mental illness or diagnosable problems; rather, it may reflect a 'deficiency in positive development' (p. 171). Positive youth development research has focused on relationships between connectedness and positive indicators of wellbeing such as optimism, hope, coping, happiness, and life satisfaction (Anderman, 2002; Camfield et al., 2009; Gillison et al., 2008). Understanding the role of music within these complex relationships and developmental processes led me to explore further the theoretical concepts in this chapter.

Multimodality, music, and wellbeing

Within multimodal literacy theory and research, little attention has been given to the meaning making potential of sound. And yet, the sonic potential of multiliteracies has grown in the digital age as more people are encountering sound through new technologies and their own exploration and consumption of Web 2.0 opportunities. There is still, however, a long way to go in terms of multimodal literacy research giving music its due. According to Ruth Finnegan (2014), sound in human communication from Plato onwards has been associated with 'emotion rather than the "higher" cognitive faculties' (p. 59). She argues that, as a result, sound compared to other literacies 'has seldom been extensively considered as a significant dimension of human communicating' (p. 60).

Together with my colleague Rachel Heydon, we examined links between wellbeing and the affordances of multimodality in our book *Why Multimodal Literacy Matters* (Heydon and O'Neill, 2016). We began with a critical post-structural treatment of the concept of wellbeing based on Watson et al. (2012). Our review of wellbeing revealed it to be a multidimensional concept with a long genealogy in the literature from Aristotelian ethics through to the 1990s' constructions of subjective and psychological wellbeing and more recently to contemporary notions of positive development and flourishing. Psychologists have tended to focus on individual aspects of wellbeing; sociologists and anthropologists have attempted more broadly defined sociocultural theorizing. Still, the concept of wellbeing continues to challenge researchers. Most of the literature on wellbeing is complex with multiple layers of conceptualizations existing across fields simultaneously. Much of the literature is instrumental in nature; thus, there is a dearth of socioculturally derived conceptions of wellbeing and conceptions that can reflect complexity, such as those stemming from post-structuralism, for example.

Watson et al. (2012) argue that wellbeing is 'contextual and embedded' (p. 7) and enacted and realized through circumstances and constituent 'encounters' (p. 7). This means that any concept of wellbeing must emphasize that it is 'relational' (p. 7). Proposing that wellbeing is relational acknowledges that it is produced between and among people, but it also requires an ethical posturing where one does not absolutely decide for the other what wellbeing means. Watson et al. (2012) reject a totalizing conceptualization of wellbeing where the alterity of the other is compromised. At the same time, they recognize that young people may need to be in 'co-relation' (p. 226) with an adult to bring wellbeing into being. This co-relation is a complex ethical encounter with the other which Watson and colleagues identify as being 'mediated' by 'human flourishing' (p. 227).

By way of illustration, consider what 15-year-old Marcus had to say about why music mattered to him:

It's important to be able to voice your opinion through music. The message we need to share about the music is that it contributes to a greater sense of community focus. Like, if you're doing music and sharing it online you're in a community of like-minded individuals who want to be doing the same thing. So, if you're in a community of musicians playing music with them and they all understand each other, you share the same ideas and it's not a judgemental environment, so you're living in an environment that's free living so you can be like I feel like this needs to be expressed and you're not being judged on your ideas. It makes you feel good about yourself.

Marcus' connection with music and wellbeing or 'feel[ing] good about yourself' is embedded in his ability to have a voice within an online community of 'like-minded individuals'. This is reminiscent of participatory cultures that encourage distributed knowledge and emphasize the importance of mediators that connect people so that they can access more knowledge and expertise than they could otherwise access within existing structures and practices (Gee, 2005). James Paul Gee (2004, 2005) refers to 'affinity spaces' as places where individuals from a variety of backgrounds and with different kinds of knowledge (e.g. tacit, intensive, extensive) come together to pursue a common endeavour: one that offers various pathways to participation, informal mentorship, and a shared sense of status in supporting each other's growth, artistry, and creativity. They become places to share expertise and knowledge without the barriers of age, class, race, gender, and education. To understand these connections further, it is helpful to conceptually enfold theoretical perspectives from new materialism, which allow for the interdisciplinary study of two dimensions of music making in their entanglement—meaning and materiality—with the aim of opening up more possibilities for young people's wellbeing to be conceptualized and to flourish.

The material turn and wellbeing

At the centre of complexity theorizing is what is referred to as the 'material turn' or the umbrella term 'new materialism' and theories associated with critical work on materiality. John Law (2004) defines materiality as 'a way of thinking about the material in which this is treated as a continuously enacted relational effect. The implication is that materials [such as music] do not exist in and of themselves but are endlessly generated and at least potentially reshaped' (p. 161). Giuliana Bruno (2014) refers to materiality as 'a refashioning of our sense of space and contact with the environment, as well as a threading of our experience of temporality, interiority, and subjectivity' (p. 8). And, Tim Ingold (2014) argues that materiality refers to 'leaky things' or 'an interchange of materials across the ever-emergent surfaces by which they differentiate themselves from surrounding medium'

(p. 65). This emphasizes a 'gathering of materials in movement … so to touch or observe a thing is to bring the movements of our own being (or rather becoming) into correspondence with the movements of the materials' (p. 65). In each of these explanations, the term new materialism requires us to rethink the relationship between the human and the non-human. We are asked to recognize that all entities and processes are composed of—or are reducible to—matter, material forces, or physical processes. Applying these insights to our understanding of how young people navigate and negotiate musical spaces require us to no longer privilege connectedness as a solely human form of interaction. Instead, we need to reassert music into the embodied practices of young people's music engagement—the material bodies of composers, musicians, and singers—as they co-collaborate in correspondence with the movement of instruments and other technologies in spaces that enable music, connectedness, and wellbeing to emerge.

To focus on critical conceptualizations of entangled musical lives in relation to young people's music engagement, I drew on the work of Karen Barad and her 2007 book *Meeting the Universe Halfway: Quantum Physics and the Entanglement of Matter and Meaning*. Barad starts from the position that matter and meaning are not separate; rather, they are 'inextricably fused together, and no event, no matter how energetic, can tear them asunder' (p. 3). Barad wants us to recognize that contemporary physics is an 'entanglement of matters of being, knowing, and doing, of ontology, epistemology, and ethics, of fact and value' (p. 3). I suggest that when this understanding is applied to today's adolescent engagement in music making, with its integral connections to new technologies and multimodal sense making, there is an opportunity to recognize the nature of music making as simultaneously about substance and significance and to seek holistic or 'lifeworld' ways to explore these components to make sense of their affordances for adolescent wellbeing.

Let's return to Grace, the 15 year old who described the value of music as replete with shared relationships, communication, emotion, meaning, and passion that are sympathetic and enduring. For Grace, the question of values or what matters about music was framed within the stance of social practices that were clearly located within spaces where interactions or transactions occurred between music and people. She struggled to convey the nuances and textures of these transactions or complex entanglements of how people can and do make meaning and the affordances of music for what she referred to as 'sympathetic' connection. She explained further:

I believe that I can give the audience something and make a connection with them. I think if they have that connection, they know what music is. So, I think that it would be a good idea—it doesn't have to be me, I'm sure there's other people—if they have a way of reaching out to the audience and then obviously, they're going to give back so that's what really music is, it's about connecting.

In describing her beliefs about music and connection, Grace engaged in what Barad (2007) refers to as the 'lively dance of mattering' (p. 37) where the material processes of life (in this case Grace's notion of 'music') intermingle with social systems (Grace's subjects 'performer' and 'audience') through a non-linear, relational process through which meaning and form are realized through 'different agential possibilities' (p. 141).

As a young encultured, embodied, moral, and aesthetic being, Grace was attempting to capture how music is not merely transmitted from performer to audience; rather, how it is an assemblage where the affordances of connectedness are inextricably tied to the mutually interdependent and co-constituted assemblage of human/non-human performer-music-audience. Another way to represent this assemblage is to imagine it 'intra-actively' (p. x) enacted in the same way as writing—not 'interactively since writing is not a uni-directional practice of creation that flows from author to page, but rather the practice of writing is an iterative and mutually constitutive working out, and reworking' (Barad, 2007, p. x). Considering music in a similar way provides a lens for making sense of how the affordances of space provide emergent opportunities for connectedness and wellbeing as the non-human agency of things (music) interacts with Grace as much as she interacts with it. According to Barad (2007) this 'intra-acting; it is an enactment, not something that someone or something has' (p. 826). Thus, this intra-acting, that emerges in spaces, is affording opportunities for connectedness and wellbeing.

Gary Ansdell and Tia DeNora (2012), who quote Havi Carel (2008), argue, 'wellbeing is the invisible context enabling us to pursue possibilities and engage in projects. It is the condition of possibility enabling us to follow through aims and goals, to act on our desires, to become who we are' (p. 11). Ansdell and DeNora go on to say that 'wellbeing involves our flourishing together, within our sociocultural community' (p. 110) and 'for many people wellbeing emerges in the spaces made between people and music' (p. 111).

How might we conceptualize the spaces that Ansdell and DeNora (2012) are referring to? Thinking about the affordances of spaces and the notion of entangled musical lives seems important in an exploration of how music contributes to young people's sense of connectedness and wellbeing, particularly in today's technology and media-infused world. I hope the discussion in this chapter offers some furture directions for researchers who are interested in young people's music engagement and how we might apply these insights to our understanding of how young people navigate and negotiate musical spaces in ways that enable connectedness and wellbeing to emerge.

References

Anderman, E. M. (2002). School effects on psychological outcomes during adolescence. *Journal of Educational Psychology*, **94**, 795–809.

Andersen, L. (2016). Critical terms: entanglement. **Making worlds: Art, materiality and early modern globalization.** Available from www.makingworlds.net/entanglement (accessed 6 December 2018).

Ansdell, G. and DeNora, T. (2012). Musical flourishing: Community music therapy, controversy, and the cultivation of wellbeing. In R. A. R. MacDonald, G. Kreutz, and L. Mitchell (Eds), *Music, health, and wellbeing* (pp. 97–112). New York: Oxford University Press.

Association of School and College Leaders (2016). Keeping young people in mind—findings from a survey of schools across England. National Children's Bureau. Available from www.ascl.org.uk/

utilities/document-summary.html?id=D91C5B0A-72A6-4117-96A9B343E51FB296 (accessed 6 December 2018).

Barad, K. (2007). *Meeting the Universe Halfway: Quantum Physics and the Entanglement of Matter and Meaning*. Durham, NC: Duke University Press.

Barnett, R. (2010). Life-wide education: a new and transformative concept for higher education? e-Proceedings from the Enabling a More Complete Education Conference, April 2010. Available from https://lifewidelearning.pbworks.com/f/RON%2BBARNETT.pdf (accessed 6 December 2018).

Barnett, R. (2012). The coming of the ecological learner. In P. Tynjälä, M.-L. Stenström, and M. Saarnivaara (Eds), *Transitions and Transformations in Learning and Education* (pp. 9–20). New York: Springer.

Bauman, Z. (2000). *Liquid Modernity*. Cambridge, MA: Polity Press.

Bukatman, S. (1996). *Terminal Identity*. Durham, NC: Duke University Press.

Bruno, G. (2014). *Surface: Matters of aesthetics, materiality, and media*. Chicago: University of Chicago Press.

Camfield, L., Choudhury, K., and Devine, J. (2009). Wellbeing, happiness, and why relationships matter: Evidence from Bangladesh. *Journal of Happiness Studies*, 10, 71–91.

Carel, H. (2008). *Illness: the Cry of the Flesh*. Stocksfield: Acumen.

Engeström, Y. (2003). The horizontal dimension of expansive learning: Weaving a texture of cognitive trails in the terrain of health care in Helsinki. In F. Achtenhagen and E. G. John (Eds), *Milestones of Vocational and Occupational Education and Training. Volume 1: The Teaching Learning Perspective* (pp. 153–180). Bielefeld: Bertelsmann.

Fenwick, T., Edwards, R., and Sawchuk, P. (2011). *Emerging Approaches to Educational Research: Tracing the Sociomaterial*. London: Routledge.

Finnegan, R. (2014). *Communicating: The Multiple modes of Human Communication* (2nd edn). New York: Routledge.

Gauntlett, D. (2007). *Creative Explorations: New Approaches to Identities and Audiences*. Abingdon: Routledge.

Gee, J. P. (2004). *Situated Language and Learning: a Critique of Traditional Schooling*. London: Routledge.

Gee, J. P. (2005). Learning by design: Good video games as learning machines. *E-Learning*, 2(1), 5–16.

Gibson, J. J. (1979/1986). *The Ecological Approach to Perception*. Hillsdale, NJ: Lawrence Erlbaum Associates.

Gillison, F., Standage, M., and Skevington, S. (2008). Changes in quality of life and psychological need satisfaction following the transition to secondary school. *British Journal of Educational Psychology*, 78, 149–162.

Heydon, R. and O'Neill, S. A. (2016). *Why Multimodal Literacy Matters: (Re)conceptualizing Literacy and Wellbeing through Singing-infused Multimodal, Intergenerational Curricula*. Rotterdam: Sense.

Ingold, T. (2008). When ANT meets SPIDER: social theory for arthropods. In C. Knappett and L. Malafouris (Eds), *Material Agency: Towards a Non-anthropocentric Approach* (pp. 209–215). New York: Springer.

Ingold, T. (2010). Bringing things to life: Creative entanglements in a world of materials. NCRM working Paper Series. ESRC National Centre for Research Methods. University of Manchester. Available from http://eprints.ncrm.ac.uk/1306/1/0510_creative_entanglements.pdf (accessed 6 December 2018).

Ingold, T. (2014). An ecology of material. In S. Witzgall and K. Stakemeier (Eds), *Power of Material/ Politics of Materiality* (pp. 59–65). Zurich: Diaphanes.

Jackson, N. J. (2012). Lifewide learning: History of an idea. E-book. Available from www. normanjackson.co.uk/uploads/1/0/8/4/10842717/lifewide_learning_history_of_an_idea.pdf (accessed 6 December 2018).

Larson, R. W. (2000). Toward a psychology of positive youth development. *American Psychologist*, **55**(1), 170–183.

Larson, R. W. (2011). Positive development in a disorderly world. *Journal of Research on Adolescence*, **21**(2), 317–334.

Law, J. (2004). *After method: Mess in social science research*. New York, NY: Routledge.

Mynatt, E. D., O'Day, V. L., Adler, A., and Ito, M. (1998). Network communities: something old, something new, something borrowed.... *Computer Supported Cooperative Work: The Journal of Collaborative Computing*, 7(1–2), 123–156.

O'Neill, S. A. (2014). Music and media infused lives: An introduction. In S. A. O'Neill (Ed.), *Research to Practice: Vol. 6. Music and Media Infused Lives: Music Education in a Digital Age* (pp. 1–15). Waterloo, ON: Canadian Music Educators' Association.

O'Neill, S. A. (2017a). Young people's musical lives: Learning ecologies, identities and connectedness. In R. A. R. MacDonald, D. J. Hargreaves, and D. Meill (Eds), *Oxford handbook of musical identities* (pp. 79–104). New York: Oxford University Press.

O'Neill, S. A. (2017b). Music and social cognition in adolescence. In R. Ashley and R. Timmers (Eds), *The Routledge Companion to Music Cognition* (pp. 441–452). New York: Routledge.

Rose, N. (2007). *The Politics of Life Itself: Biomedicine, Power, and Subjectivity in the Twenty-first Century*. Princeton, NJ: Princeton University Press.

Sefton-Green, J. (2008). From learning to creative learning: Concepts and traditions. In J. Sefton-Green (Ed.), *Creative Learning, Creative Partnerships* (pp. 15–26). London: Arts Council of England.

Urry, J. (2007). *Mobilities*. Cambridge: Cambridge University Press.

Warschauer, M. and Matuchniak, T. (2010). New technology and digital worlds: Analyzing evidence of equity in access, use, and outcomes. *Review of Research in Education*, **34**(1), 179–225.

Watson, D., Emery, C., and Bayliss, P. (2012). *Children's Social and Emotional Wellbeing*. Bristol: The Policy Press.

Chapter 17

Wellbeing, young people, and music scenes

Andy Bennett and Lisa Nikulinsky

Introduction

The sociocultural connections between young people and music have long been acknowledged and studied as an object of academic enquiry (Chambers, 1985). Within this, scene
has become a popularly applied concept in both theoretically and empirically focused
work on the significance of music in the everyday lives of youth and young adults (Straw,
1991; Bennett and Peterson, 2004). Conventionally, such work has tended to cluster into
three main, interrelated areas that can broadly be described as production, performance,
and consumption. Although each of these themes could, in essence, be linked to aspects of
wellbeing, little work has been done in this area. When emphasis is placed on music scenes,
in relation to notions of wellbeing among young people, this is often with respect to the
more potentially pathological effects of musical taste. This is seen, for example, in litera-
tures examining the relationship between genres such as rap and metal and a propensity
for violence among fans of these musics (see, for example Epstein et al., 1990), and connections between music and drug use (Forsyth et al., 1997). Drawing on empirical data collected among young people between the ages of 18 and 30 years in south-west Australia, this
chapter will offer a different perspective by considering some of the more positive effects on
the wellbeing of young people that membership of music scenes can foster. Specifically, the
chapter will consider the significance of music scenes for young people in relation to issues
such as social inclusion, feelings of positive belonging, and the promotion of self-esteem.

The history of music, youth, and identity

*... People's heaviest investment in popular music is when they are teenagers and young adults .... People do
use music less, and less intently, as they grow up.*

(Frith, 1987, p. 143)

While at one level this observation from Simon Frith has been challenged by more recent
work on popular music and ageing (see, for example, Bennett, 2013) it remains relevant
for our understanding of music as a key resource for many young people in terms of

their identity-making at both individual and collective levels. Ever since the emergence of rock and roll, the first definitively branded 'youth' music, during the early 1950s, successive generations of young people have grown up with genres, artists, and songs that they identify as being of their generation. In essence, since the mid-twentieth century, music, and more specifically popular music styles including rock, punk, rap, indie, and dance, has been an important part of the way in which young people have sought to forge cultural identities for themselves, such identities being pivotal to the aesthetic and lifestyle distinctions young people have used to mark themselves off from the parent culture (Bennett, 2000). Official responses to the 'youthquake' (Leech, 1973) of the post-war era and its metamorphosis over the next few decades were predominantly negative in outlook and tone. Attempts to censor the television performances of Elvis Presley in the USA during the mid-1950s because of the singer's allegedly over-sexualized movements (see Shumway, 1992) were a precursor to increasingly negative forms of reaction to youth cultures that would occur in the 1960s, 1970s, 1980s, and 1990s. During this time a succession of youth cultures, including mods, rockers, punks, rappers, and ravers became the focus of what Stanley Cohen (1987) has described as a moral panic. As Cohen observes, central to such moral panic has been the stereotyping of youth cultures as 'folk devils'; that is, 'the gallery of types that society erects to show its members which roles should be avoided' (1987, p. 10).

It was only during the later 1960s and the emergence of the hippie counterculture, a movement that appeared more middle class and, to some degree intellectualized, that some social commentators began to reflect on the more culturally meaningful aspects of young people's reactions to popular music (Hall, 1968/2016). Key musical events of the era, such as the Woodstock Music and Arts Fair in August 1969, graphically illustrated the cultural importance of popular music for youth at this time as some 400 000 people gathered at a greenfield site near the town of Bethel in upper New York state to watch performances by some of the biggest and most culturally significant artists of the time, among them The Who, Jimi Hendrix, and Janis Joplin (Bennett, 2004). Certainly, official reactions to the counterculture often remained negative. However, the range of 'non-violent', if sometimes over-romanticized, solutions suggested by the counterculture for social change opened up different ways of looking at the significance of popular music and its influence on youth, and their sense of belonging and 'community'. Such a discourse has remained ongoing in some of the more recent literature on youth and music, for example in work on rap, where the value of street art and dance serve as creative solutions to urban issues (Rose, 1994), and straightedge, a music and style that promotes a core ideology of abstinence from drugs, alcohol, and sexual promiscuity (Haenfler, 2006). It remains the case, however, that overall the more positive benefits to youth of being involved in music scenes remain under-examined in academic research.

Music scenes

Initial attempts to theorize the collective response of youth to popular music and its associated stylistic resources made use of the term 'subculture', a model that had previously been applied in the work of Chicago School sociologists during the first part of the twentieth century to provide sociological explanations for youth deviance (see, for example, Matza and Sykes, 1961). During the early 1970s, cultural theorists in Britain took the subcultural framework and applied it to spectacular post-war youth cultures, such as the teddy boys, mods, skinheads, and punks, as a means of interpreting the stylized responses of the latter to issues of class inequality and socioeconomic dislocation (Hall and Jefferson, 1976; Hebdige, 1979). The concept of subculture was variously criticized because of its reliance on a class-based analysis of youth's collective appropriation of music and style, an approach that was claimed not to bear up to empirical scrutiny (Muggleton, 2000). Critical responses to subculture included the application of music scene as an alternative and more flexible framework for studying the collective importance of music and style for youth.

Thus, whereas subculture's structuralist approach insists on the importance of class and community as indices of musical taste, scenes invariably transcend particular localities and class-based communities 'reflect[ing] and actualiz[ing] a particular state of relations between various populations and social groups, as these coalesce around particular coalitions of musical style' (Straw, 1991, p. 379).

The concept of music scene thus becomes useful in a number of ways when attempting to uncover the everyday significance of music in the collective cultural practices of young people. First and foremost, it allows for an understanding of such cultural practices as forged through a series of shared experiences, which may or may not reflect a common experience of class, ethnicity, gender, etc., but also extends to other issues such as association through shared aesthetics and lifestyle practices and politics, as these work across different social groups and communities. Scene is also a useful framework for studying the various kinds of practices and activities that inform musical involvement, a process identified by ethnomusicologist Christopher Small (1998) as 'musicking'. In addition to performing in a band and/or attending live gigs, such practices extend to things such as the production and promotion of bands and artists, providing artwork for recordings and/or concert promotion, writing critical reviews of concerts and albums, and so forth. The scenes literature also extends to an understanding of the more affective and virtual aspects of scene participation (Bennett and Peterson, 2004), the latter having additional important resonances for our understanding of music scenes as fostering an important sense of belonging and wellbeing among young people. This is considered in further detail in the following sections of this chapter.

Methodology and research context

The following data were collected during a study focusing on young people in the southwest Australian coastal township of Margaret River between September 2016 and April 2017. A total of 11 young people, six male and five female participants between the ages of 15 and 25 years, were invited to contribute to the research project. The principal research method applied in the study involved the conducting of semi-structured, in-depth interviews using open-ended conversations as a means to elicit thick description and nar-ratives about popular music culture and its impact on wellbeing, scene membership, and identity. All interviews were recorded and, subject to the consent of the participants, were later transcribed for the purposes of analysis.

This study is concerned with both youth identity, wellbeing, and music scene member-ship (including music consumption and music practices) among young people living in the Margaret River township in Western Australia. According to Bennett (2014) Perth, the nearest major city to Margaret River, 275 km away, is often described as one of the most isolated cities in the world. Perth has an image and perception that radiates beyond the city to its outer regions, which permeate their own brand of rural isolation. Margaret River has particular sociocultural nuances. Its rural locale provides an out-migration of young people overlaid with counter-flows of in-migrants seeking lifestyle changes, with rural and coastal amenities as well as wine and surfing industries. David Farrugia (2015) promotes 'peripheral' youth identities as offering significant sites for analysis. This study pays particular attention to how young people invest in music (consumption, creation, and listening practices) and how they form allegiance or membership to specific music scenes. Building on the current conception of scenes as entities that can be simultan-eously local, translocal, and virtual (Bennett et al., 2008), the research findings drawn on in this chapter provide insights as to how participants in this community understand and define scene. Consideration of how participants construct and invest in scenes through interaction with each other, and in doing so shape their identities, will also be explored.

A music scene as the family you choose

Within this ethnographic research situated in a rural localized location, participants were asked if they considered themselves as being part of a local or virtual music scene. A key motive for this was to pay attention to the micro-processes that come together to produce scenes. Jeremy described how he believes that a strong local DIY punk scene exists and permeates the local community in Margaret River. He richly described how the event Day in the Dust (a local one-day DIY punk and skate event) had established a space for punk, temporally transforming a rural farm site into a punk place. This one-day festival ma-nipulated the natural environment and aesthetics of a local farm setting in order to create something unique for people affiliating with local punk and skate culture.

Jeremy (25 years old) describes his active participation and sense of community mem-bership in a local hardcore scene:

What attracted me was first the music and the second you start meeting people with the same interests, the same bands and it's just a big community. You might fall down at a hardcore show and you get picked up. You can crowd surf and people catch you. It's really just a massive family, which forms out of listening to the music that you love. It is just unreal ... to be able to listen to this heavy abrasive music, and it just opens you up once you start going to the shows, start meeting other people in the scene and you just get into it. And it's just a big community, a big family ... the community is a reward that comes with the music.

This example adds to our understanding about how participants create and sculpt specific sites and spaces to preserve scenes, as well as how they construct their identities and scene membership within spatial contexts. As Ola Johansson and Thomas Bell explore, music scenes 'range from local, i.e. based on proximity, to non-local in which fans and performers of a genre are scattered geographically but cohesive in their allegiance to the genre' (2009, p. 220). All participants, but especially those who identified with punk and metal scenes, drew attention to local scenes as involving face-to-face interactions and therefore typically taking place in localized spaces which become associated with a scene, for example venues, record shops, public spaces, and tattoo parlors.

The sociogeographic 'spatial' element is also recognized by participants within the social spaces of music. Participants all made reference to Margaret River's environment and geography: both to its geographical isolation and visually captivating 'awesome' and 'iconic' coastline and landscape. They made reference to the direct influence of their geographical location as influencing the dominant local scenes they identified with and perceived as existing. Sienna (21 years old) made particular reference to locality, claiming:

I see my local scene, particularly when I am with friends that aren't from here. I think I am definitely part of the scene down here, like the weather and the beach here, it's just the way we live ... you know ... we are all really laid back. We dress laid back, chilled, a little bit hippy, not too hippy. Yeah I really notice it when I am with people that aren't from here. Like, if I take myself out of here, like when I go to the Gold Coast or Byron Bay, where I have been quite a lot over the last couple of years, I see myself as 'oh yeah, that's my scene'. Like south-west WA is my place, and that's the people I belong to.

Pepper Glass (2012) references this local focus as advantageous to the idea of a scene in that it locates networks of people who are in actual times and places. This expands upon the monolithic restrictive conceptualizations of youth, subcultures, and identity as discussed earlier in this chapter (see also, Muggleton, 2000; Chaney 2004). Providing an alternative lens, studies of scene consider how members identify and connect with each other and how those connections then offer and inspire new identities, spaces, and forms of expression and counterculture. What Sienna's narrative identifies is the notion of being laid back as a subjective melding of identity. Identifying with her town, Sienna points out the specific stylistic references connecting her with her chosen scene.

Scene membership was also recognized by participants as existing within translocal and virtual spaces. The Internet, social networking, and music streaming applications and platforms all assisted participants in being able to access and consume music, providing kinship and affiliation with specific music scenes. Sunny (18 years old) described how virtual scene membership provided many opportunities for global connectivity. Sunny identified positive benefits in his access to the Internet assisting him to participate in a scene regardless of geographical location, which he describes as 'isolating'. This lack of local scene membership did not hinder his virtual ability to access music, making him part of something he perceived as both powerful and connective:

Being able to use the Internet to view video clips, stream music, and watch music live on Facebook ... being able to talk on line about music, yes bloody oath, it's made a big difference ... sometimes it feels like its my only way of being connected in a sense really ... YouTube and Spotify, they're the two big things that I use to get connected to other people and find new bands.

Sonny's description identifies the unifying qualities of the Internet, supporting and enabling individuals from diverse locations to join together in virtual spaces accessing music, thus facilitating the growth of meaningful communities and identities beyond those that manifest in their physical localities (Williams, 2006).

The connectivity of music

Music was noted by all participants as rich material with which to express themselves, forging connection with both self and others. Here work by Tia DeNora (2000), which conceptually explores music as a technology of self, is particularly relevant and we expand on this idea through framing music as a technology of identity work during adolescence. This supports research from Tarrant (2002), Saarikallio and Erkkila (2007), and McFerran (2010), who argue that music is especially meaningful and pertinent during the life trajectory of adolescence. Certain genres, bands, and songs provide ideas or narratives which young people identify and value about themselves. At the same time, these representations provide a context for images of self. The sense of self is locatable in music: 'Musical materials provide terms and templates for illustrating self-identity' (DeNora, 2000, p. 79). This is illustrated by Lily, aged 18, who defines herself as '... kind of hardcore, intense, strong willed, and I like, I love that kind of music'. Similarly, through acknowledging self in relation to music, and music in relation to self, Jeremy was able to identify the meaning of each:

I was into rap and hip-hop and I went through all the stages like that and I loved all that sort of stuff and built my way up, got into the punk scene and yes found metal, which I now believe to be me, at the end of it. Metal and punk is me. It takes care of me and I take care of it.

Here lies the recursive circle. Music is perceived as an ally, a personal forum to articulate connectivity with self and others. Music, as a mirror, enables one to recognize one's self. Music can be embedded in conversation facilitating a young person's perception of himself or herself, illustrating a personal identity claim. Jeremy's description enables insight into how a range of diverse musical tastes mark all the different aspects of self and supports post-modernist perspectives of identity being 'variable, multifarious and fluid' (Thurlow, 2005, p. 5).

Another research participant, Jim (24 years old), described music as being a vehicle to assist and inform life decisions. In the following interview extract he looks back reflectively over time, attributing these decisions to the specific genre of hardcore:

Interviewer: Do you feel in terms of who you are as a person, your values … say loyalty, trust, openness, all those things you have spoken about which you say are referenced in hardcore, do you find that directly connects with you as a person?

Jim: Yes, definitely. I've picked myself up on it quite a few times. I think … I've done … who I am is reflected by the music I listen to. Where I haven't done it on purpose, it's just happened naturally. I've done something, or made a decision, and I'm proud of that decision and I'm like where did that come from and I think back, and it certainly comes directly from the music that I listen to.

Jim expressed what other participants also referenced in their interviews; that is, that music has transformative powers. It 'does' things, can change or inspire decision-making processes, it actually makes things happen. Engagement with music identifies connections between ongoing musical influences and one's subjective outlook on the world. Through the narratives of all participants who were connected to a multiplicity of musical genres, styles, and scenes whether it be hardcore, punk, metal, or indie-folk, all expressed the deep connection between music and self, and the ways in which this relationship impacted on them as individuals. It enables them to critically reflect upon their decisions and choices, identifying the direct capacity of music to engineer personal agency. At the same time, participants also reference the more subtle effects of music and membership of music scenes influencing their ability to articulate social and personal values in their day-to-day lives. As Alex, (22 years old), observes;

I use music for so much. So it's like a person—if you say … 'Okay a person is music', you would say 'I'm feeling like this', they (it) just gets me and reacts the way I want it to and then goes away when I'm done. Music being the perfect mate!

Music: an essential tool for wellbeing

The research results discussed thus far reveal that participants use music in both personal and unique ways and that music for them can be a method of both measuring and maintaining a sense of wellbeing. Another significant theme that emerged from the findings was the way in which research participants were able to express vulnerability through the prism of musical tastes and scene affiliation. Dylan (17 years old) described his appreciation of music that he perceived as taking risks in terms of composition and lyrical content. This in turn enabled him to feel more open to express narratives of vulnerability about himself to his band members and peers. As a result of appreciation and love of the band Radiohead and specific lyrics, Dylan describes:

Yeah ... Radiohead. Thom Yorke's lyrics. I think they've made me ... um, er ... I'm not very good with words .... It's made me think about more than just myself, the bigger picture ... sort of like his vulnerability has given me things ... you know the track 'Day Dreaming' on the new album? ... there's this lyric (singing) 'This goes beyond me'. I love that lyric.

Dylan attributes the vulnerability in this song providing him with a personal catharsis. An ability to document or access something that deeply resonates with him. This demonstrates an awareness of how to utilize music to arrive at, alter, and describe experiences or aspects of self. The vocabulary of using music to achieve what you 'need' was identified in all 11 interviews conducted for the study that informs this chapter. This 'need' was linked to expression of feelings and documenting interactions with others. These findings are consistent with research by Suvi Saarikallio and Jaakko Erkkila (2007) where eight young Finnish people described that they had a sense of the kinds of music they needed to listen to and when.

Later in the interview, Dylan takes this theme even further, describing how Radiohead had influenced decisions he had made in personal relationships, gaining self-reflexive insights. Music has not only been an inspiration for Dylan, but he believes 'it's just who I am'. Elaborating on this point, Dylan says music is a bridge and offers connection to things that are 'beyond me' including insights and theories he otherwise would not be able to access. Dylan strongly believes that Radiohead deeply impacts his life, offering solace and comfort:

Dylan: I guess it's like having someone reaffirm what you are feeling I guess .... It's like ... you know that (Radiohead) song 'There, There'? ... That song was definitely the one that got me through ...

Interviewer: What was it about that song?

Dylan: Probably the lyrics ... you know the chorus (singing) 'Just cos you feel it, doesn't mean it's there' ... Actually, it's probably helped me a lot more than I thought—that lyric. Going after you know, relationship things ... and him saying 'doesn't mean it's there'. That really made me think ... yeah I probably would have made some pretty big mistakes if it weren't for that lyric.

Interviewer: Isn't that beautiful though? I love how lyrics can do that. They can soundbyte your life.

Dylan: It did that for me. I play that track again and again and that lyric nailed it.

This specific Radiohead lyric assisted Dylan; it documented a high-intensity cathartic experience, which he cites was unique to his relationship with Radiohead and that particular song. Dylan went on to acknowledge that 'Radiohead might not be for other people' in so far as his original reasons for being attracted to the band documented uncertainties about the world and himself and his struggle to socially assimilate.

Nina (19 years old) describes how the band Midnight Oil was able to assist with documenting a sense of injustice perpetrated against her within her part-time job. She remarks:

Whenever in my life ... and recently I've had a lot of work stress and I play Midnight Oil when I'm feeling angry or when I'm feeling like ... there's this issue going on, cos I feel they [Midnight Oil] are the ones that speak out about issues, and there's this part of me that's um ... I might cry ... there's this part of me that wanted to lately take on that Midnight Oil stance and be vocal....

Nina is able to utilize the lyrics of Midnight Oil as apparatus enabling her to access courageousness as a direct response to the injustice of micro-management she experiences in her workplace. As she describes her love of Midnight Oil, it leads her to make direct interrelation, between her own personal account of injustice drawing fortitude from the lyrical content and message.

Conclusion

This chapter has examined the relationship between young people, membership of music scenes, and aspects of emotional and physical wellbeing. As we have sought to illustrate, delving into the research participants' narratives of how they perceive, associate with, and identify with specific scenes can help and inform our nuanced understanding of youth cultures which are continuously being negotiated in the local, global, and virtual nexus. The adolescent life stage, which is now understood as spanning the ages of 10–24 years, is a period of significant personal development in which feelings of vulnerability and isolation are frequently experienced. In presenting the results of our research on a small sample of adolescent youth in the Margaret River region of south-west Australia, we have explored ways in which association with a music scene or scenes provides a form of deep connectivity through which these young people can feel a sense of self-fulfillment and belonging.

References

Bennett, A. (2000). *Popular Music and Youth Culture: Music, Identity and Place*. London: Macmillan.

Bennett, A. (Ed.) (2004). "Everybody's happy, everybody's free": Representation and nostalgia in the Woodstock film. In A. Bennett (Ed.), *Remembering Woodstock* (pp. 41 - 54). Aldershot: Ashgate.

Bennett, A. (2013). *Music, Style and Aging: Growing Old Disgracefully?* Philadelphia, PA: Temple University Press.

Bennett, A. (2014). Popular music, cultural memory and the peripheral city. In A. Barber-Kersovan, V. Kirchberg, and R. Kuchar (Eds), *Music City: Musikalische Annäherungen an die »kreative Stadt«* (pp. 105–119). Bielefeld: transcript.

Bennett, A. and Peterson, R. A. (Eds) (2004). *Music Scenes: Local, Trans-Local and Virtual*. Nashville, TN: Vanderbilt University Press.

Bennett, A., Stratton, J., and Peterson, R. A. (2008). The scenes perspective and the Australian context. *Continuum: Journal of Media & Cultural Studies*, 22(5), 593–599.

Chambers, I. (1985). *Urban Rhythms: Pop Music and Popular Culture*. London: Macmillan.

Chaney, D. (2004). Fragmented culture and subcultures. In A. Bennett and K. Kahn-Harris (Eds), *After Subculture: Critical Studies in Contemporary Youth Culture* (pp. 36–48). Basingstoke: Palgrave.

Cohen, S. (1987). *Folk Devils and Moral Panics: The Creation of the Mods and Rockers*, 3rd edn. Oxford: Basil Blackwell.

DeNora, T. (2000). *Music in Everyday Life*. Cambridge. Cambridge University Press.

Epstein, J. S., Pratto, D. J., and Skipper Jr, J. K. (1990). Teenagers, behavioral problems, and preferences for heavy metal and rap music: A case study of a Southern middle school. *Deviant Behavior*, **11**, 381–394.

Farrugia, D. (2015). The mobility imperative for rural youth: The structural, symbolic and non-representational dimensions of youth mobilities. *Journal of Youth Studies*, **19**(6), 836–851.

Forsyth, A. J. M., Barnard, M., and McKeganey, N. P. (1997). Musical preference as an indicator of adolescent drug use. *Addiction*, **92**(10), 1317–1325.

Frith, S. (1987). Towards an aesthetic of popular music. In R. Leppert and S. McClary (Eds), *Music and Society: The Politics of Composition, Performance and Reception* (pp. 133–149). Cambridge: Cambridge University Press.

Glass, P.G. (2012). Doing scene: Identity, space and the interactional accomplishment of youth culture. *Journal of Contemporary Ethnography*, **14**(6), 695–716.

Haenfler, R. (2006). *Straight Edge: Clean-Living Youth, Hardcore Punk, And Social Change*. Rutgers University Press: Piscataway, NJ.

Hall, S. (1968/2017). The hippies: An American "moment". In A. Bennett (Ed.), *Youth Cultures*, vol. **1** (pp. 107–138). London: SAGE Publications.

Hall, S. and Jefferson, T. (Eds) (1976). *Resistance Through Rituals: Youth Subcultures in Post-War Britain*. London: Hutchinson.

Hebdige, D. (1979). *Subculture: The Meaning of Style*. London: Routledge.

Johansson, O. and Bell, T. L. (2009). Where are the new US music scenes? In O. Johansson and T. L. Bell (Eds), *Sound, Society and the Geography of Popular Music* (pp. 219–244). London: Routledge.

Leech, A. (1973). *Youthquake: The Growth of a Counter-culture Through Two Decades*. London: Littlefield and Adams.

Matza, D. and Sykes, G. M. (1961). Juvenile delinquency and subterranean values. *American Sociological Review*, **26** (5), 712–719.

McFerran, K. (2010). *Adolescents, Music and Music Therapy: Methods and Techniques for Clinicians, Educators and Students*. London: Jessica Kingsley Publishers.

Muggleton, D. (2000). *Inside Subculture: The Postmodern Meaning of Style*. Oxford: Berg.

Rose, T. (1994). *Black Noise: Rap Music and Black Culture in Contemporary America*. London: Wesleyan University Press.

Saarikallio, S. and Erkkilä, J. (2007).The role of music in adolescents' mood regulation. *Psychology of Music*, **35**(1), 88–109.

Shumway, D. (1992). Rock and roll as a cultural practice. In A. DeCurtis (Ed.), *Present Tense: Rock and Roll and Culture* (pp. 117–133). Durham, NC: Duke University Press.

Small, C. (1998). *Musicking: The Meanings of Performing and Listening*. Middletown, CT: Wesleyan University Press.

Straw, W. (1991). Systems of articulation, logics of change: Communities and scenes in popular music. *Cultural Studies*, **5**(3), 368–388.

Tarrant, M. (2002). Adolescent peer groups and social identity. *Social Development*, **11**(1), 110–123.

Thurlow, C. (2005). Deconstructing Adolescent Communication. In A. Williams and C. Thurlow (Eds.), *Language as social action. Talking adolescence*: Perspectives on communication in the teenage years ((pp. 1–20). New York, NY: Peter Lang.

Williams, J. P. (2006). Authentic identities: Straightedge subculture, music, and the Internet. *Journal of Contemporary Ethnography*, **35**(2), 173–200.

Chapter 18

'There is a good spot in my heart': A story of a music therapy group that enables young sex offenders to reconnect with themselves, their stories, and their communities

Helen Oosthuizen

The process begins

'We're all here because of something to do with sex, right?'

A group of five young men sit around me in a circle, looking down, shifting in their seats. They don't know each other, speak different languages and are from different race groups and communities. Sitting in this group is also a statement that 'I am a sex offender'. It's humiliating.

These young South Africans have been referred to the Support Programme for Abuse Reactive Children (SPARC) by courts, social workers, or schools. SPARC is a diversion programme initiated by a non-governmental organization, The Teddy Bear Clinic for Abused Children, as a response to increasing numbers of child-on-child offences (Teddy Bear Clinic, 2019). Young people who have committed an offence for the first time (between the ages of 7 and 17 years) commute from their home communities to attend 12 weekly group sessions that include music therapy followed by cognitive behavioural and psycho-educational therapies facilitated by social workers. The programme aims to divert participants away from the court system and provide them with alternative possibilities for their lives, to prevent recidivism.

Whereas their offences may have been motivated by concurrent drug or alcohol abuse, peer pressure, an exploration of sexuality, or even a learned normalization of sexually inappropriate behaviour, a significant number of programme participants also bring with them personal experiences of abuse or neglect, fragmented or dysfunctional family systems and violence within their communities and homes (Prentky et al., 2009). Many have received little support to cope with traumatic experiences. SPARC is not just about a sexual offence; it's about supporting young people struggling to define their identities and relationships within challenging circumstances.

Music, music therapy, and young offenders

'Now, here I am … a white woman, rather older than the rest of you, with all these instruments. Some of you may be wondering what this has to do with you and what I'm expecting?' A few smiles.

Music is an important part of SPARC. Group members often walk into sessions with earphones in their ears, and don't forget to put them back in again before they leave. Music is a coping mechanism, it can help young people to regulate their emotions (Miranda, 2013) and music is a statement of who they are, who they are not, where they belong, and perhaps also that they belong somewhere (Tarrant et al., 2001).

Young people are generally intrigued to encounter music in our diversion programme. Documented literature, however, supports the value of music therapy within similar contexts in addressing goals that include enhancing the self-esteem of participants; encouraging appropriate expressions of emotions; helping young people to gain insight into their personal life experiences and fostering healthy social skills (Ierardi and Jenkins, 2012; Skaggs, 1997; Smeijsters et al., 2011).

The SPARC music therapy programme draws from an eclectic approach, including both active (drumming, improvising, or songwriting) and receptive (music listening along with reflection or exploration of imagery) music therapy techniques to address similar goals that also align with themes covered within the cognitive behavioural programme. Whether our music sounds like a product of accomplished musicians or more like a deafening noise, the focus is on para-musical affordances such as the potential of musical experiences for enabling and containing the release of powerful emotions or exploration of social interactions (Ansdell, 2014). In this way, the overall diversion programme motivates young people to engage cognitively, physically, emotionally, and socially, without being limited by what they can verbalize (Omar et al., 2012). As the therapist I facilitate music-based activities and encourage contributions that support, challenge, and offer insight to group members. These experiences may help to transform how participants construct their lives both within and beyond the programme. Further, SPARC participants, perhaps awaiting a 'punitive' programme, have expressed that they particularly enjoy creative programmes such as music therapy that focus on their strengths and potential apart from their offence (Omar et al., 2012).

The following case story reflects my experience of a group of five young men and the music we explored in the SPARC programme.

I don't fit in here: finding a place to belong

Once initial greetings are over, I ask each group member to take a djembe drum. Ashwin[1] smiles. He's a drummer in his church band. Others appear a little nervous, but welcome the opportunity of playing rather

---

[1] All names of group members have been changed to protect their confidentiality

than talking. My directive lead of a few simple beats ensures that all can participate. Slowly, the group is drawn together, beating, moving as one unit, even if there is little eye contact, little explicit connection with one another.

Structured drum beats can offer a predictable and thus safe space to begin our process as group members focus on their own beats as well as entraining to the sounds and expressions of others (Camilleri, 2002). As a therapist I carefully time my beating, decreasing the tempo to include a group member struggling to manage a beat, increasing dynamics to meet the spiralling energy and excitement of the group. Participants are physically, mentally, and emotionally drawn into a musical community, necessitating the contributions of every member, regardless of prior musical training or skills. We all have an innate drive towards belonging and the so-cial bonds formed as we drum together are a powerful motivator for participation (Pavlicevic, 2010).

Once the group is comfortable with drumming, I introduce a new beat, with rests where I invite each group member to offer a short sequence of their own to be imitated by the others. Those more musically competent rush at the opportunity, beating confidently and clearly. Others are hesitant. Sandile starts off, then stops, shakes his head.

The opportunity to contribute a new beat offers each member a non-verbal means of introducing themselves. This introduction is a culmination of both personal character-istics and learned cultural norms (Stige, 2002). Ashwin's beating expresses his personal confidence and musical skills. Tshepo's playing is tentative, though his beat reflects that of a popular hip hop song. As group members follow the beats initiated by their peers, these expressions are heard and affirmed, while the group explores positive social interactions through listening and working together (Skaggs, 1997). I listen, and reflect. Taking into account musical ability and learning, these musical introductions offer important feed-back about who and how these young people are.

I ask what it felt like to offer our own beats. Ashwin and Joe burst out that it was great. No one else makes eye contact. I choose to comment on what I've noticed: 'Wow, some of you played really fast with cool beats. But some of you struggled.' I explain how music can sometimes express how we are, then con-tinue: 'I wonder if some of you actually feel like you're not quite fitting in, perhaps even with this group as a whole?' Suddenly Sandile looks up: 'Yeah', he says, 'I don't fit in with this music, this group, this stuff.' He's been quiet up until this moment and now we understand that this is possibly more than an anxiety about beating a drum.

Sandile's anxiety was expressed and so transformed into something meaningful for himself and others. His music voiced what he may not have been aware of within himself, never mind finding words or courage to state it. After this point, others began to acknowledge

Sandile. There was more eye contact and time was allowed for him to find a beat. Ashwin and Joe sometimes jumped in to support the attempts Sandile made. This also motivated the initially quiet Tshepo and Xolani to offer beats of their own with slightly more confidence. Through positive experiences of affirmation and support, group members began to trust a little more, try new ideas and discover themselves within the group.

Building a supportive community is particularly important for young people who have committed sex offences. In their own residential or social communities (or even within themselves) these young people may have been shunned, responded to with shock or disdain, or alternatively encouraged to keep quiet and deny their behaviour. They need to find a space to openly explore the nature of their offences and life experiences. For this group, perhaps it was our drumming that opened this space.

Connecting through stories: the story of a man and a cup

It's the third session. Group members are getting to know one another and are slightly less self-conscious. I offer that today we'll make a story, a 'movie', based on a 'soundtrack' that includes five short excerpts of music. I have selected music that has no lyrics and will most likely not be well known to group members to allow space for creative ideas to emerge rather than only pre-existing associations.

In response, some eyes roll. Others lean forward. 'Cool!', they say. I play the first excerpt, then ask for ideas. The group starts off slowly: 'um, there's a man driving …' … 'and it's late at night …'. I play the second piece. Ideas come faster. Some group members get animated … 'The man's exhausted, he tries to pour himself a whisky' … 'Ya … but as he gets a cup the cupboards crash down on him' … (a lot of laughing) … 'and his cup keeps running away, pouring out his whisky'. I encourage everyone to offer something and negotiate with the group when many ideas are offered at once, but otherwise allow the story to move in any direction, no matter how bizarre the plot may appear. The third excerpt: 'The cup hides under the man's bed, and as he tries to get at it he falls asleep.' Joe stops and says: 'This is just a story right?' Less laughter now. 'In his dream the cup takes the man to a very dark and scary part of his house he didn't know about.' The fourth excerpt: 'He feels frightened and alone' … 'but then discovers that this was a dream. His cupboards haven't fallen'. The fifth excerpt: 'He goes to the piano and plays, expressing how he felt in his dream.'

Most groups I've worked with love creating stories. Stories and myths are embedded in all cultures and communities. Through our identification with a hero or heroine we can connect with aspects of our inner selves and explore different perspectives and possibilities (Pearson, 2012). In this case, the group's only (human) character is not even given a name, and is thus distanced from the group, de-personalized. This might make any connections between his experiences and those of the group more bearable. It's a way of articulating the 'unspeakable' (Errington et al., 2013).

Young people are generally familiar with the way music works in movies. The music elicits a wide range of imagery (Wesley, 2002). Some excerpts offer a spacious palette to work from, others suggest an entry of more intense or emotional content, before progressing towards a comforting or triumphant resolution. The music calls the group to embark on their own hero's journey along with challenges and rewards.

In the fourth session, I read the story back to the group, and ask questions. Why is the man so tired? What is the dark space? And what might this all have to do with their offences? This elicits an intense discussion. After some time, I suggest that the group draw their discussion together around major themes. They describe these as circumstances surrounding their offences:

◆ *being in a dark or difficult place*

◆ *pressure (peer pressure, or pressure from alcohol)*

◆ *bad decisions (referring to the actual offence).*

One of the group members suddenly asks, 'But where do we get help? As young guys, who can we talk to about these things?' Most group members struggle to think of any kind of support system. We add a last theme:

◆ *help to escape.*

This is one aspect I will stress when giving the social worker feedback. He may offer practical suggestions, and will be supporting group members beyond this process.

Working through parts of this story became a means through which group members gained deeper insight into aspects of themselves and their past experiences. They could also help one another as peers grappling with similar issues. The themes related directly to their lives and offending behaviour, so I continued to work with these, moving from verbal exploration towards active music making.

As the fourth session draws to a close, we move back to the music instruments to embody our themes through improvisation. My sense is that this will wrap up our discussion in a meaningful way, and enable a release of the intensity of emotions experienced through the session. Group members place themselves around an array of instruments they have chosen: guitars, keyboard, drums, and percussion. I explain that they can play as they like to 'let out' what each theme sounds or feels like to them. They know by this stage that there's no need to try and form the music into any kind of aesthetic product.

I call out the first theme: 'A dark space'. The music starts. It's sparse, awkward, and unpredictable. A muffled drum beat, a few taps on claves, tentative strums on a guitar. Joe starts vocalizing, moaning almost as if he is in pain ... I am not sure how to join the group and decide to just listen, to see where the music might lead.

I call the second theme: 'Pressure'. The music intensifies. It's still unpredictable, but loud now, with fewer moments of silence. More group members try out vocal sounds. The music accentuates a feeling of chaos ...

I call the following theme: 'Bad decisions.' The group ignores me. I call again. Still no change. I need to stop the group entirely before we can move to this theme. The group does not want to re-experience what it was like to commit an offence.

The music gets even louder and feels heavy. The sounds fill the space, there's not a chance to breathe. There is still no sense of tempo or phrasing and the vocal sounds seem to wander about. It's completely fragmented, yet not without a sense of group members trying to hold things together. It feels exceptionally tense. I'm uncomfortable and have to work hard not to move on immediately.

I call out the last theme, with some relief: 'Help to escape'. But the group struggles to change their music. As they had asked earlier, I now wonder from where and whether they could possibly 'get help', even musically. I then take a large djembe and bring in a strong basic beat. Slowly, the group finds a beat around this. They listen and fit their beats in with one another so that I can draw back and leave my drum. The music feels lighter and eventually becomes quite jubilant. The group is playing as a unit with a catchy, strong rhythm. Two group members get up and start dancing.

As we end, a group member comments: 'Yo, that dark space ... that was hectic.' There's some discussion around how hard it felt, and how hard it was to escape. Another group member says: 'Wow, I never knew we could get all of this out of just playing music!'

I am not sure whether this group may have explored this sequence of events in such depth cognitively as they did non-verbally; individually as they did collaboratively. Music-making is a flexible means of communicating ourselves to others, enabling adolescents to express themselves honestly. Through music this group could physically re-enact and work through the awkward internal experiences surrounding their offences without necessarily disclosing 'secret' information (McFerran, 2010; Skaggs, 1997).

Concurrently to this process, together with the social worker, group members had written letters to the children they had abused[2], acknowledging their remorse and hopes to do better in the future. This began a process of moving outwards, beyond the relative safety of the group space.

I wanna know what it's like: a rap

The fifth session: remaining with our themes, I ask group members to imagine what they might say to someone they could trust to provide 'help to escape'. Joe writes out the lyrics and then recites a rap by the artist Lecrae (2006). It's about a man who's really messed up and needs help. This inspires Sandile to recite a rap he knows in Zulu and I ask him to translate. 'It's about a boy who steals stuff because he's so poor, but he then goes to jail,' he says.

Some therapists challenge the use of rap music in a therapeutic context due to explicit, violent, or negative content. However, these lyrics articulate difficult life experiences or feelings about sexuality that a number of young people connect to (Tyson et al., 2012). The content of some raps also express healthy values and themes such as hopes for the future, joy, 'the importance of family, positive role models, perseverance/resiliency', or 'positive self-image', among others (Yancy and Hadley, 2012, p. xxvii). The group find support beyond the context of this group through their music.

The process of sharing rap lyrics initiates a decision to create an original rap. The group want to write something that could help young people in similar situations to theirs. In this way they become the 'help' they longed for in their own lives, a significant part of owning their experiences. Group members negotiate, rework, and finally loosely base their rap around a hook: 'I wanna know what it's like', describing their temptation to

---

[2] Letters would only be given to these children in cases where this would be helpful and healing for both parties. The purpose of writing letters was more for group members to develop empathy for those impacted by their actions

commit sexual offences. Over the next few sessions, the group works on their rap, as we continue to discuss the meanings evoked through the hook (which included spontaneous phrases such as 'I wanna be taller, just a lil' bit older, I wanna fly higher') and through individual verses of group members. Some lines are from raps the boys know well, others are original.

The rhythmic structure of a rap serves to organize ideas offered by young people into an aesthetic and clear format. Perhaps this helped group members to manage the chaotic aspects of their lives they had expressed through our improvisation. Perfecting and then performing a rap offers an experience of mastery within a medium many young people share and connect with deeply (Lightstone, 2012). Both the process of creating the rap and the focus on a final performance became significant factors in these young people's therapy process.

As the rap evolves, group members take on distinct roles. Ashwin sets a steady rhythm that forms a basis for the whole rap. Joe appears to be the most 'lyrical' rapper and draws from raps he knows well to tell his story. Each week, Sandile comes up with some new material, then shrugs and says it won't work even when offered the chance to rap in his first language, Zulu. Joe offers help and Ashwin changes his rhythms to fit with Sandile's attempts, but still his lines don't come together as he'd like. Tshepo looks very self-conscious and keeps his head down but the way he's moving a little to the music shows some interest. Xolani smiles but does not participate at all.

One of the goals of SPARC is to motivate programme participants to take responsibility for their futures. It was important for group members to decide how they would contribute to this process, trying out and negotiating different ways of relating and being. In this way, they could consider their potential to contribute meaningfully within a community.

Xolani's lack of participation was difficult to align with the group process, and yet he needed the space to choose this role. In a compulsory programme such as SPARC, the only form of control a group member may have is to choose not to participate (Ierardi and Jenkins, 2012). This in itself might express an ability to choose to abstain from further offending behaviour. Xolani does not simply 'play' along as expected.

My role in the group is now less directive and flexible even though I need to remain very aware of the group as they interact personally and musically. I mediate between group ideas, then fill in a musical accompaniment. I notice Tshepo tentatively moving his body with the rapping, and teach him a simple bass line on the keyboard. He practises over and over, and starts to work together with the others. He's finding a way to belong. I notice Sandile's attempts to add his own rap and make sure the group give him ample space to offer something. The fact that he is trying so hard is important. His life is filled with many difficulties, and the ability to master a challenge such as this may help him to build resilience in other contexts. Xolani offers nothing despite attempts to involve him in rapping, playing supportive drum rhythms or learning a keyboard line. I move between offering options for his participation and allowing his non-participation.

As the therapist in this process I was very aware of my lack of expertise within the hip hop genre, and poor grasp of the first languages of some group members. The group needed the freedom to work within languages and genres with which they were familiar, validating their identities and enhancing opportunities for them to express themselves freely (Ahmadi and Oosthuizen, 2012). As the group took ownership of their creative process, preparing to move out towards the broader community, my role was increasingly that of a supportive witness.

Performing as a means of connecting to the broader community

For our last session, parents and clinic staff have been invited to a performance of our rap. I am rather nervous. I feel that I need to ensure that the group is able to adequately perform their product, offering something they are proud of. I start directing the group, but they're not following my lead. The group huddles together to chat (without me—that is). Then Ashwin explains that he doesn't like the echo of the djembe drums he's playing in this room, so he'll need to use the keyboard. This means I need to split the keyboard into drum kit and bass sounds for Ashwin and Tshepo. There's no longer room for my accompaniment. I also have a sense that the group's saying to me ... thank you, we'll take it from here.

I sit in an audience of a few staff members and two parents. Ashwin nods to bring the group in. There's the hook, and some spontaneous improvised phrases. The group gets more energized, louder, and confident. Even Xolani is playing along with some shakers. Ashwin is pushing his arm against Tshepo to make sure Tshepo stays in time. Tshepo's looking very cool, his hoodie over his head, moving with each beat. The group perform the verses we've practised. But then the music goes on. After a slight, awkward silence only filled by the constantly repeated drum rhythm, Sandile stands up and takes from his pocket a rap he's written. I thought he had resigned himself to just being a 'percussionist'. I am taken aback. Sandile raps:

> *I am a person I want to be*
> *But never tried to believe*
> *My soul will never be seen like the waves of the sea*
> *I may look good but I am not*
> *But there is a good spot in my heart*
> *Yes I pray, I pray to God*
> *But patience is needed*
> *Whether I like it or not*
> *How am I an evil spirit*
> *I hope not 'cos I don't feel it ...*
> *...*
> *... Stand out and shout*
> *You will be known about*
> *That's how I am*

Sandile found his voice! After the performance, he comes up to me. He hasn't come to say goodbye, or thank you, or await affirmation. All he wants to know is: 'When do we get copies of the DVD?' This is the group's product. He wants to take it with him, maybe to remember our group, or to show this to the people he chooses, those significant to him who he hopes will witness his potential.

Privacy is of exceptional importance within the diversion process. The mere possibility of a community member sharing some knowledge about crimes committed could have implications for the entire futures of both perpetrators and survivors of abuse. And yet, offences are committed within communities that must be considered (Errington et al., 2013). These communities will encourage or discourage group members, hold them accountable, accept or reject them, support or neglect them. Without the support of a community, these young people will find it difficult to continue to develop healthy identities. Thus, while most of the therapy process is kept private, a space for group members to confidentially share their difficult feelings and experiences, the process culminates in a performance. It's recorded so that group members can choose who needs to see it. Through their performance, group members can communicate their potential and desire to take responsibility for their future lives and decisions (Ahmadi and Oosthuizen, 2012). 'That's how I am', they are saying.

Conclusion

A group of five young men leave the room. Each holds a DVD recording of their rap, a reminder of a group music therapy process where they could experience belonging and support from one another as they explored their life experiences. Five young people return to their communities free of a criminal record, accountable to take ownership over their lives. They will continue to meet many challenges presenting difficult choices but through music have experienced alternative ways of connecting and being with others. They leave with an opportunity to consider futures that hold hope.

Acknowledgement

The author would like to acknowledge the advice and support of Katrina McFerran and Lauren Gower.

References

Ahmadi, M. and Oosthuizen, H. (2012). Naming my story and claiming myself. In S. Hadley and G. Yancy (Eds), *Therapeutic Uses of Rap and Hip-Hop* (pp. 191–210). New York: Routledge.

Ansdell, G. (2014). *How Music Helps in Music Therapy and Everyday Life.* Aldershot: Ashgate.

Camilleri, V. (2002). Community building through drumming. *The Arts in Psychotherapy, 29,* 261–264.

Errington, K., Errington, S., Oosthuizen, H., and Sangweni, N. (2013). Dancing, drumming and drawing the unspeakable. *Matatu: Journal for African Culture and Society, 44,* 55.

Ierardi, F. and Jenkins, N. (2012).Rap composition and improvisation in a short-term juvenile detention facility. In S. Hadley and G. Yancy (Eds), *Therapeutic Uses of Rap and Hip-Hop* (pp. 253–274). New York: Routledge.

Lecrae. (2006). After the Music Stops. Reach Records.

Lightstone, A. (2012). The importance of hip-hop for music therapists. In S. Hadley and G. Yancy (Eds), *Therapeutic Uses of Rap and Hip-Hop* (pp. 39–56). New York: Routledge.

McFerran, K. (2010). *Adolescents, Music and Music Therapy: Methods and Techniques for Clinicians, Educators and Students.* London: Jessica Kingsley.

Miranda, D. (2013). The role of music in adolescent development: Much more than the same old song. *International Journal of Adolescence and Youth*, **18**(1), 5–22.

Omar, S., Steenkamp, E. and Errington, S. (2012). *Children who Sexually Abuse other Children: A South African Perspective*. Bloemfontein: Sun Press.

Pavlicevic, M. (2010). Playtime at work. In M. Pavlicevic, A. D. Santos, and H. Oosthuizen (Eds), *Taking Music Seriously: Stories From South African Music Therapy* (pp. 155-169). Cape Town: Music Therapy Community Clinic.

Pearson, C. S. (2012). *Awakening the Heroes Within: Twelve Archetypes to Help us Find Ourselves and Transform our World*. London: Harper Collins.

Prentky, R., Pimental, A., Cavanaugh, D. and Righthand, S. (2009). Understanding the treatment needs of adolescents. In A. R. Beech, L. A. Craig, and D. Kevin (Eds), *Assessment and Treatment of Sex Offenders: A Handbook* (pp. 430-450). Oxford: Wiley Blackwell.

Skaggs, R. (1997). Music-centred creative arts in a sex offender treatment programme for male juveniles. *Music Therapy Perspectives*, **15**(2), 73–78.

Smeijsters, H., Kil, J., Kurstjens, H., Welton, J., and Willemars, G. (2011). Arts therapies for young offenders in secure care—A practice-based research. *The Arts in Psychotherapy*, **38**, 41–51.

Stige, B. (2002). *Culture-Centred Music Therapy*. Gilsum, NH: Barcelona.

Tarrant, M., North, A. and Hargreaves, D. (2001). Social categorisation, self-esteem and the estimated musical preferences of male adolescents. *The Journal of Social Psychology*, **141**(5), 565–581.

Teddy Bear Clinic (2019). Home. Retrieved 09/01/2019 from http://ttbc.org.za/

Tyson, E., Detchkov, K., Eastwood, E., Carver, A. and Sehr, A. (2012). Therapeutically and socially relevant themes in hip-hop music: A comprehensive analysis of a selected sample of songs. In S. Hadley and G. Yancy (Eds), *Therapeutic Uses of Rap and Hip-Hop* (pp. 99–115). New York: Routledge.

Wesley, S. (2002). Guided imagery and music with children and adolescents. In: K. Bruscia and D. Grocke (Eds), *Guided Imagery and Music: The Bonny Method and Beyond* (pp. 137-149). Gilsum, NH: Barcelona.

Yancy, G. and Hadley, S. (2012). Introduction. In S. Hadley and G. Yancy (Eds), *Therapeutic Uses of Rap and Hip-Hop* (p. xxiii). New York: Routledge.

Chapter 19

Social media, adolescent developmental tasks, and music

Roseann Pluretti and Piotr S. Bobkowski

Introduction

Social media platforms (e.g. Facebook, Snapchat) debuted in the first decade of the twenty-first century, and have since become important channels through which many young people experience music. Like older media, such as radio, records, CDs, and MP3 files, social media facilitate young people's engagement with music. Unlike previous media, social media merge a number of previously disparate music-related functions, allowing young people to engage with music more efficiently. Young people today can use social media not only to consume music, both in audio and video formats, but also to convey their affinity for music genres or artists, to receive music recommendations from network connections, to communicate directly with artists, and to share their personal music remixes and covers. In this chapter we discuss how social media and music intersect in the lives of young people, focusing on three key developmental tasks.

Social media use

Young people use social media frequently. Seventy per cent of European young people (14–17 years old from six countries) said that they used social media every day (Tsitsika et al., 2014) and 45% of US young people (13–18 years old) likewise reported daily use (Common Sense Media, 2015). Forty per cent of European young people said that they spent 2 hours or more each day using social media, and that they used social media more than any other online tool like instant messaging or email (Tsitsika et al., 2014). Young people from the United States who used social media likewise reported spending an average of 2 hours a day with these platforms (Common Sense Media, 2015). Older adolescents reported spending more time with social media than younger ones, and girls reported greater social media use than boys (Common Sense Media, 2015). What is less clear is how much of their time with social media young people spend listening to music. Young people from the United States said that they most frequently accessed music via smartphones, radios, iPods, and computers (Common Sense Media, 2015). Any of these devices other than the radio can host social media, and many social media platforms can be used to stream music. It is likely, therefore, that many young people listen to music and watch music videos via social media.

The activities in which young people engage on social media shape the potential outcomes of these media. Eline Frison and Steven Eggermont (2015) distinguished between passive and active, and private and public social media uses. They showed that Flemish young people (12–19 years old) who engaged more frequently in passive Facebook practices (e.g. browsing profiles) subsequently perceived less friend support than those who engaged more frequently in active public practices (e.g. posting public messages). According to this study, therefore, active and public social media practices relate to greater social benefits than passive practices. While young people can use social media not only to communicate but also to create and distribute their own media, content creation does not appear to be frequent. On average, young people from the United States devoted only 3% of the time they spent with digital devices to content creation, while spending 26% of this time communicating and 39% of the time consuming content passively (Common Sense Media, 2015). While many young people undoubtedly use social media to create and share their music with others, these figures suggest that the average adolescent is more likely to interact with, and to communicate about, content on social media including music, than they are to create and disseminate their own original music content via these platforms.

Developmental tasks

Our discussion of how social media and music intersect in young people's lives focuses on three broad developmental tasks. Psychologists theorize that developmental tasks emerge at specific points in the life course, mark moments of potential growth, and serve as gateways to subsequent successful functioning and development (Havighurst, 1972). The tasks around which we structure our discussion are the reorganization of social relationships, the crystallization of an identity, and physical maturation. Although in the following sections we discuss unique phenomena separately, these three tasks, and the experiences that cluster around them, are closely entwined in young people's lives.

Social development

Social media provide young people with tools and environments for enacting social exchanges that can both advance and stymie their social development. Sharing music and music preferences in social media is part of the currency of these social exchanges (Davis, 2012); that is, one of the badges used to communicate social affiliation and one of the markers with which young people embody online spaces (Taylor et al., 2014).

The social connections and processes that happen in social media largely reflect offline networks and processes, but also can extend these in new ways. A content analysis of young people's Facebook profiles, for instance, showed that they largely used social media to anchor their offline contacts by displaying their offline relationships, locations, and tastes (Zhao et al., 2008). These included the young person's favourite music genres, artists, and songs. Social media have also redefined some of the conventional social functions of adolescent life. In ethnographies, interviews, and content analyses, danah boyd (2010) found that social media not only provided young people new ways to communicate with friends, but also that social media compelled the publicly visible performance of friendship through friend lists and feedback on content. This suggests that when a young person posts something about a newly released single on social media, they and members of their friendship group may expect that their friends will engage with their post. Such exchanges about music and all other important topics thus publicly affirm adolescent relationships, while their absences potentially signal relationship breaches.

How young people use social media and, conversely, how this use relates to the social outcomes they experience appears to be shaped by their social needs. One group of Bermudan young people (13–18 years), for instance, reported using social media to communicate with peers and to increase their sense of belonging (Davis, 2012). Social media use appears to be related positively to social functioning. Dutch young people (11–14 years) who used social media more and with greater intensity were more satisfied with their friendships than those who used social media less (Antheunis et al., 2016). Artemis Tsitsika et al. (2014) also found that European young people (16–18 years) who used social media more reported greater social competence than those who used social media less.

Although much of the evidence connecting social media use with positive social outcomes is correlational, leaving open the possibility that more socially adjusted young people simply use social media more than their less well-adjusted peers, some research does illustrate how social media facilitates positive social development. Social media allows young people to connect easily with their favourite celebrities or musicians by following these individuals' social media accounts. Through these celebrities' social media messages, followers get 'backstage access' to the famous individuals' personal lives (Marwick and boyd, 2011). Such direct communication between celebrities and fans can profoundly impact the fans' perceived level of connection to the artists, even if the fans only observe such artist–fan exchanges. Lady Gaga, for instance, has used social media extensively to connect directly with her followers. Interviews with Lady Gaga's fans from six continents illustrated the positive psychosocial effects that social media can facilitate (Click et al., 2013). The fans, many of them adolescents, called themselves Little Monsters and reported feeling like they were in an intimate, familial relationship with Gaga, their Mother Monster. Through direct contact, Lady Gaga affirmed and celebrated these followers' outsider status, thus assisting them to develop a positive identity, increase their self-worth, and successfully negotiate their offline relationships.

Social challenges and risks

One challenge that some adolescent social media users face is the collapsing of multiple social contexts in one space. Whereas offline, unique social environments, such as family, school, and work, allow individuals to tailor their behaviours and the tastes they communicate to unique social contexts, a social media audience can include representatives of all current and past social environments. Collapsed social contexts may prompt young people to monitor and negotiate their social media activity (boyd, 2014), or to use certain platforms exclusively with distinct social groups (e.g. Facebook for family, Snapchat for friends). This means, for example, that parents and other adults may be privy on social media only to some of the music that young people like and consume. To mitigate against collapsed social contexts, they may compartmentalize the social media platforms on which they share their music tastes.

Cyberbullying and other unsolicited online contacts constitute more serious social media use risks. Across 36 studies about cyberbullying among 12–18-year-olds, Michele Hamm et al. (2015) found that a median of 23% of young people reported being cyberbullied. Among European young people from 25 countries, Elisabeth Staksrud et al. (2013) found that 8% of 9–16-year-olds who used social media reported being bullied. Specific social media practices appear to increase a young person's risks of experiencing cyberbullying and other undesired online contacts (Staksrud et al., 2013). These practices include using publicly accessible profiles, chatting with online-only contacts, and sharing private information. It is possible that the public sharing of music lists on Spotify or video song covers on YouTube, for instance, may expose young people to unsolicited comments and harassment from strangers or anonymous online contacts.

Social identity development

Young people pursue the development of a coherent and stable sense of self by looking to peers and adults for culturally acceptable roles, behaviours, and attitudes to incorporate into their developing identities. They are also self-conscious about how others view them and reflective about how they view themselves. Social media can facilitate a young person's identity development by helping them learn about identity elements, and by offering them a platform for their identity presentations and subsequent feedback.

Music can perform an important socializing role in a young person's identity development, which social media can facilitate. Young people can use social media to draw identity cues from music lyrics, musicians, and from groups of fans who follow specific artists or music genres. For instance, US young people (13–18 years) reported that YouTube music videos taught them about new ways of being and acting, prompted them to reflect on their behaviours, and gave them hope (Roux, 2012).

While individuals largely use social media to connect with their offline friends and acquaintances (Zhao et al., 2008), some young people also value social media's virtual connections outside their offline social circles (Anderson and McCabe, 2012). College-aged gay, lesbian, and bisexual individuals who reflected on their adolescence, for example, agreed that the Internet and social media were important tools in their identity development, allowing them to communicate with other gay, lesbian, and bisexual individuals and to access information not available in their offline environments (Bond et al., 2009). Participation in music-oriented online forums on platforms such as Reddit, for instance, can expose young people to ideas, individuals, and lifestyles with which they are not familiar in their offline lives, and thus expand the repertoire of identity cues on which to draw in constructing their own identities.

Although social media can expand a young person's worldview, its overall contribution to identity exploration may be limited. Many young people may prefer online spaces like social media for identity work because these spaces are away from the gaze of parents and other adults (Anderson and McCabe, 2012). Family and friends, however, continue to provide the overarching context for adolescent identity development. Bermudan adolescents (11–19 years), for instance, who engaged in online identity explorations and experiments understood their identities less clearly than those who did not engage in such online explorations (Davis, 2013). Those who understood their identities more clearly had better relationships with their mothers and friends than those who understood their identities less clearly. For many young people social media may serve only as an ancillary source of identify cues and ideas.

The identity elements that young people project in social media, including their music tastes, can reproduce or challenge prevalent cultural norms. One study, for instance, illustrated the reproduction of gender norms in adolescents' online profiles (Ringrose and Barajas, 2011). British girls (14–16 years) reflected societal standards of feminine beauty in their social media presentations by featuring photos of highly sexualized female bodies, and by using sexual usernames like 'whore'. Counter to this, some young people use social media to present identities that oppose cultural norms. Carla Stokes (2007) found that some US black girls (14–18 years) resisted black hypersexual cultural scripts in their social media profiles and instead presented empowering sexual scripts appropriated from hip hop music. Some of the girls identified as 'down-ass chicks,' for example, and emulated female rappers through confrontational personas, while others used hip hop forms to self-present both power and femininity while eschewing sexual and violent content.

The audiences that young people imagine to be viewing their social media play a crucial role in shaping their presentations. Their social media disclosures, including their music tastes and favourites, are calibrated to elicit an approving response from these audiences. Egle Oolo and Andra Siibak (2013) found that Estonian adolescents (13–16 years) were aware of their extensive social media audiences when creating posts but said that only their close friends' feedback mattered to them. boyd (2014) found that young people tailor their social media presentations to fit their imagined audiences. One adolescent whom she observed, for example, who was vying for a university athletic scholarship, treated his Facebook profile like a professional resume for sports recruiters, while another crafted a profile filled with crass language and inappropriate humour, explaining that the friends who were allowed to see his private profile would appreciate his humour.

Social media audiences play such an important role that the feedback that young people receive on their social media presentations can affect their wellbeing. European young people who received more positive social media feedback had higher social self-esteem and felt greater friend support than those who received less positive feedback (Frison and Eggermont, 2015; Valkenburg et al., 2006). The music and music tastes that young people share and endorse in their social media profiles and music lists are constructed with an audience in mind. It is likely that young people share their music only with those audiences who they expect to endorse their tastes. The audience's reaction to and engagement with music content can affect their self-perceptions and the extent to which they continue to show affinity for this content.

Physical development

Social media can facilitate what young people know about the physical changes they undergo, how these changes affect them, and how they respond to these changes. Social media content, including music-related content like music videos and artists' profiles, can contribute to how young people navigate these physical changes and the associated risks.

Adolescent physical development can usher in a heightened awareness of one's body and questions about being satisfied with it. Critics have blamed the media, including music videos, advertising, and television shows, for promoting a narrow and unattainable standard of beauty. Social media tend to reinforce this standard, contributing to many young people's negative perceptions of their bodies. In a longitudinal survey, Dian de Vries et al. (2016) found that Dutch young people (11–18 years) who initially used more social media ended up being more dissatisfied with their bodies 18 months later than their peers who initially used social media less.

Young people sometimes take unnecessary risks because the regulatory functions of their brains, which control impulsive responses, have not yet fully developed (Steinberg, 2008). Concerns about conventional media (i.e. music, movies, television shows, video games) modelling undesirable or risky behaviours like sexual promiscuity and substance use for young people are well documented. Music content in social media also can be a vehicle for risk behaviour portrayals. An analysis of the 40 most popular music videos on YouTube showed that 45% of these videos featured alcohol-related images and 22% featured tobacco-related images (Cranwell et al., 2014). In an associated survey, 81% of British young people (11–18 years) had watched at least one of these videos and the average adolescent watched seven of them. Most of these young people had watched these videos more than once. Given that popular music often deals with mature themes and that some of it glorifies what are considered risky behaviours, it may not be surprising that music-related social media messages that young people consume often include portrayals of risky behaviour.

There is a correlation between the risky themes that young people present in their social media and how much they identify with these risks. In one study that illustrated this, adolescents in the United States (14–17 years) were asked to construct social media profiles using a variety of content elements, and also to rate themselves on a sexual maturity scale. Young people who rated themselves as more sexually mature chose to represent themselves with images and statements, including music lyrics that were sexually more intense than young people who self-rated as less sexually mature (Bobkowski et al., 2016). For example, sexually more mature young people were more likely to use in their profiles Bruno Mars' lyric 'Yeah, your sex takes me to paradise' than less sexually mature young people. While such portrayals of risk-related symbols and text may reflect young people' identities, these messages also appear to have an inflated effect on how other young people perceive these behaviours. Young people who viewed risk behaviour presentations in social media overestimated the extent to which their peers engaged in these risky behaviours (Black et al., 2013), thus likely developing skewed risk behaviour norms and increasing their likelihood of engaging in them.

The peer context of risk behaviour portrayals on social media may render young people especially vulnerable to being influenced by them. This concern is rooted in social cognitive theory (Bandura, 2001), which suggests that the likelihood of adopting observed behaviours increases when observers identify with their behavioural models, and when these models are rewarded. Because young people primarily use social media to connect with their peers, it is likely that they identify more with their social media connections than they do with more remote models such as characters in music videos or television shows. Most social media platforms also have built-in reward systems wherein users 'like' or re-share specific content, thus communicating their approval of specific messages and their posters. Thus, it is likely that a risky behaviour like substance use modelled in social media by a peer will have greater influence on an adolescent's attitudes and behaviours than the same behaviour modelled by a more remote model like a musician or a music video character. Meanwhile, a music video featuring a risky behaviour that is endorsed by peers on social media is likely to have a greater effect on an adolescent's attitude toward this risky behaviour than the same music video that is not immediately endorsed by a network of peers.

Social media in context

The process by which young people are affected by their consumption of social media content containing risky behaviours may be oversimplified in many social media studies, and in the public imagination. The news media tends to characterize adolescent social media use as unhealthy, dangerous, secretive, and damaging to conventional relationships (Stern and Odland, 2017). Adolescent agency, creativity, and the benefits that can accrue to young people from social media use are rarely discussed. The reinforcing spirals theory (Slater, 2007) reminds us that media consumption and effects take place within a broader offline social context of the family, peers, and neighbourhoods. These agents can condition young people to search out or avoid certain media messages, and to be more or less susceptible to the effects of these messages.

Michael Slater and Kimberly Henry (2013) illustrated this in a longitudinal study of 7th and 8th grade US students, aged between 12 and 14 years old, that focused on music tastes, friendship groups, and risky substance use (i.e. alcohol, cigarettes, marijuana). In this study, young people who initially spent more time consuming specific types of music were more likely than those who consumed less of this music to associate more over time with friends who shared similar music tastes. This increase in time spent with friends was related, in turn, to an increase in the likelihood of adopting risky substances that were normative within these friendship groups. This study illustrates that the link between consuming risk behaviour portrayals in social media, including music-related social media, and enacting these behaviours, tends not to be direct but mediated by friendships and friends' behavioural norms.

Conclusion

Social media platforms have redefined how young people engage with music. In the past, young people expressed their affinity for music through posters, mix tapes, band apparel, and fan letters. Today, young people only need social media to perform all of the same tasks. They also can do this collectively with, and in view of, friends and potentially more extensive audiences. Music-related social media practices can solicit feedback that, depending on its valence, further can shape their music tastes and affiliations.

In this chapter we discussed how social media assists young people in their social, mental, and physical development, and how music intersects social media's functions in these developmental tasks. Adolescents can learn about new identity cues from their favourite musicians by watching their music videos or following their personal social media accounts. They can signal elements of their developing identities to their audiences by presenting music tastes and related social affiliations in their social media. They can receive feedback on their music interests via comments and 'likes', and incorporate this feedback into their music tastes and identities. Young people can use social media to connect with others who share their musical interests, potentially developing friendships or a sense of belonging. Young people also can use music-related social media to develop positive or negative impressions of their bodies, and to learn about how members of the music fan cultures with which they identify relate to risky behaviours like substance use. Our discussion is not exhaustive but aimed to identify the key points at which social media and music can impact adolescent development.

Social media will continue to play an important role in how young people experience music, and in how they complete their developmental tasks. With relatively little research thus far examining the interplay between music, adolescent development, and social media, scholars interested in building a research agenda at the intersection of these three phenomena have an almost blank canvas with which to work. Such research can continue not only to explicate current cultural processes, but also to advance theoretical development on the uses and effects of digital media.

References

Anderson, L. and McCabe, D. (2012). A coconstructed world: Adolescent self-socialization on the internet. *Journal of Public Policy & Marketing*, **31**(2), 240–253.

Antheunis, M., Schouten, A., and Krahmer, E. (2016). The role of social networking sites in early adolescents' social lives. *The Journal of Early Adolescence*, **36**(3), 348–371.

Bandura, A. (2001). Social cognitive theory of mass communication. *Media Psychology*, **3**(3), 265–299.

Black, S., Schmiege, S., and Bull, S. (2013). Actual versus perceived peer sexual risk behavior in online youth social networks. *Translational Behavioral Medicine*, **3**(3), 312–319.

Bobkowski, P., Shafer, A., and Ortiz, R. (2016). Sexual intensity of adolescents' online self-presentations: Joint contribution of identity, media consumption, and extraversion. *Computers in Human Behavior*, **58**(1), 64–74.

Bond, B., Hefner, V., and Drogos. K. (2009). Information-seeking practices during the sexual development of lesbian, gay, and bisexual individuals: The influence and effects of coming out in a mediated environment. *Sexuality & Culture*, **13**(1), 32–50.

boyd, d. (2010). Friendship. In I. Mizuko (Ed.), *Hanging Out, Messing Around, and Geeking Out: Kids Living and Learning with New Media* (pp. 79–116). Cambridge, MA: MIT Press.

boyd, d. (2014). *It's Complicated: The Social Lives Of Networked Teens*. New Haven, CT: Yale University Press.

Click, M., Lee, H., and Holladay, H. (2013). Making monsters: Lady Gaga, fan identification, and social media. *Popular Music and Society*, **36**(3), 360–379.

Common Sense Media. (2015). *The Common Sense Census: Media Use by Tweens and Teens*. San Francisco, CA: Common Sense Media.

Cranwell, J.,Murray, R. Lewis, S., Leonardi-Bee, J., Dockrell, M., and Britton, J. (2014). Adolescents' exposure to tobacco and alcohol content in Youtube music videos. *Addiction*, **110**(4), 703–711.

Davis, K. (2012). Friendship 2.0: Adolescents' experiences of belonging and self-disclosure online. *Journal of Adolescence*, **35**(6), 1527–1536.

Davis, K. (2013). Young people's digital lives: The impact of interpersonal relationships and digital media use on adolescents' sense of identity. *Computers in Human Behavior*, **29**(6), 2281–2293.

de Vries, D., Jochen P., de Graaf, H., and Nikken, P. (2016). Adolescents' social network site use, peer appearance-related feedback, and body dissatisfaction: Testing a mediation model. *Journal of Youth and Adolescence*, **45**(1), 211–224.

Frison, E. and Eggermont, S. (2015). Toward an integrated and differential approach to the relationships between loneliness, different types of Facebook use, and adolescents' depressed mood. *Communication Research*. doi:10.1177/0093650215617506.

Hamm, M., Newton, A., Chisholm, A., Shulhan, J., Milne, A., Sundar, P., Ennis, H., Scott, S., and Harting, L. (2015). Prevalence and effect of cyberbullying on children and young people: A scoping review of social media studies. *JAMA Pediatrics*, **169**(8), 770–777.

Havighurst, R. (1972). *Developmental Tasks and Education*. New York: David McKay Company.

Marwick, A. and boyd, d. (2011). To see and be seen: Celebrity practice on Twitter. *Convergence: The International Journal of Research into New Media Technologies*, **17**(2), 139–158.

Oolo, E. and Siibak, A. (2013). Performing for one's imagined audience: Social steganography and other privacy strategies of estonian teens on networked publics. *Cyberpsychology: Journal of Psychosocial Research on Cyberspace*, 7(1), 48–59.

Ringrose, J. and Barajas, K. (2011). Gendered risks and opportunities? Exploring teen girl's digitized sexual identities in postfeminist media contexts. *International Journal of Media and Cultural Politics*, 7(2), 121–140.

Roux, M. G. (2012). *Adolescent Experience af the Effect of Watching YouTube Videos on Sense of Self*. Boston, MA: Massachusetts School of Professional Psychology.

Slater, M. (2007). Reinforcing spirals: The mutual influence of media selectivity and media effects and their impact on individual behavior and social identity. *Communication Theory*, **17**(3), 281–303.

Slater, M. and Henry, K. (2013). Prospective influence of music-related media exposure on adolescent substance-use initiation: A peer group mediation model. *Health Communication*, **18**(3), 291–305.

Staksrud, E., Ólafsson, K., and Livingstone, S. (2013). Does the use of social networking sites increase children's risk of harm? *Computers in Human Behavior*, **29**(1), 40–50.

Steinberg, L. (2008). Risk-taking in adolescence: New perspectives from brain and behavioral science. *Current Directions in Psychological Science*, **16**(2), 55–59.

Stern, S. R. and Odland, S. B. (2017). Constructing dysfunction: News coverage of teenagers and social media. *Mass Communication and Society*, **20**(4), 505–525.

Stokes, C. (2007). Representin' in cyberspace: Sexual scripts, self-definition, and hip hop culture in black American adolescent girls' home pages. *Culture, Health, & Sexuality*, **9**(2), 169–184.

Taylor, Y., Falconer, E., and Snowdon, R. (2014). Queer youth, Facebook and faith: Facebook methodologies and online identities. *New Media & Society*, **16**(7), 1138–1153.

Tsitsika, A., Tzavela, E., Janikian, M., Olafsson, K., Iordache, A., Schoenmakers, T., Tzavara, C., and Richardson, C. (2014). Online social networking in adolescence: Patterns of use in six European countries and links with psychosocial functioning. *Journal of Adolescent Health*, **55**(1), 141–147.

Valkenburg, P., Peter, J., and Schouten, A. (2006). Friend networking sites and their relationship to adolescent's wellbeing and social self-esteem. *Cyberpsychology & Behavior*, **9**(5), 584–590.

Zhao, S., Grasmuck, S., and Martin, J. (2008). Identity construction on Facebook: Digital empowerment in anchored relationships. *Computers in Human Behavior*, **24**(5), 1816–1836.

Chapter 20

Globalizing adolescence: Digital music cultures and music therapy

Michael Viega

Introduction

Adolescents across the globe connect and engage in shared music experiences via digital technology. Music content is being listened to, created, and shared instantaneously on a variety of online platforms, typically using mobile technology. Making music using new technologies have allowed for increasingly egalitarian digital spaces that provide teenagers with the opportunity to discover, invent, and generate new musical identities. Music composers and writers of the twentieth century, such as John Cage (1961), R. Murray Schafer (1977/1994), and Brian Eno (1993), professed that musicians of the future would not need to be virtuosos, taking years of lessons to be technically proficient. Instead, musicians would be allowed to express their individuality and uniqueness using the raw elements of sound afforded by music technology. As a music therapist, I have seen philosophical assumptions come alive within my direct music encounters with adolescents using digital technology in a music therapy context.

I began my career in music therapy at the start of the new millennium, working primarily with adolescents in a variety of clinical settings who have experienced adversity and trauma. Since that time, I have been aware of how evolving digital platforms have impacted that way adolescents receive, experience, create, and listen to music. This in turn has shaped my own practice, forcing me to develop competencies in using drum machines, recording software, samplers, and synthesizers. I did not want to simply co-opt new technologies as a means of engaging teenagers but rather find ways for them to be used as the primary vehicle towards meeting therapeutic goals and enhancing musical relationships. In addition, how I listened to music deepened as I began to focus on the timbre and texture of the music production, hearing the imagery potential within the soundscapes of various popular music styles. In essence, the ways in which I work and listen as a music therapist are intrinsically linked to how music production and consumption have evolved in the twenty-first century. These shifts often became apparent for me in moments when the young people I worked with introduced me to new and innovative digital music platforms.

The purpose of this chapter is to highlight how advances in digital technology have impacted the ways adolescents connect to themselves and others within the context of music therapy. To do this, I will chronologically share my own digital adventures as a music therapist working with adolescents in a variety of clinical settings; beginning with the rise of Napster and MP3 file sharing in 2000, to the current accessibility of streaming and mobile technology. I have chosen to share my own stories to demonstrate how advancing technologies intersect with clinical practice in ways that can enhance therapeutic process and relationship. To conclude, I will discuss the ethical challenges of using digital technologies with adolescents and make suggestions for music therapists to enhance its use in therapy.

The rise of digital music culture from 2000 to 2004

The 1990s were a transitional decade in which foundational structures and technologies of the Internet solidified. However, it was the next decade that saw a dramatic shift in how people consumed, experienced, and interacted with it on a daily basis. In July 1999, Napster became one of the first peer-to-peer file-sharing Internet sites, and went on to transform a wide range of conversations about copyright law and the ethical consumption of music, ulitmatley transforming the music industry. It is no coincidence that 1999 marked the peak of CD sales, which then dramatically dropped by 2002 giving way to the exploding market of digital downloads (Kot, 2009). However, in the early days of Napster's existence, its ethical use within a clinical setting was ambiguous and new ways of listening and experiencing music were unfolding.

In the autumn of 2000, I was starting my clinical music therapy internship in a suburb of Washington DC with youth who were transitioning from a prison and/or psychiatric setting back into public school. At that time, the facility's Internet connection was much faster than a typical home modem, which made the computer in the music room a primary site for new songs to be heard and shared. The adolescents there were introducing each other to music not accessible through mainstream channels. This impacted our music therapy sessions because the teenagers were bringing in culturally specific songs to be performed and listened to. This necessitated me to develop competencies by learning music styles and cultural histories of which I was unfamiliar.

Many of the adolescents I worked with in Washington DC spent evenings at clubs experiencing go-go music, a sub-genre of African American music that blends '70s funk with modern Hip Hop sensibilities, focusing on syncopated drumming rhythms and interactive call-and-response experiences (Lornell and Stephenson, 2009). As an intern, I wanted to immerse myself in go-go music, to learn about it and understand what the experience was like for the adolescents I was working with. Before Napster, my access to go-go music would have been very limited, as it was only available for people who actively participated in its culture, which was localized to specific neighbourhoods that shared cassette tapes created during live events. Listening with the adolescents I was working with, I was able to learn about the rhythmic structure of go-go music, its interactive participatory rituals, and the subtle aesthetic preferences people had for certain groups and performances. This led to extended go-go jam sessions with groups of adolescents that were from rival gangs, much to the astonishment of the other counsellors. In addition, access to Napster allowed me to indulge in my own independent listening, which caused me to be a more reflexive listener and participate in music cultures that I was not indigenous too. The ethical ramifications of this, including issues of cultural appropriation and colonization of music cultures in therapy, continue to reverberate into present.

Looking back, the primary shift of this time was the increased ease with which we had to access music. The subversive nature of peer-to-peer file sharing seemed to fit in with a long history of youth music cultures that sought new ways of experiencing music by bypassing traditional avenues of consumption and distribution. File sharing allowed the adolescents I was working with to download music from anywhere around the world without the limitations and boundaries of music categories from a record store. This period marked a change in how the teenagers and I listened, accessed, and experienced music together. Within the next few years, new sampling and recording technology took centre stage in my sessions, allowing the young people I worked with to cut and paste any sound or song found on the Internet and construct new music worlds in the songs they created.

Recording and remixing from 2005 to 2009

Today all sounds belong to a continuous field of possibilities lying within the comprehensive dominion of music. *Behold the new orchestra: the sonic universe!*
And these new musicians: anyone and anything that sounds!

(Schaffer, 1994, p. 5)

Being a music therapist often means having to get used to travelling with a large cargo of instruments. It was always an adventure to walk into various clinical settings with a guitar in my right hand, a bag full of percussion being held by two fingers in my left hand, a djembe slung over my back and held by the other fingers, an electric keyboard under my right arm, and any extra fingers devoted to other musical odds and ends. With perfect balance, I would walk into a room of adolescents who would typically reject these instruments, calling them 'childish' and 'corny'. In 2006, I bought my first drum machine/synthesizer and also began using GarageBand, recording software for Apple's iMac laptop computer. Equipment that had seemed foreign, complicated, and for professional producers or DJs only suddenly became user-friendly, accessible, and egalitarian. This resulted in a defining moment in which I lightened my load, carrying a backpack with a laptop and drum machine, and a guitar in my hand. I began to approach various music therapy methods, like songwriting, differently in terms of the use of the therapeutic space and relationships. This included creating a studio environment in sessions and being called a 'music producer' by many of the young people I was working with during this time.

The digital technology I used was chosen for two reasons. First of all, I had developed competency in the equipment I was using, which allowed for fluid therapeutic moments to go unhindered by technological mishaps. Secondly, the young people I was working with could approach and create music on this equipment at any level with which they felt comfortable. My therapeutic studio at this time consisted of the following equipment, many I continue to use:

1) Tascam US-122L: an audio interface, so that acoustic and electronic instruments could be captured in the recording software.

2) GarageBand Apple Loops: Apple Loops are pre-recorded music files, created and designed for use on Apple computers, which contain a few seconds of music from a variety of individual instruments, vocals, and sound effects.

3) Korg EMX1 Electribe Music Production Station: this electronic instrument is both a drum machine and synthesizer.

4) Korg ESX1 Electribe Music Production Sampler: similar to the EMXI, this electronic instrument can record, sequence, and manipulate any sound from an outside source and turn that sound into a musical instrument.

5) Synthesizer Vocoder: this is a synthesizer keyboard, which mimics electronic analogue sounds from various modern genres of dance and popular music.

6) Korg Midi Keyboard: this keyboard connects to the USB interface of the computer, providing more choices in keyboard sounds and effects.

7) Korg Kaossilator Dynamic Phrase Synthesize: this is a handheld synthesizer/drum pad with a touch-screen interface.

Out of all the emerging technology of this time, I began to rely on two techniques for therapeutic songwriting: looping and remixing.

Looping

Apple's GarageBand, introduced in 2004, allowed people to capture sound from any source—a moment from a pre-recorded song, environmental ambiance, a vocalization, or live instrumentation—manipulate and layer it to create new musical worlds; one did not have to have a music engineering degree to do this! GarageBand also included built-in, preset sound effects to enhance instrumentation and a digital interface that was easy to navigate, even for first-time users. However, it was the pre-recorded Apple Loops, musical phrases, and patterns that could be repeated for extended amounts of time that was a game changer for helping the adolescents I worked with during this time to create their own innovative sonic environments.

During this time, I began working at a children's hospital with children and adolescents who had acquired a spinal cord injury following a traumatic accident. I found that Apple Loops allowed the patients to have autonomous choice, self-efficacy, and agency in creating their own individualized soundscape. GarageBand was not just a means to record a finished product, but was the primary compositional tool used in the creative process. Patients were able to continuously fine tune the composition depending upon how they felt each time they listened to it. Once completed, there was the additional benefit of being able to share the song directly with others online, usually family and friends in other areas around the world. Many adolescents I worked with felt marginalized and alienated due to their social, psychical, and/or psychological turmoil. Composing their inner worlds, and sharing them though sound and song, appeared to provide validation that their voice mattered, and in turn could teach others about their lives and experiences through songs.

Remixing

Remixing has been described as the formal act of using copying/cut and paste (sampling) music technology to re-contextualize a pre-existing sound or pre-composed song towards the creation of a new composition (Navas, 2009). Remix culture is a global community of artists and fans who see the Internet as an open-source digital environment that is central to creating new works of art using sampling hardware and software. It is used widely in Hip Hop, electronic dance music, electronica, and other dance-oriented popular music styles. Remixing as a creative act appears to be well suited for rebellious adolescent art in the twenty-first century, as it can be a paradoxical mix of political activism and lackadaisical creativity. A composer can recycle and appropriate material outside of their immediate experience, incorporate it within their own context, discover new meaning within the art, and (re)present it in a way that makes the discourse more complex. Remixing appears well suited to help an adolescent explore various identities and create something new to share with the world.

For the adolescents I worked with at the hospital, new digital online patforms like YouTube (which debuted in 2005) allowed sound to be gathered from any source around the world and remixed towards therapeutic aims. For instance, one young man who lost his sight following a neurological surgical procedure recycled sounds from his favourite video games and popular YouTube videos to represent his own experience of dealing with his subsequent blindness and depression. He first created a drumbeat by sampling sound effects from the popular Nintendo video game *Super Mario Brothers*. Then he added vocal samples from his favorite YouTube videos, which created a narrative that represented his lived experience of his recent trauma. It was apparent to me that this experience was rewarding for him, as evident through his enthusiastic participation, providing him a sense of agency and self-determination in the midst of his current medical condition.

Concurrently, remixing could also be used by patients dealing with stressful sounds from their environments such as noises from bedside monitors, nurses talking loudly outside the door, and cries from other rooms. Patients could appropriate those sounds and transform them into something aesthetic. The new compositions created by these adolescents allowed them to connect to and reclaim a sense of agency amidst a medical crisis. Subsequently, these compositions began to find digital forums in which these creations could be shared, first through Myspace and soon after via Facebook and Twitter.

Social media and the digital self from 2010 to today

Youth are not merely influenced by their digital world; they are the creators—actively and interactively constructing and reconstructing their identities; establishing, re-connecting, or "de-friending" relationships; as well as challenging and transforming cultural norms in online and offline contexts.

(Michikyan and Suárez-Orozco, 2016, p. 411)

With the advent of Spotify, Pandora, and other music streaming services, users have been able to personalize music preferences, share playlists with their online community, and gain instantaneous access to songs. In addition, platforms like SoundCloud, Mixtape, and Dafpiff have created an egalitarian online space for people to curate playlists, share personal songs, and build an online music community. When these services began to make their way into my music therapy sessions, I remember thinking that the possibilities introduced by Napster and peer-to-peer file sharing at the start of the twenty-first century had now become a reality. During this time, I was able not only able to access young people's favourite songs quickly to meet a therapeutic need, I was able to help them individualize and create new musical identities through these social media platforms.

Lil' j, a patient who was hospitalized for a corrective orthopaedic surgery, used rapping and beat-making in music therapy to enhance coping and engage in culturally meaningful experiences. He had an extensive family unit that visited and kept in constant contact through digital technology. One session, Lil' j was discussing how his cousin made beats. Using text messaging on his mobile device, Lil' j asked for, and quickly received, an instrumental rap beat from his cousin, which consisted of a rhythm track with added sound effects and synthesized harmonic elements. Lil' j immediately uploaded the beat into GarageBand and improvised lyrics on top of the track. He then uploaded the track to SoundCloud for his family and extended to hear. Lil' j was proud of his creation and wanted to make the song public for anyone to hear.

For Lil' j, digital technology allowed him to stay connected with his family while hospitalized. What stands out most in this example is the family's ability to participate and support Lil' j's creation from a distance, demonstrating digital technology's ability to help people engage in meaningful, culturally relevant experiences. In addition, Lil' j wanted to create an anonymous digital identity on SoundCloud, likening it to being able to create a 'superhero version' of himself. His performance can be heard here: https://SoundCloud.com/latin50).

Another example is Katherine, an African American adolescent in foster care who loves to listen to rap music but, at first, did not show interest in sharing her preferences within the therapeutic relationship. The ability to quickly access some of her favourite neighbourhood rappers using various streaming platforms (especially www.datpiff.com) created a space for Katherine to share and reflect on her preferences. She then began to create playlists on www.mixcloud.com of her favourite music, which she categorized by her various moods and life circumstances. Then using a DJ app for the iPad, she blended the music and added sound effects to personalize her creation. Moving from receptive to creative music experiences allowed Katherine to share her uniqueness within our relationship at a level and pace comfortable for her. She could explore her cultural identity through her favourite local rappers and then share her mixes with others through digital media platforms.

Ethical considerations for using digital technology

Although the benefits of using digital media within a music therapy environment have been explored above, there are several ethical considerations to consider. First, having instant access to music from anywhere in the world means that the historical, biographical, and cultural context can get lost. This may lead to appropriating music for use in therapy without developing cultural competencies. Hadley and Norris (2016) suggest that music therapists should seek competencies to understand the potential risks of appropriating and colonizing music cultures in therapy. The ability to access new music cultures may lead to an increased empathy of the social, cultural, political, and historical contexts that impact the lives of marginalized people (Viega, 2016). This may help therapists use music that may be outside of their own experience in a way that honours the cultural identities of the adolescents they are working with, while also presenting themselves as an authentic and reflexive listener.

Second, the legality of file sharing and cut-and-paste digital technology is often raised in relation to remix culture. Activists such as Lawerence Lessig (2008), a Harvard Law School professor and an expert of intellectual property in the Internet age, have argued against outdated copyright laws in the United States by noting that it criminalizes youth cultures and how young people consume, create, and participate in digital media. This raises a conflict between what is ethical and what is lawful, especially in relation to engaging in music experiences that require sampling technology. When engaging youth in remixing, mash-ups, and digital manipulation of pre-composed music are music therapists infringing on copyright or are they providing ethical and evidence-based treatment? This is an ethical dilemma that is ambiguous and in need of future exploration.

Finally, digital software and social media platforms offer many benefits as described above. However, reflexivity must be used to account for potential ethical dilemmas. For instance, Baker (2015) notes that sharing songs created in therapy could make people vulnerable to social ridicule such as cyberbullying. These issues can be exacerbated with adolescents who are susceptible to digital stress such as those who experience increased anxiety and depression after using social media (Best, Manktelow, & Taylor, 2014). If an adolescent decides to share a song they wrote in therapy using a social media platform, it would be good for therapists to discuss not only the potential dangers of online harassment, but also issues related to confidentiality. Overall, with all the various digital media platforms available to adolescents, their clinical use and contraindication in therapy will need continued exploration.

Conclusion

This chapter has highlighted the impact of digital technologies that have shaped my practice with adolescents in various settings since the beginning of the twenty-first century. The primary benefits discussed have been increased egalitarian access to music, exploration of identity through sonic digital environments, creating group belonging through digital technology, and empowering autonomous choice and creativity. In addition, as a music therapist my ways of listening to popular music styles has expanded, hearing the imagery possibility their soundscapes (Viega, 2014). However, adolescents are also facing increased digital stress on a daily basis, which must be considered when bringing technology into a therapeutic space.

New digital inventions sprout every day and it is youth culture that turns these technologies into challenging and subversive art forms. As a music therapist, this is what I find most interesting working with adolescents. There is a continuous innate drive for youth to reinvent the world around them and create something new, exciting, and beautiful. I feel that a conscientious approach to using digital technology with adolescents is warranted: one that recognizes its inherent benefits while also being reflexive about its potential harm. Digital technology is not just a means to engage adolescents in therapy but also a medium that offers endless opportunities for innovation and discovery.

References

Baker, F. (2015). *Therapeutic Songwriting: Developments in Theory, Methods, and Practice.* London: Palgrave.

Best, P., Manktelow, R., and Taylor, B. (2014). Online communication, social media and adolescent wellbeing: A systematic narrative review. *Children and Youth Services Review*, **41**, 27–36.

Cage, J. (1961). *Silence: Lectures and Writings.* Hanover, NH: Wesleyan University/University Press of New England.

Eno, B. (1983). The studio as compositional tool. *Down Beat*, **50**(7), 56–57.

Hadley, S. and Norris, M. S. (2016). Musical multicultural competency in music therapy: The first step. *Music Therapy Perspectives*, **34**(2), 129–137. DOI: doi.org/10.1093/mtp/miv045

Kot, G. (2009). *Ripped: How the Wired Generation Revolutionized Music.* New York: Scribner.

Lessig, L. (2008). *Remix: Making Art and Commerce Thrive in the Hybrid Economy.* New York: Penguin.

Lornell, K. and Stephenson, C.C. (2009). *The Beat: Go-go Music from Washington DC.* Jackson, MI: University Press of Mississippi.

Michikyan, M. and Suárez-Orozco, M. (2016). Adolescent media and social media use: Implications for development. *Journal of Adolescent Research*, **31**(4), 411–414. doi:10.1177/0743558416643801.

Navas, E. (2009). Remix: The bond of repetition and representation. In S. Sonvilla-Weiss (Ed.), *Mashup Culture* (pp. 157–178). New York: SpringerWien.

Schafer, R. M. (1977/1994). *The Soundscape: Our Sonic Environment and the Tuning of the World.* Rochester, VT: Destiny.

Viega, M. (2014). Listening in the ambient mode: Implications for music therapy practice and theory. *Voices: A World Forum for Music Therapy*, **14**(2). doi:10.15845/voices.v14i2.778.

Viega, M. (2016). Exploring the discourse in Hip Hop and implications for music therapy. *Music Therapy Perspectives*, **34**(2), 138–146. doi:10.1093/mtp/miv035.

Chapter 21

My iPod, YouTube, and our playlists: Connections made in and beyond therapy

Carmen Cheong-Clinch

Introduction

According to the National Mental Health Commission's Second Australian Child and Adolescent Survey of Mental Health and Wellbeing, one in seven young people aged between 4-17 years experience a mental health condition (Lawrence et al., 2015). An average of one young person aged between 15 and 24 years dies from suicide every day. It is made worse by recent surveys that indicate there has been a significant increase in the number of young people who meet the criteria for serious mental illness over the past 5 years, rising from 18.7% in 2012 to 22.8% in 2016 (Mission Australia, 2017) and the suicide rate for young Australians was the highest in 10 years in the same year (Longbottom, 2016).

There has been considerable investment from government that has seen an increase in a range of prevention strategies. However, it appears that current treatments and approaches do not produce the much needed gains and do not have a good alignment with the needs of the young person (MacKee, 2016). It is time to think differently about how youth mental health is approached, the perspective of both mental health literacy and promotion, and early intervention and recovery.

Preferred music and young people with mental illness

When I began my work as a music therapist in 2008 at an acute adolescent mental health facility, I was warned that these young people were 'hard to reach'. Staff on the ward described the patients as uninterested, hostile, aggressive, and generally not responsive to any kind of engagement. Yet if I asked young people 'what kind of music do you like?' (McFerran, 2010, p. 87), I could be met with a flicker of surprise or disbelief, and a hint of interest in the young person's eyes, before they would offer a reply. This often led to discussions about attending a concert, the latest track, or a favourite song. These interactions with young people who are allegedly 'hard to reach' did not match the grunt or sullen responses I had been told to expect.

Young people listening to music with earphones is not an uncommon sight. Hearing young people say 'I won't be able to live without my music' (Cheong-Clinch, 2013) is particularly pertinent to those with whom I work in the adolescent inpatient facility. They often describe their engagement with their preferred music as incredibly important and even a lifeline to them. So it is unthinkable for the young people who would generally listen to their music on their mobile telephones not to have access to their music during their hospital stay, as the current hospital regulations do not permit the use of mobile telephones and/or listening devices with a built-in camera.

Technology has changed since I began work at that facility. Engaging with social media, video games, and music listening is personalized, portable, easily available, and readily accessible. Young people are used to listening to music on palm-size devices, via YouTube or streaming sites like Spotify. As part of a service improvement initiative at the adolescent facility in 2017, young people are now able to access and listen to their preferred music on a digital tablet accessed through Spotify. This new provision by the facility ensures access to young people's preferred music has kept up with technological advances, as well as align with their current means of engagement.

Andrew Bennett (2008) describes young people's engagement with music as a dynamic and interactive process that is steeped in a complex interplay between their preferred music and everyday lives. As found in my research study, which examined the preferred music of young people with mental illness (Cheong-Clinch and McFerran, 2016), preferred music enabled young people to express their emotions and to define and regulate their emotional experiences in different contexts and conditions on an everyday basis. This is not a surprising finding, and appears to be similarly reported in another study of healthy young people (Bosacki and O'Neill, 2015). The young people in that study report that their music is a way for them to express themselves, especially when they find it hard to do so using words. Their song choices relate to their own experiences, reflect their inner life, resonate with their identities, search for meaning, and declare that music is their best friend. As one young person described:

Music means a lot to me because you know you always, like, listen to it, it sometimes helps you through really hard times and yeah I just think it's really important, it helps to express who you are.

Music therapy in an acute adolescent mental health facility

In the adolescent facility, both individual and group music therapy sessions are conducted with the aim of meeting the goals of a young person's hospital stay to contribute to his/her diagnosis formulation, treatment, recovery, and safety planning. The latter two admission goals involve working with the young person to identify their primary coping strategies and circumstances that are possible triggers for their distress, and reflect on the impact of the coping strategy to manage the distress. With music being identified by many young people as a primary coping strategy, a group music listening session is conducted specific to meeting the recovery and safety planning goals. The session consists of listening to their preferred music on YouTube, followed by facilitated reflection and discussion about the impact of their music choice on their current emotional state.

Young people who took part in my study described the experience of sharing music in group music therapy as being of warmth and friendship, fun, and acceptance. I use the analogy of the musical campfire to explain the therapeutic engagement and experience of young people sharing and listening to their preferred music (Cheong-Clinch and McFerran, 2016). Listening to music with a music therapist and with peers also provides a significant change from their usual everyday routine of solitary music listening (Larson, 1995). Unless they have a music listening device without a built-in camera to listen to music, many of the young people will have no access to music. A hospital admission is an emotionally critical and vulnerable time, so for many young people listening to their preferred music is a much needed as well as familiar engagement for them.

Young people with severe mental and emotional difficulties can struggle to find emotional words to adequately express and communicate their pain (Cohen et al., 2013; Venta et al., 2013). I regularly observe that young people who have mental health difficulties use simple emotional words to describe their emotions and situations that underpin their hospital stay. Their vocabulary does not reflect the severity of the emotional and mental health conditions that have caused them to be admitted to an acute adolescent inpatient psychiatric facility. Many of the emotional words and descriptions appear to be the normal 'ups and downs' of adolescent life and are not adequate when describing their mental and emotional difficulties and complexities. However, their preferred music is an intimate medium for their emotional experience and a familiar means for emotional expression in group music therapy. Often they listen to music to 'reflect' their feelings, as one young person in the study explained:

If you're having a bad day, having a down day, you listen to softer acoustics, piano, lyrics where there's singing and if you're really energetic you listen to up-tempo motivating stuff.

It is perhaps not surprising that young people use music to express themselves, as described by one young person who said '[It's] easier to express myself without using too many words through music'. A young person who struggled with suicidal thoughts might have few words to describe the challenges that have led to that distress. However, a number of preferred songs might help to describe and explain their emotional state. Hearing the young people's stories on their terms is a crucial aspect of any therapeutic relationship. Sharing the young person's favourite song is a way to directly engage with the young person (McFerran, 2010). So sitting together with a young person to listen to music that reflects their inner turmoil has the potential to enable the therapist to become more attuned to the young person's experience of emotions and vulnerability, which in turn cultivates trust (Griffith and Larson, 2016).

A number of the young participants in my study reported experiencing acceptance of their preferred music. They also found it surprising, as they often perceived judgement from adults. This is not an unusual perception, as young people's preferred music is often not well received. This may have stemmed from a number of studies that offer a binary view to correlate music with negative behaviours and emotional states (Baker and Bor, 2008; Bushong, 2002). As a result, young people's preferred music has at times been restricted by adolescent mental health providers for fear that certain genres of music might be detrimental to young people's mental states. However, this is neither my observation nor clinical experience in the adolescent facility where I work. A service improvement survey in 2015 revealed overwhelming and positive feedback from both young people and nursing staff about the use of preferred music and the role of music therapy during their hospital stay (Cheong-Clinch et al., 2015).

As a young person's mental health declines, so often does their engagement and interaction with their friends, family, and school (Al-Yarman et al., 2002). The therapeutic process of sharing and listening to their music preferences is also a way for each group member to share and connect with each other's emotional stories. It is possible that through the shared means of their preferred music they have the opportunity to express themselves, and connect with others' stories in a similar way.

Some young people in my study reported that sharing music preferences had the ability to reveal and enable them to 'see' and 'hear' the emotional circumstances of the other young people in the group music listening session. One young person observed insightfully:

When you gather around to watch YouTube [to listen to music] you really get to know them, you don't even have to talk to them.

It appears that listening to music with peers also has the potential to normalize the experience of having mental health difficulties, which may result in social re-engagement.

Music playlists are currently popular with young people, but playlist creation was a relatively new thing in 2008. There were restrictions to access personal devices (and therefore preferred music) during a young person's hospital stay, so the young person and I would work together to put a playlist of their chosen songs onto a CD so that they could have access to it at any time. Quite naturally, the young people also shared their personal playlists with each other in the hospital. During a group music therapy session, the young people would create and burn a playlist onto a CD consisting of their own personal favourite songs, all together. These were often later shared or gifted to each other prior to their hospital discharge as a token of friendship, connection, and support.**

Integrating music in youth mental health literacy and wellbeing

Research has shown that young people regularly use online services to find out about mental health topics (Kauer et al., 2014). In fact, young people report they are already using technology as an informal complement to treatment (Montague et al., 2015) and finding out about general health knowledge (Uhrig et al., 2010). A number of studies have shown a range of uses of social media platforms from sexual health promotion (Jones et al., 2012; Rice, 2010) to providing avenues of support to those who self-injure (Kaukiainen and Martin, 2017). It suggested that these platforms have limitations (Bobkowski and Smith, 2013; Kaukiainen and Martin, 2017) and reveal modest effects (Brown and Bobkowski, 2011). Regardless, it is important that they facilitate pathways to increasing mental health literacy, help-seeking, and therapeutic engagement for young people who are struggling (Rickwood et al., 2007)

Youth mental health literacy and promotion needs to align with young people's developmental needs (Velardo and Drummond, 2017) to reach out and meet their search for meaning, relevance, autonomy, and agency. Their desire to seek help correlates with their mental health literacy. Young people are more likely to seek help when they recognize they have a problem, and have positive attitudes and perceptions about mental health difficulties (Rickwood et al., 2007).

The findings from my research also revealed the dualistic nature of the impact of young people's music listening. In spite of the young people's firm beliefs and perceptions that their music engagement would take away the pain of their emotional and mental health difficulties, their music engagement did not always meet these expectations. In fact, their music had the potential to make them feel worse. In addition, the degree of transformation from their music engagement depended on their awareness of it, and its impact fluctuated in relation to the complexity of their mental illness. Another study (McFerran and Saarikallio, 2014), which explored the beliefs of 40 young Australians aged between 13 and 20 years, also reported that at times the consequences of their music listening had been unhelpful.

This is a crucial finding as music listening has been suggested to be a natural coping strategy for young people (Frydenberg, 2008; Miranda, 2013). I have often observed many acutely unwell young people to be either oblivious to the negative impact of their music listening, and/or continue to engage with their preferred music despite its detriment. As their music listening has the ability to exacerbate their deteriorating emotional and mental states, emotional competence about their own music engagement is particularly necessary in times of acute distress. It is also a way to build mental health literacy as improving their awareness to identify their emotional states and abilities to self-regulate using music may be an important first step towards help-seeking (Rickwood et al., 2007).

Therefore, music therapy sessions in the adolescent facility have the specific aim of raising awareness and developing an insight into music listening in relation to feeling better. Many young people often list music listening as their primary coping strategy or the first thing they turn to in their emotional distress so this is an essential treatment goal as part of their hospital stay.

Developing a music-based e-platform

In 2011, in response to the national campaign Making Music Being Well that was conducted at the time, I created Tune Your Mood (TYM) to use music to facilitate emotional literacy and to encourage young people to think about and identify the positive ways and impact of their everyday music listening engagement. At the same time I collaborated with award-winning youth health portal Tune In Not Out (TINO) to develop a web-based platform that engages with young people through their preferred music. At the time, 'cool' youth health websites were few and far between, and the young people I met and worked with at the hospital showed little interest in engaging with them. TINO's multimedia delivery captured my attention, and inspired me to take what young people were already doing—that is, creating playlists and sharing—beyond music therapy to the online world.

TINO is a web portal consisting of information sourced from the main youth mental health agencies on a wide range of youth health topics, ranging from mental health conditions, sexual health, relationships, alcohol, and other drugs to school-related topics. This 'one-stop shop' is youth-friendly and easy to navigate, which eliminates confusion and difficulty for young people to easily explore and access the information in a variety of formats such as videos, blogs, factsheets, and music.

TINO also provides opportunities for young people to participate where they are invited to contribute and share their own stories of how they address, negotiate, and overcome life's challenges. In a similar way TYM invites young people to submit and upload their playlist and a short description of the positive impact and/or significance of the playlist on TINO. The aim is not to relive or retell stories of pain through their music, but to observe and put into words the transformative power of their music. Similar to group music therapy where young people listen to each other's stories through one another's song choices, sharing their own positive playlist and a short description helps young people to safely mirror and be mirrored by others' playlists and descriptions.

The interactive digital media content underlies the success and effectiveness of TINO as a site that provides '24hr TV for life's challenges' (TINO); in particular, the interaction helps them to develop reflective capacity and build on their existing strengths. It is visually appealing and easy to navigate, with content and language that are accessible to young people. At the same time, it provides information about the major youth mental health services and how to access and engage with them to promote health, prevention, and early intervention.

Engagement is a term much used in youth mental health circles as it is well recognized that receiving appropriate early intervention support for prevention and treatment are vital during adolescence (Rickwood et al., 2007). Unfortunately, in addition to young people's declining mental health and general disengagement they can also be reluctant to seek professional help for mental health problems. They can find it difficult to maintain engagement with services and mental health professionals, however well intentioned they are. Perhaps mental health services and professionals also find it difficult to engage with these young people, as found by some of my colleagues in the adolescent inpatient facility. There appears to be a disjunction between young people and professionals, which may be attributed to young people's developmental need for autonomy and agency. They may see professionals as 'paid to do our jobs', to exert power over them, or being motivated to 'change' them (Hughes, 2009, p. 123). Their preferred music has the potential to do this. Dave Miranda (2013) suggests that music-based prevention initiatives can be useful for young people as they recognize relevant elements of their youth culture within it. danah boyd describes music as the 'cultural glue among youth' (boyd, 2007, p. 4). So it is not surprising that there is positive feedback when we share and listen to their and other young people's preferred music and read the stories about music listening on TYM in group music therapy. The following clinical vignette of a session illustrates the use of TYM on TINO.

It had been a rough day for the four young people with an eating disorder. It was the end of first week for Jodi, and the beginning of the third week of their hospital stay for Chloe, Erin, and Gabbi. They had their weight measured in the morning which showed an increase in their respective weights, much to their disgust. They had specific instructions to finish all of their meals and snacks as per their meal plans. Chloe and Gabbi had also been told that a nasogastric tube would be inserted to assist in their re-feeding process as part of their recovery.

I found them in their bedrooms before lunch, looking anxious and distressed, and informed them that I would be doing a group music therapy session for their post-meal support. They were accepting of this temporary relief. After lunch we walked to the music room where music listening sessions on YouTube are held. They were looking visibly uncomfortable. Erin even asked her nurse for a warm pack to place on her stomach.

I explained the aim of the session was about using specific music listening choices to feel better. I asked them what they did when they felt upset. Jodi shrugged her shoulders and announced that she did not feel upset until she was admitted to hospital a week ago. Chloe agreed with her, and added that having to eat all of her lunch made her more upset. She began to cry as she was adamant that the nasogastric tube over-night feeding was unnecessary and made her feel 'more depressed'. Both Erin and Gabbi looked on while maintaining a flat affect, but said nothing. I asked Erin about the warm pack she had asked to put on her stomach. She said that the nurse had told her that it was a way to help her feel better after lunch, and so she had asked for it. When I asked her if it made a difference, she quietly replied, 'A little'.

This was going to be tough session, as they did not demonstrate much responsiveness. I had expected it, as often in the early stage of recovery during a hospital stay young people with an eating disorder are either un-aware of how they are feeling or do not know how to manage their distress. Research (Money et al., 2011) tells us that those with an eating disorder have little recognition and vocabulary of how they are feeling and are generally avoidant of negative emotions.

I directed the young people to the playlists found on the music page of TINO, and showed them the young people's submissions and descriptions of their playlists. I chose 'boost my mood' category of playlists and picked a playlist, Mixtures, to continue the session. The first line in the description of the playlist caught Gabbi's attention, which she read aloud 'I listen to songs so that I don't need to think—that's what I do, it takes my mind off things'. This was a good start. I looked around and asked the others if they listened to music so that they did not need to think about their day. All of them nodded. So I asked them if this was what they wanted to do and if they wished to listen to a song of their choice to do that. They nodded more enthusias-tically this time. Gabbi asked to listen to her song first. While listening to Gabbi's song, I observed that they were paying attention to the song. Gabbi was mouthing the words of the song, while Chloe was tapping her fingers on the table along with the beat of the song. After the song, I asked them what they had experienced. Gabbi replied that she had missed that song, and that listening to it helped her temporarily forget that she was in hospital.

After we listened to the next song, I turned to the description of Mixtures again, and asked the group, 'so does listening to music change your mood?' I read the next line in the description which was 'songs can change my mood when I'm feeling down'. The young women began to open up about their need to listen to music, and that they missed listening to music during their hospital stay. They admitted that listening to music after lunch was helpful as they were feeling physically unwell. We proceeded to listen to each person's song choice and discussed how the song helped them to feel better. They were asked to reflect and describe other ways they had felt unwell—whether it was a physical discomfort or a general sense of being upset, and then the impact of the music listening on that sensation. Being able to recognize and identify negative aspects of sensation, rather than avoiding it, was an important step towards mental health literacy. During the session, I asked them if they would be happy to share their playlist and a short description of the discussion from the music therapy session with other young people on TINO. They were excited by the prospect that their playlist and story would be beneficial to other young people who were looking at TINO.

Young people's significant relationships with music and technology provide a youth-centred rationale for their uses in and beyond therapy. This aligns with current mental health strategies that encourage developmentally appropriate ways of thinking and working with young people who have a mental illness. The focus here is to identify strengths and facilitate intentional opportunities to 'feel good and function well' (Keyes and Annas, 2009, p. 197). This is of particular significance to adolescent mental health, as the success of strategies for their mental health recovery during adolescence has implications for adult development and wellbeing (Keyes, 2006).

Conclusion

To summarize the process of sharing preferred music in group music therapy and connecting young people to help-seeking and participation in their own recovery beyond therapy, through their engagement with uploaded playlists on TYM, I will draw on the principles of Martin Seligman's wellbeing construct (Seligman, 2011).

Positive emotion

Around the musical 'campfire', young people intentionally select and listen to their preferred music with the music therapist and others in the group, which generates emotions such as acceptance and fun. Creating and uploading intentional playlists consisting of music that have a positive impact in their everyday lives can assist in being deliberate in engaging in pleasurable tasks, as it is easier for people to engage in these tasks when given the goal of doing so (Westgate et al., 2017). Over time, engaging in positive emotions and experiences has the potential to transform negative experiences and build psychological capital (Czikszentmihalyi, 1997).

Engagement

Even Ruud (2002) has suggested that music listening may be a technology of health where young people engage with their music to personalize their environment and actively use music to make themselves feel better. So music listening can be a relevant and intrinsically motivated engagement (Ryan, 2007) that has the potential to propel (Larson, 2000) young people towards greater participation in their ongoing mental health literacy and recovery.

Relationships

Engaging with a music-based e-platform like TYM in a multimedia youth health portal has the potential to build relationships in a number of ways. It builds on young people's existing intrapersonal relationships with music and online engagement. For example, during a group music therapy session, sharing music listening and playlists to the TYM music webpage is a way to build a therapeutic relationship, as well as being an interpersonal process of re-establishing connections with peers in the group. At a systemic level, it is also a way of showing respect (Epstein, 2010) to the young person, to reflect and acknowledge the central role of both music and technology in their everyday lives.

Meaning

Preferred music has been shown to be a crucial emotional language for young people. Hence, shared and preferred music listening is a meaningful way for young people to identify and express their emotions (Cheong-Clinch and McFerran, 2016).

Achievement

Through their participation in music therapy, young people can become more aware and intentional about what to do musically and what might work for them when they deal with difficult things. Young people have an incredible capacity to become emotionally competent, especially through their music. They may also gain a sense of accomplishment in being able to effectively manage their distress.

Young people's significant relationships with preferred music and technology provide a rationale for TYM as an outreach to, and between, young people. Connecting with their preferred music provides a meaningful emotional engagement, and has the potential to raise their awareness of how they are engaging with music to feel better or not. It is also crucial to reinforce positive adaptive resources, such as their music listening, as part of ongoing recovery and wellbeing beyond therapeutic engagement, and vital for building youth self-esteem, self-efficacy, and civic engagement (Flicker et al. 2008). Understanding the emotional engagement and relationship young people have with their music and technology is necessary to develop meaningful and relevant resources and services. The creation of TYM in a youth health portal provides the necessary glue to connect young people to build youth mental health literacy and wellbeing, and improve help-seeking behaviour.

References

Al-Yarman, F., Bryant, F., and Sargeant, H. (2017). *Australian Children 2002: Their Health and Wellbeing*. Canberra: Australian Institute of Health and Welfare.

Baker, F. and Bor, W. (2008). Can music preference indicate mental health status in young people? *Australasian Psychiatry: Bulletin of Royal Australian and New Zealand College of Psychiatrists*, 16(4), 284–288. doi:10.1080/10398560701879589.

Bennett, A. (2008). Towards a cultural sociology of popular music. *Journal of Sociology*, 44(4), 419–432.

Bobkowski, P. and Smith, J. (2013). Social media divide: characteristics of emerging adults who do not use social network websites. *Media, Culture & Society*, **35**(6), 771–781. doi:10.1177/0163443713491517.

Bosacki, S. L. and O'Neill, S. A. (2015). Early adolescents' emotional perceptions and engagement with popular music activities in everyday life. *International Journal of Adolescence and Youth*, **20**(2), 228–244. doi:10.1080/02673843.2013.785438.

Boyd, D. M. (2007). Why youth (heart) social network sites: The role of networked publics in teenage social life. In *MacArthur Foundation Series on Digital Learning – Youth, Identity, and Digital Media* (pp. 1–26). Cambridge, MA: The MIT Press.

Brown, J. and Bobkowski, P. (2011). Older and newer media: Patterns of use and effects on adolescents' health adn well-being. *Journal of Adolescent Research*, **21**, 95–113.

Bushong, D. (2002). Good music/bad music: Extant literature on popular music media and antisocial behaviour. *Music Therapy Perspectives*, **20**, 69–79.

Cheong-Clinch, C. (2013). *Musical Diaries: An Investigation of Preferred Music Listening by Young People with Mental Illness in Various Contexts and Conditions*. Melbourne: The University of Melbourne.

Cheong-Clinch, C., Burke, C., and Hatherill, S. (2015). What they said—Perspectives from young people and nursing staff about the role of music therapy in an adolescent inpatient unit. Poster presented at: Princess Alexander Hospital Health Symposium, Brisbane, QLD.

Cheong-Clinch, C. and McFerran, K. S. (2016). Musical diaries: Examining the daily preferred music listening of Australian young people with mental illness. *Journal of Applied Youth Studies*, **1**(2), 77–94.

Cohen, N., Farnia, F., and Im-Bolter, N. (2013). Higher order language competence and adolescent mental healt. *Journal of Child Psychology and Psychiatry*, **54**(7), 733–744.

Czikszentmihalyi, M. (1997). *Finding Flow: The psychology of Engagement with Everyday Life*. New York: Basic Books.

Epstein, R. (2010). *Teen 2.0: Saving our Children and Families from the Torment of Adolescence*. Fresno, CA: Quill Driver Books.

Flicker, S., Maley, O., Ridgley, A., Biscope, S., Lombardo, C., and Skinner, H. 2008. Using technology and participatory action research to engage youth in health promotion. *Action Research*, **6**(3), 285–303.

Frydenberg, E. (2008). *Adolescent Coping: Advances in Theory, Research and Practice*. Hove: Routledge.

Griffith, A. N. and Larson, R. W. (2016). Why trust matters: How confidence in leaders transforms what adolescents gain from youth programs. *Journal of Research on Adolescence*, **26**(4), 790–804.

Hughes, D., Brisch, K. H., Bomber, L., Batmanghelidjh, C., Delaney, M., Heyno, A. et al. (2009). *Teenagers and Attachment—Helping Adolescents Engage with Life and Learning*. London: Worth Publishing.

Jones, K., Baldwin, K., and Lewis, P. (2012). The potential influence of a social media intervention on risky sexual behavior and chlamydia incidence. *Journal of Community Health Nursing*, **29**, 106–120.

Kauer, S. D., Mangan, C., and Sanci, L. (2014). Do online mental health services improve help-seeking for young people? A systematic review. *Journal of Medical Internet Research*, **16**(3), 1–15.

Kaukiainen, A. and Martin, G. (2017). Who engages with self-injury related Internet sites, and what do they gain? *Suicidology Online*, **8**, 66–77.

Keyes, C. L. M. (2006). Mental health in adolescence: Is America's youth flourishing? *American Journal of Orthopsychiatry*, **76**(3), 395–402.

Keyes, C. L. M. and Annas, J. (2009). Feeling good and functioning well: Distinctive concepts in ancient philosophy and contemporary science. *The Journal of Positive Psychology*, **4**(3), 197–201. doi:10.1080/17439760902844228.

Larson, R. (1995). Secrets in the bedroom: Adolescents' private use of media. *Journal of Youth and Adolescence*, **24**(5), 535–550.

Larson, R. W. (2000). Toward a psychology of positive youth development. *American Psychologist*, **55**(I), 170–183.

Lawrence, D., Johnson, S., Hafekost, J, Boterhoven, De Haan K., Sawyer M., Ainley, J., and Zubrick, S.R. (2015). *The Mental Health of Children and Adolescents.Report on the Second Australian Child and Adolescent Survey of Mental Health and Wellbeing*. Department of Health, Canberra.

Longbotoom, J. (2016). Suicide rates for young Australians highest in 10 years. Retrieved from https://www.abc.net.au/news/2016-11-30/system-for-suicide-prevention-rates-highest-10-years/8076780

MacKee, N. (2016). No gain from rise of antidepressants. *Medical Journal of Australia*, Issue 18, 16 May. Retrieved from https://insightplus.mja.com.au/2016/18/no-gain-rise-antidepressants/.

McFerran, K. S. (2010). *Adolescents, Music and Music Therapy: Methods and Techniques for Clinicians, Educators and Students*. London: Jessica Kingsley Publishers.

McFerran, K. S. and Saarikallio, S. (2014). Depending on music to feel better: Being conscious of responsibility when appropriating the power of music. *Arts in Psychotherapy*, **41**(1), 89–97.

Miranda, D. (2013). The role of music in adolescent development: Much more than the same old song. *International Journal of Adolescence and Youth*, **18**(1), 5–22.

Money, C., Genders, R., Treasure, J., Schmidt, U., and Tchanturia, K. (2011). A brief emotion focused intervention for inpatients with anorexia nervosa: A qualitative study. *Journal of Health Psychology*, **16**(6), 947–958.

Montague, A. E., Varcin, K. J., Simmons, M. B., and Parker, A. G. (2015). Putting technology into youth mental health practice: Young people's perspectives. *SAGE Open*, **5**(2). doi:10.1177/2158244015581019.

Rice, E. (2010). The positive role of social networks and social networking technology in the condom-using behaviors of homeless young people. *Public Health Reports*, **125**, 588–595.

Rickwood, D. J., Deane, F. P., and Wilson, C. J. (2007). When and how do young people seek professional help for mental health problems? *The Medical Journal of Australia*, **187**(7), 35–39.

Ruud, E. (2002). Music as a cultural immunogen: Three narratives on the use of music as a technology of health. In I. M. Hanken, S. Graabaek, and M. Nerland (Eds), *Research in and for Higher Music Education. Festchrift for Jarald Jorgensen*. Oslo: NMH-Publications.

Ryan, R. (2007). Motivation and emotion: A new look and approach for two reemerging fields. *Motivation and Emotion*, **31**, 1–3.

Seligman, M. (2011). *Flourish: A Visionary New Understanding of Happiness and Wellbeing*. New York: Free Press.

Uhrig, J., Bann, C., Williams, P., and Evans, W. D. (2010). Social networking websites as a platform for disseminating social marketing interventions: An exploratory pilot study. *Social Marketing Quarterly*, **16**, 2–20.

Velardo, S. and Drummond, M. (2017). Emphasizing the child in child health literacy research. *Jorunal of Child Health Care*, **21**(1), 5–13

Venta, A., Hart, J., and Sharp, C. (2013). The relation between experiential avoidance, alexithymia and emotion regulation in inpatient adolescents. *Clinical Child Psychology and Psychiatry*, **18**, 398–410.

Westgate, E. C., Wilson, T. D., and Gilbert, D. (2017). With a little help for our thoughts: Making it easier to think for pleasure. *Emotion*, **17**, 828–839.

Author Index

Tables and figures are indicated by an italic *t* and *f* following the page/paragraph number.

Subject Index

Tables and figures are indicated by an italic *t* and *f* following the page/paragraph number.